ALLE ZEIT WACH
SJ
1842

Monographien aus dem Gesamtgebiete der Psychiatrie **41**

Herausgegeben von
H. Hippius, München · W. Janzarik, Heidelberg
C. Müller, Prilly-Lausanne

Band 32 **Drogenabhängigkeit und Psychose.** Psychotische Zustandsbilder bei jugendlichen Drogenkonsumenten
Von B. Bron

Band 33 **Ehen depressiver und schizophrener Menschen.** Eine vergleichende Studie an 103 Kranken und ihren Ehepartnern
Von D. Hell

Band 34 **Psychiatrische Aus- und Weiterbildung.** Ein Vergleich zwischen 10 Ländern mit Schlußfolgerungen für die Bundesrepublik Deutschland
Von W. Mombour

Band 35 **Die Enkopresis im Kindes- und Jugendalter**
Von A. Wille

Band 36 **Alkoholismus als Karriere**
Von F. Matakas, H. Berger, H. Koester, A. Legnaro

Band 37 **Magersucht und Bulimia.** Empirische Untersuchungen zur Epidemiologie, Symptomatologie, Nosologie und zum Verlauf
Von Manfred M. Fichter

Band 38 **Das Apathiesyndrom des Schizophrenen.** Eine psychopathologische und computertomographische Untersuchung
Von C. Mundt

Band 39 **Syndrome der akuten Alkoholintoxikation und ihre forensische Bedeutung**
Von D. Athen

Band 40 **Schizophrenie und soziale Anpassung.** Eine prospektive Längsschnittuntersuchung
Von C. Schubart, R. Schwarz, B. Krumm, H. Biehl

Band 41 **Towards Need-Specific Treatment of Schizophrenic Psychoses.** A Study of the Development and the Results of a Global Psychotherapeutic Approach to Psychoses of the Schizophrenia Group in Turku, Finland
By Y. O. Alanen, V. Räkköläinen, J. Laakso, R. Rasimus, A. Kaljonen

Yrjö O. Alanen, Viljo Räkköläinen,
Juhani Laakso, Riitta Rasimus, Anne Kaljonen

Towards Need-Specific Treatment of Schizophrenic Psychoses

A Study of the Development and the Results of a Global Psychotherapeutic Approach to Psychoses of the Schizophrenia Group in Turku, Finland

With 7 Figures and 108 Tables

Springer-Verlag
Berlin Heidelberg New York
London Paris Tokyo

Yrjö O. Alanen
Viljo Räkköläinen
Juhani Laakso
Riitta Rasimus
Anne Kaljonen
Department of Psychiatry
Institute of Clinical Sciences
University of Turku
Kurjenmäentie 4
20700 Turku 70
Finland

ISBN-13:978-3-642-82824-9 e-ISBN-13:978-3-642-82822-5
DOI: 10.1007/978-3-642-82822-5

Library of Congress Cataloging-in-Publication Data
Alanen, Yrjö O.
Towards need-specific treatment of schizophrenic psychoses.
(Monographien aus dem Gesamtgebiete der Psychiatrie ; 41)
Bibliography: p.
Includes index.
1. Schizophrenia–Treatment–Finland–Turku.
2. Schizophrenia–Prognosis. 3. Psychotherapy.
I. Title. II. Series.
RC514.A39 1986 616.89'82 86-13109
ISBN-13:978-3-642-82824-9 (New York)

Softcover reprint of the hardcover 1st edition 1986

Typesetting: Fotosatz & Design, 8240 Berchtesgaden

2125/3130-543210

Acknowledgements

The planning and accomplishments of the earlier phases of this study were based on a research contract between the University of Turku and the Academy of Finland within the period from April 1st, 1976 to March 31st, 1980. The analysis of the research data and the writing of this monograph were greatly forwarded by the appointment of the leader of the study team as a Research Professor of the Academy from September 1st, 1982 to August 31st, 1985. It also secured the economic support necessary for the later phase of the study. Without this support from the Academy of Finland, the study would have been impossible to carry through; therefore, we want to express our gratitude.

Among our colleagues, we want to thank especially Dr. Ritva Järvi, M. D., then Psychiatrist of the Parainen Mental Health Office, now Medical Director of the Turku Mental Health District, who acted as the independent investigator while the 2-year follow-up was carried out in 1978–79. Our warmest thanks are also due to the psychiatrists in charge of the different units of the Turku Mental Health District for their collaboration during the time of our study, as well as to many physicians, psychologists, nurses and social workers who acted as therapists, supervisors and staff members treating the patients. We also want to thank the patients themselves and their family members for their willing attitude in participating in the investigations of the various phases of the study. We also thank the units outside our own district who gave information on the treatments, as well as the National Pension Bank of Finland and especially its regional office in Turku for providing us permission for gathering information.

Our special thanks are due to Mrs. Sirkka-Liisa Leinonen for the translation of the text into English, and to Mrs. Mari Hakkala and Mrs. Tuula Tiihonen, who typed the manuscript, for their skillful cooperation. Mr. Lars-Runar Knuts, Lic. Phil., assisted in the planning of the statistical analyses in the beginning of the study and Mrs. Merja Kronström and Miss Johanna Kytölä participated in the execution of some of the analyses.

Turku, April 1986

Yrjö O. Alanen
Viljo Räkköläinen
Juhani Laakso
Riitta Rasimus
Anne Kaljonen

Contents

1	**Background and Goals of the Study**	1
1.1	Illness Models of Schizophrenia	1
1.2	The Goals of the Study and Their Connection with the Local Health Care System	6
2	**Prognosis of Schizophrenia and the Research on Psychosocial Modes of Therapy**	12
2.1	General View of the Prognosis and Factors Contributing to It	12
2.2	Effect of Neuroleptic Medication on the Prognosis	15
2.3	Studies on the Effect of Psychotherapy and Other Psychosocial Modes of Treatment	16
2.3.1	Individual Psychotherapy	17
2.3.2	Family Therapy	22
2.3.3	Group Therapy	25
2.3.4	Other Studies	26
3	**Study Project, Material and Methods**	31
3.1	Beginning of the Project and the Patient Series	31
3.1.1	The Research Team and the Planning of the Project	31
3.1.2	Diagnostic Criteria for Inclusion in the Series	32
3.1.3	Inclusion of the Patients in the Series	36
3.2	Course of the Project	38
3.2.1	Psychiatric Basic Examination	38
3.2.2	Psychologic Basic Examination	38
3.2.3	Action Research by the Team	39
3.2.4	Two-Year Psychiatric Follow-up	40
3.2.5	Two-Year Psychologic Follow-up	41
3.2.6	Five-Year Psychiatric Follow-up	42
3.3	Data Analysis and Statistical Methods	44
4	**Findings of Psychiatric Basic Examination. Indications of Therapeutic Plans**	46
4.1	Psychosocial Background of Patients	46
4.1.1	Sex and Age	46
4.1.2	Family Background	46

4.1.2.1 Mental Health of Members of Primary Family 46
4.1.2.2 Atmosphere and External Structure of Primary Family . 47
4.1.2.3 Social Background of Primary Family 48
4.1.3 Prepsychotic Development of Patients 49
4.1.3.1 Physical and Psychologic Development 49
4.1.3.2 Social Development 53
4.1.3.3 Data on the Patients' Secondary Families 56
4.1.3.4 Relatives' Attitudes Towards the Patient 57
4.2 Admission for Treatment and the Clinical Background Variables 58
4.2.1 Previous Treatments. Admission for Present Treatments 58
4.2.2 Clinical Pictures 60
4.2.3 Categories Constructed on the Basis of the Quality of Ego Dysfunctions (Ego-Dynamic Sub-Grouping) . . 64
4.3 Case-Specific Therapeutic Plans 67
4.3.1 Intervention in Crisis 69
4.3.2 Individual Therapies 69
4.3.3 Family Therapies 69
4.3.4 Group Therapy of Out-Patients 70
4.3.5 Psychotherapeutic Community on a Hospital Ward . . 70
4.4 Summary and Discussion 71

5 Implementation of Therapies and Factors Influencing It 78
5.1 Use of In-Patient and Out-Patient Treatment 79
5.1.1 In-Patient Treatment 79
5.1.1.1 The Length and Number of the In-Patient Periods . . . 80
5.1.1.2 Did a Longer First Hospital Period Lessen the Need for Later Hospital Treatments? 84
5.1.2 Out-Patient Care 88
5.2 Implementation of Psychotherapeutic Treatments . . . 91
5.2.1 Initial Intervention in Crisis 94
5.2.2 Individual Therapies 95
5.2.2.1 The Therapeutic Orientation 95
5.2.2.2 Number and Frequency of the Sessions 98
5.2.2.3 Connections with the Background Variables 99
5.2.3 Family Therapy 101
5.2.3.1 The Therapeutic Orientation 101
5.2.3.2 Number and Frequency of the Sessions 103
5.2.3.3 Connections with the Background Variables 104
5.2.3.4 Supportive Contacts with Family Members 105
5.2.4 Treatment in a Psychotherapeutic Community 106
5.2.4.1 Therapeutic Orientation 106
5.2.4.2 Connections with the Background Variables 107
5.2.5 Group of Psychotherapy Cases 109
5.2.5.1 Criteria of Inclusions. Combinations of Different Therapeutical Models 109
5.2.5.2 Connections with the Background Variables 111

5.2.6 Patients Remaining Excluded from the Psychotherapeutic Treatments . . . 113
5.2.7 Occupational Groups, Psychotherapeutic Training and Supervision of the Therapists . . . 114
5.2.8 Discontinued Therapies . . . 117
5.3 Somatic Treatments . . . 118
5.3.1 Neuroleptic Medication . . . 118
5.3.2 Other Somatic Treatments . . . 122
5.4 Social and Rehabilitative Measures . . . 122
5.5 Selection of the Mode of Therapy in the Light of the Psychologic Basic Examination . . . 124
5.5.1 Internal Object World and Motivation to Therapy . . . 124
5.5.2 Inclusion in and Exclusion from the Group of Psychotherapy Cases . . . 126
5.5.3 Implementation of Individual Therapy . . . 126
5.5.4 Selection for Family Therapy . . . 127
5.5.5 Selection for Community Therapy . . . 128
5.5.6 Selection for Pharmacotherapy . . . 129
5.5.7 Summary . . . 130
5.6 Summary and Discussion . . . 132

6 Prognosis and the Effect of Therapies on It . . . 144
6.1 How Was the Prognosis Measured? . . . 145
6.1.1 Implementation of the Prognostic Study . . . 145
6.1.2 Sub-Areas of the Prognostic Study . . . 145
6.1.3 Credibility of the Prognostic Findings: Comparison of the Two-Year Follow-up Findings Made By the Team and the Independent Examiner . . . 146
6.2 Clinical Prognosis . . . 149
6.2.1 Patients Who Died Or Were Not Reached for the Follow-up Examination . . . 149
6.2.2 Occurrence of Psychotic Symptoms . . . 149
6.2.3 Occurrence of Nuclear Symptoms of Schizophrenia . . . 152
6.2.4 Suicidal Tendencies and Violence . . . 154
6.2.5 Other Observations on the Patient's Clinical Status. Phenomenon of Defencelessness . . . 155
6.2.6 Summary and Discussion . . . 156
6.3 Psychodynamic Prognosis . . . 160
6.3.1 Psychosexual Development . . . 161
6.3.2 Development of Interpersonal Relationships . . . 164
6.3.3 Insight and Sense of Illness . . . 169
6.3.4 Summary and Discussion . . . 172
6.4 Psychosocial Prognosis . . . 175
6.4.1 Working Capacity . . . 176
6.4.2 Social Role and Disability Pensions . . . 179
6.4.3 Dwelling Conditions . . . 182
6.4.4 Occupational Identity and Its Development . . . 183

6.4.5 Maintenance or Loss of the Grip on Life 185
6.4.6 Summary and Discussion 187
6.5 Prognosis in the Light of Hospital Treatments 190
6.5.1 In-Patient Days During the Follow-up Years 191
6.5.2 Patients Treated in Hospital During the Last Two Follow-up Years 195
6.5.3 Summary and Discussion 197
6.6 Development of Families and Family Relationships . . 200
6.6.1 Psychic Health and Family Members 200
6.6.2 Follow-up of the Marital Relationships 201
6.7 Effects of Psychotherapy and Medication on Prognosis: Statistical Analysis 202
6.7.1 Inclusion in the Group of Psychotherapy Cases and Medication 203
6.7.2 Intensive Individual Therapy and Treatment in a Psychotherapeutic Community 209
6.7.3 Global Prognostic Assessment According to Strauss and Carpenter Outcome Scale 210
6.7.4 Summary and Discussion 215
6.8 Prognosis and the Factors Affecting It: Summary and Discussion 217
6.8.1 Comparison of the Different Sub-Areas of Prognosis . 218
6.8.2 Patient-Specific Background Factors As Predictors of the Prognosis 220
6.8.3 Conclusions of the Effect of Treatment 225

7 Development of Need-Specific Treatment of Schizophrenic Psychoses 232
7.1 Need-Specificity of Treatment As Concept 232
7.2 Implementation of Need-Specific Treatment in Our Project and the Factors Affecting It 233
7.3 Need-Specificity and Prognosis of Treatment 237
7.4 Indications of Psychotherapeutic Treatments: Five Patient Groups Differentiated on the Basis of Primary Therapeutic Concern 239
7.4.1 Primary Treatment Long-Term Individual Therapy . . 239
7.4.2 Primary Treatment Couple Therapy Or Conjoint Therapy of the Patient's Procreated Family 240
7.4.3 Primary Treatment Conjoint Therapy of the Patient's Family of Orientation 242
7.4.4 Primary Treatment Flexible Family- and Environment-Oriented Intervention in Crisis 243
7.4.5 Primary Treatment Extensive Support to the Patient to Help Him Cope in His Social Environment 245
7.4.6 Discussion 246
7.5 Prerequisites for Developing Need-Specific Treatment . 248

8 Towards Need-Specific Treatment of Schizophrenic Psychoses: Summary . . . 253
8.1 Goals of the Study and Methodologic Planning . . . 253
8.2 Findings of the Initial Psychiatric Examination . . . 255
8.3 Implementation of Treatments . . . 256
8.4 Prognosis and Factors Contributing to It . . . 258
8.5 Development of Need-Specific Treatment of Schizophrenic Psychoses . . . 263

Appendices 1 – 10 . . . 266

References . . . 284

1 Background and Goals of the Study

1.1 Illness Models of Schizophrenia

The risk of schizophrenic psychosis is generally considered to be about 1 % for the part of the population reaching the age of 40–45 years. Some recent American studies based on three epidemiological catchment areas have shown the lifetime prevalence of schizophrenia to be even higher, 1.0–1.9 % (Robins et al. 1984).

In the Mini Finland survey carried out on a nation-wide representative sample of the population aged over 30 in Finland in the late 1970's (Lehtinen 1983) 0.9 % prevalence of schizophrenia was obtained in the sickness insurance districts of southern and southwestern Finland, while the district of northern Finland had 2.2 % and the district of eastern Finland 2.1 %. Another survey suggests that the regional differences might be due to differences in the chronicity of schizophrenia rather than be caused by differences in the incidence (Hakkarainen and Salokangas 1985).

Of the working age population of Finland, 0.78 % were on disability pension because of schizophrenia on December 31, 1981. Schizophrenia was the cause for 10.4 % of the pensions granted to working age population in Finland, the corresponding percentage for the age group of 16–44 years being as high as 23.9 %.

Figures of this kind clearly illustrate the significance of schizophrenia for public health as well as the national economy but say little of the amount of human tragedy and suffering, the broken hopes and the shattered human relations involved in every serious psychosis.

What, then is schizophrenia, what do we know of its causes, and how to treat it?

We can define *schizophrenia as a mental disease usually manifested at a relatively early age and characterized by at least partial disintegration of the intact complex of personality functions, developmental regression, and a tendency to withdraw from interpersonal relationships to a subjective mental world frequently coloured by-delusions and hallucinations.* Schizophrenia is no uniform illness as regards either the symptoms or the progress. Its boundaries are disputable, and its prognosis may be highly variable in different cases.

Researchers in the field of psychiatry do not agree on the essence and causes of schizophrenia, but present highly contradictory notions on that point. This is due to the differing research traditions, the methodologic commitments and modes of thinking related with these, and even – it sometimes seems – the mutually different views on the world, Weltanschauungen, held by the investigators. The therapeutic approaches to schizophrenia, in turn, are influenced by these different ways of scientifically defining schizophrenia, or *the illness models:* they determine the practical therapeutic measures applied to schizophrenic patients. *As far as we can see, the development of the treatment of schizophrenic patients has greatly suffered from the lack of an integrated illness model combining different approaches,* or at least of the inadequate application of such a model (Alanen et al. 1982 a).

Below, we will present a brief review of the most important illness models of schizophrenia and their effects on treatment. These are the scientific-medical or biomedical model, the individual-psychologic model and the transactional model, supplemented by the sociologic and ecologic approach. All of these models have their own justification based on research data obtained, their own contributions to the therapeutic methods, and their own limitations, too. These illness models and the treatment modes based on them are shown in a somewhat simplified scheme in Figure 1.

The *biomedical model* is founded on the assumption that schizophrenia is a process of illness affecting the cerebral functions at the organic level. This model is deeply embedded in the general medical tradition and our scientifically oriented research culture, and it continues to hold the dominant position in the study and treatment of schizophrenia. New hypotheses on the anatomic-physical and/or biochemical causes of schizophrenia and findings interpreted as supporting these hypotheses have been proposed constantly over the past few decades.

It is not possible to examine in detail the findings related to the various biomedical hypotheses here. Notable support for the research carried out along the biomedical model was naturally obtained from the alleviating effects the neuroleptic drugs

1. *Biomedical model*
   "The illness is comprehended as an organic brain process" or at least the biological dimension of it is uniformly emphasized
   - psychopharmacological treatment
   - other "organic" treatments
2. *Individual psychological model*
   "The illness is based on a deep-rooted disorder of the personality development"
   - individual psychotherapy
3. *Transactional (systemic) model*
   "The illness is part of a disordered interactional network"
   - family therapy
   - group and community based treatment systems

---

4. *Sociologic and ecologic approach*
   "The patients must have support as members of community"
   - environment-centered mental health activities
   - rehabilitation

---

5. *Integrated model*
   "Various illness models are variously justified in various cases"
   - therapy should be planned globally, according to case-specific needs

Fig. 1. Illness models of schizophrenia

introduced in the 1950's had on the symptoms of mental diseases. Their effect has been found to be based on the blocking of the effect of dopamine at post-synaptic membrane receptor sites (Carlsson and Lindqvist 1963). Psychologic and clinical studies have demonstrated that one important influence of medication is the strengthened protection against stimuli, both internal and external, which helps the patient to protect himself better from experineces too anxiety-provoking for him. But the studies on the potential effects of dopamine or the metabolic changes of other transmitter agents on the onset of psychosis still remain at the level of hypotheses (Carlsson 1978, Bowers 1980, Wyatt et al. 1982). The same is true of the etiological significance of the enlargement of cerebral ventricles, which has been found particularly in older patients (e.g. Tanaka 1981) and appeared not to be specific to schizophrenic disorder (Rieder et al. 1983).

The notions on the part of hereditary factors in the etiology of schizophrenia also remain partly conflicting. The investigations carried out by Kety and Rosenthal et al. (Kety et al. 1971, Rosenthal et al. 1971, Wender et al. 1974) in Denmark and the United States on the children of schizophrenic mothers placed in adoptive families speak heavily in favour of their significance. The extensive study of adopted children conducted by Tienari and his co-workers in Finland focusses particularly on the study of the family environment (Tienari et al. 1983, 1985). The results also seem to indicate the significance of genetic predisposition, but simultaneously demonstrate that a disturbed rearing environment is another important predisposing factor for development resulting in schizophrenia. Healthy family environments, in turn, protect even the adoptive children genetically predisposed to schizophrenia from psychic disturbances.

At present controlled use of medication is an integral part of the treatment of most schizophrenic patients. Drugs have helped to make the schizophrenic symptoms less deep, the periods of hospital therapy shorter, and the possibilities of treating patients on an out-patient basis better. The studies to be reviewed in Chapter 2 however, indicate that their contribution to the improvement of the long-term clinical prognosis of schizophrenia is relatively restricted.

Treatment of schizophrenia accordant exclusively with the biomedical model also has adverse consequences, especially the superficiality of the therapeutic policy. When the therapeutic efforts focus on the alleviation of the psychotic symptoms by means of heavy medication, the characteristic quality of the patient's personal problems easily remains outside of the therapeutic interest leading to a neglect of the naturally existing potentials for personal growth. The support of the patient in his social environment may also lack the necessary persistence.

We further know that abundant neuroleptic medication of long duration has its direct harmful effects. A particular cause of worry that has emerged over the past few years is the observation of frequently irreversible tardive dyskinesia appearing in 10–40 % of the patients given neuroleptic therapy for several years (e.g. Gerlach 1977, Tepper and Haas 1979, Jeste and Wyatt 1981). Equal attention should also be given to the psychologically negative effects of pharmacotherapy – anhedonia, general lack of motivation, social isolation- which have been referred to by e.g. Carpenter et al. (1977). The patients themselves often complain of these.

The *individual-psychologic* model considers schizophrenia a disorder that can be approached and treated in psychological terms. Predisposition to it is crucially dependent on a weakness of personality, either congenital and/or it has come about through early traumatic experiences leading to a lack of individualization and of the capacity to relate with other people at a differentiated level. The illness is manifested later, often as a consequence of the conflicts faced in adolescence. They need not, in themselves, be any different from the problems encountered by all people upon entrance into adulthood, but for the potential schizophrenic they amount to overpowering anxiety and break down the limits of his ability to adjust (Räkköläinen 1977). The logical and integrative part of his personality becomes disintegrated under the increasingly intolerable pressure, his ability to differentiate clearly between the impulses of his internal mental world and the external sensations disappears at least partly, and he begins to withdraw into a mental world representing the discrepancy between the needs of the schizophrenic and the reality.

The individual-psychologic model of schizophrenia has evolved out of the dyadic psychotherapeutic work with these patients. Its roots lie in the psychoanalytic research developed by Freud; its first significant pioneers included Federn (1943), a student close to Freud. Several psychoanalysts have, however, followed Freud (1915) in being pessimistic as to the capability of psychotic patients to establish a stable psychotherapeutic relationship. Many of the most important developers of this field have therefore come from the margins of the main stream of psychoanalysis, e.g. Sullivan (1931, 1962), Fromm-Reichmann (1950, 1959) and Benedetti (1955, 1983).

Our possibilities to understand schizophrenic patients have been crucially improved by this mode, and it constitutes the foundation for individual psychotherapy, which has helped several patients not only to recover from their symptoms of mental illness, but also to re-obtain their faculties of mind for further intrapsychic and interpersonal development. The essential goal of psychoanalytically oriented psychotherapy is the differentation and improvement of the internal self and object representations, which, when successful, results in permanent changes of the psychological structure of personality (e.g. Pao 1979).

Even so, long and intensive psychotherapies have only been given to relatively few patients, generally in centres specialized on this therapeutic orientation, and the results of follow-up studies in large patient series have not been particularly encouraging (cf. 2.2.1.). The implementation of a comprehensive psychotherapeutic approach in the treatment of schizophrenic patients within community health care systems has also been prevented by doubts as to the availability of resources and other prerequisites (e.g. Strauss and Frader 1976).

The weakness of the individual-psychologic theory formation lies in its often highly deterministic notion of the early origin of the predisposition to schizophrenia. It is precisely this that results in the primary therapeutic pessimism, or, at least, reserve. It also involves negligible attention paid to grave and mutual dependency problems in the actual interaction network of the patient. If, for example, there exists a continuous and circular "stalemate" in the family environment, involving both the patient and his (or her) parents or spouse, the individual-centred approach cannot provide adequate opportunities for forming a psychodynamic overall view of the situation or for carrying out the necessary therapeutic interventions.

In the *transactional model* both the individual-centred and illness-oriented notion of schizophrenia have been abandoned. According to this model, both the background and the current dynamics of the psychosis are seen to be inextricably linked with the transactional situations between human beings. Schizophrenia is not seen to differ essentially from the other psychic disorders, but is rather regarded as the most extreme part of the pathology of the family system, i.e. the problems mutually shared by a family unit.

The development of this notion of illness has been promoted by the experiences of individual psychotherapy on the one hand and by family studies (e.g. Lidz et al. 1957, 1965, Wynne et al. 1958, 1977, Alanen 1958, 1980) and family therapy on the other. The findings of family research and family therapy have clearly demonstrated the persistence of deep-rooted dependence relationships and other interactional disorders in the family environments of schizophrenic patients. They often continue to exist at the time of the onset of schizophrenia and they are also of important and concrete significance for the prognosis of the illness.

For an essential part, the development of the transactional model was promoted by the theory of "interpersonal psychiatry" proposed by H.S.Sullivan (1953). Sullivan wrote as early as 1930 that the most central factors in the investigation and treatment of schizophrenia are "not the sick individuals, but the complex, specifically characteristic situations" (Sullivan 1962). Later on, the notions based on the transactional model have been influenced by particularly the systems theory (e.g. Fleck 1976, Selvini-Palazzoli et al., 1977, Stierlin 1983).

In the treatment of schizophrenia, these approaches have resulted in the development of family therapy and other environmentally oriented modes of therapy, especially the increased significance of the therapeutic communities. It has been seen, particularly in the case of young schizophrenics, that the recovery of the patient requires that a change take place even in the other family members and their relations with the patient. Through family therapy or other forms of family-oriented approach it is also possible to support the other family members and relieve their anxiety. At the same time, the positive potentials also present in the families (as well as in the other social networks of the patient) are stimulated and may become an important support to the patient's progress.

The experiences obtained of family therapy are of relatively short duration so far, which makes it difficult to assess their overall significance. Favourable experiences have been described, however (cf. 2.2.). The same also applies to the therapeutic communities, which have been developed both within the hospital and out-patient settings.

The treatment of schizophrenia on the basis of an overly one-sided transactional model also has its drawbacks and limitations. These may appear, in particular, as a disregard of the reality of the patients's individual pathology and its conjunction with the structure of his personality, expecting that the individual pathologic structures would spontaneously disappear or become unnecessary, as the transactional pathology is eliminated. This is often not the case, however, and it is often useful to combine individual therapy on the one hand and family or environmentally oriented therapy on the other to achieve the optimal results.

In Figure 1, the *sociologic and ecologic approach* has been separated from the previous illness models with a dash line, because it does not involve (at least to any important extent) an etiologic theory formation similar to those contained in the other models. The therapeutic measures based on these approaches, particularly social rehabilitation are, however, quite equally important as the modes of therapy presented above.

Rehabilitation and the other measures intended to support the patient socially can easily be related to the modes of therapy accordant with each of the etiologic illness models. Some of the pioneers of rehabilitation, e.g. Wing (1978), combine their approach with the biomedical etiologic model. From a theoretical point of view, the sociologic and ecologic approach can be conceived of as an expanded level of the transactional notions. Only it is not confined to the networks of the most intimate human relationships, but also pertains to the interactions between the individual and his more extensive social environment and his physical environment.

For the most orthodox proponents, each of the aforesaid etiologic illness models provides a sufficient basis for both theory formation concerning schizophrenia and the therapeutic measures in practice. At the same time, ways of thinking and modes of therapy based on the other illness models tend to arouse resistance in them. Particularly the notions based on the biomedical model have – owing to their dominant position – restricted the adoption of the treatment approaches created on the basis of the other models.

Although we know far from everything about the etiology of schizophrenia, we should, in our view, recognize the multidimensional nature of the origin and development of this illness. It is probable that the different etiologic factors as well as their mutual interaction are weighted differently in the different cases.

Each of the models alone is too narrow a basis for a proper plan of orientation in most actual treatment situations. The development of therapy must also be carried out along the principles of this *integrated illness model* based on diagnostic and treatment measures derived from all the four models. It must not be conceived of and applied in a superficially eclectic manner. The therapeutic needs of each patient – and his closest environment – must be considered in detail, finding out which therapeutic measures are indicated and how they can best be implemented and mutually combined.

1.2 The Goals of the Study and Their Connection with the Local Health Care System

The purpose of our study is to renovate and develop the treatment of the patients of the schizophrenia group within the framework of the public psychiatric health care system in our country by applying a global, integrated model of illness. We make a particular effort to develop the *psychotherapeutic* and *family-oriented treatment* more intensively than has been done up to date. The project was carried out within the Mental Health District of Turku, located in the southwestern part of Finland, but we hope that the experiences obtained from it can also be applied to similar developmental work to be undertaken elsewhere in Finland and in other countries.

It is important for the accomplishment of the study that the Clinic of Psychiatry in Turku – differently from the other psychiatric university hospitals in Finland – is not part of the university central hospital but belongs to the Turku City Hospital and the Turku Mental Health District. Together with the other units of this district the Clinic has been in charge of the psychiatric services (during the study, unsectorized) of the town of Turku (population 160 000). This has made it possible to launch extensive efforts towards the study and treatment of schizophrenia.

Table 1. Community psychiatric treatment units of the Mental Health District of the City of Turku

Hospitals	
Clinic of Psychiatry (University Hospital)	111 beds
Clinic of Psychiatry (University Hospital)	18 day patients
Kupittaa Hospital	364 beds
Other hospitals (chronic patients)	139 beds
Altogether 3.7 beds per 1000 inhabitants	
Open care	
The Turku Mental Health Office	17 staff members
Out-patient activity of the Clinic of Psychiatry	
Psychiatric Out-patient Clinic of the University Central Hospital (General Hospital)	6 staff members

The treatment units of the community psychiatric system in Turku and the number of their personnel are shown in Table 1. Which is based on official data collected at the initial stage of our project in 1977 (Suomen sairaalatalous 1977).

Although the Psychiatric Out-Patient Department of the Turku University Central Hospital did not belong to the Turku Mental Health District, we regarded it as being a psychiatric unit of the public health care system and hence included it in our work. When we include the Out-Patient Clinic for Alcoholics and the private sector, there were altogether 408 psychiatric out-patient visits per 1 000 inhabitants 15 years of age and over in 1977 in the Turku area (Lehtinen et al. 1979).

The number of psychiatric hospital beds is high in Finland. The number of in-patient beds in Turku was 614, which accounts for 3.7 permille of the town's population. It was somewhat lower than the mean for the whole country (4.2 permille per population). The therapeutic activities were rendered difficult by the old age of the hospital buildings and the large size of the wards. Hence the 111 patients that could be admitted into the Clinic of Psychiatry were divided between three wards with an average of 37 patients. The ward for acute psychoses had 39 beds. Functionally, it was divided into two parts, both of which were mixed wards. The two admission wards of the Kupittaa hospital, one of which was for males and the other for females, each accommodated 26 patients.

The number of personnel per 100 patients in the Kupittaa hospital was equal to the mean reported for the Finnish central mental hospitals, 52. The corresponding figure for the Clinic of Psychiatry (including the patients of the day hospital as half-time patients) was 61. The Kupittaa hospital had 6 posts for doctors, while the Clinic of Psychiatry had 4 posts for senior doctors with teaching obligations and 5 posts for resident physicians specializing in psychiatry.

The number of personnel in the Turku Mental Health Office – 17, of whom 14 were actual therapeutic staff – was exceptionally low compared with the mean for the whole country. This was also indicated by the number of visits to the mental health office, which was 14 513 in 1977. When, a few years later in 1979, the National Board of Health made a survey of the out-patient personnel of the Finnish mental health districts per 100 000 inhabitants, the Turku Mental Health District with its ratio 1.26 was the last but one in the statistics, the corresponding mean for the whole country being 2.2. and the figure for the Etelä-Savo Mental Health District, which had the best resources, as high as 4.2.

The out-patient activities of the Clinic of Psychiatry were carried out in such a way that the staff members working on the wards continued their therapeutic relationships with some patients even after their discharge. The number of out-patient visits to the clinic in 1977 was 3 753, of which about half were made by patients receiving after-care for their psychosis.

The clinic has no staff particularly for out-patient care, because the out-patients have been legislatively assigned to the mental health office, and the officials responsible for the health care in the town of Turku were unwilling to make exceptions to this rule. The work carried out in the clinic was therefore long hampered by an excessively hospital-centred orientation, whose unfavourable consequences are also shown by the follow-up study on the results of the early stages of our therapeutic approach (Salokangas 1983, 1985). The after-care of out-patients was an effort to eliminate partly this shortcoming.

As regards the development of psychotherapeutic and family oriented therapeutic activities, our project is based on the research and therapeutic tradition developed in the Clinic of Psychiatry since 1967. An intentional effort has been made to develop the wards of the clinic into psychotherapeutic communities working towards extensive therapeutic goals (Alanen 1975, Salonen 1975, Alanen et al. 1978b). Favourable experiences have been obtained from the active participation of nurses and mental nurses in therapeutic work in the form of therapeutic relationships continued beyond the in-patient period and established and maintained under supervision (Aaku et al.1980). Most of this work has been carried out as individual therapy, but efforts have been made to include even family and group therapy in its sphere.

The psychodynamic and psychotherapeutic investigation carried out at our department has concentrated on both individual therapy (Salonen 1976, 1979) and family therapy (Alanen 1973, 1976, Alanen and Kinnunen 1975, Aaltonen 1982) of schizophrenic patients as well as the life situations influencing the onset of psychosis and its prognosis (Räkköläinen 1976, 1977, Räkköläinen et al. 1979). Social-psychiatric and prognostic studies on schizophrenia have been pursued by Salokangas (1977, 1978, 1980).

Through close cooperation, the psychotherapeutically oriented approach has also been introduced in the out-patients units participating in the project: the psychiatric out-patient department of the University Central Hospital of Turku as well as the Turku Mental Health Office, whose staff attended the psychotherapeutic supervision provided within this project.

There was, however, a notable difference between the therapeutic approaches of the two hospitals of the Turku Mental Health District. The Kupittaa Hospital laid the main emphasis on psychopharmacologic treatment, and the hospital therapy was kept as short as possible; after the in-patient period the patients generally received further therapy in the mental health office, but the connection between the hospital and the out-patient therapy was loose. The Clinic of Psychiatry, in turn, emphasized the psychotherapeutic approach, and medication was considered a part of the therapeutic whole serving the purposes of psychotherapy. The in-patient periods in the Clinic of Psychiatry were often longer in duration. The planning of out-patient therapies to be given after the in-patient stage was considered important while the patient was still in hospital.

The difference in the therapeutic practices of the two hospitals provided some opportunities to compare the outcomes of the different approaches in the follow-up study. But the differences also had the consequence that our study and its results cannot be taken as representing exclusively the features and activities typical specifically of the psychotherapeutic approach. To achieve such exclusiveness would have been beyond our means and resources, anyway.

While planning our research method, we explicitly gave up the idea of dividing our population in two parts receiving different treatments. This would not have been suited to the kind of global developmental work we were aiming at. A division of this kind would have been particularly difficult to carry out in the therapeutic communities of the Clinic of Psychiatry, where most of the new patients in need of hospital therapy were admitted. Their purpose is to include all the patients in the community activities, and the possibility of both the patients and the staff to have a say on the individual with whom they are to establish their therapeutic relationship is valued.

The lack of a control series was partly compensated by the *group of psychotherapy cases* which was kept separate from the rest of the series (cf. Ch. 5.2.6.). The prognosis of this group was compared with the prognosis of the patients not included in this group and mainly treated with pharmacotherapy. The comparison was complicated by the fact that the background variables of these patient groups were weighted differently owing to different selective factors. This was taken into account, as long as possible, in the statistical analyses of the prognostic findings for both the group of psychotherapy cases and the patients given other modes of treatment.

The *research series* consists of the 100 patients 16–45 years of age and resident in Turku who were admitted successively for their first period of treatment because of psychosis of the schizophrenia group into one of the aforesaid units of community psychiatric health care system during 19 months in 1976–1977. At the time of the admission a basic examination was carried out on the patients and their family environments, and follow-up studies were carried out two and five years later.

The *central problems of the study* were as follows:

1. How widely have the different activities included in the global approach been implemented? To what extent has the succesful implementation of the therapies or failure in this been dependent on the clinical, psychosocial and psychologic background variables constructed on the basis of the patient characteristics? What other factors seem to have influenced this?
2. What is the need for different psychotherapeutic treatments, pharmacotherapy and rehabilitation on the basis of the findings, and what are their indications in a series of schizophrenic patients first admitted for therapy? In what way are the different modes of therapy indicated in the different patient groups and how should they be integrated with each other? What conclusions can be drawn concerning the relations between the psychotherapeutic treatments and pharmacotherapy and the effects of the psychotherapeutic approach on the need for medication?
3. In what way, according to the follow-up study, have the clinical, psychodynamic and psychosocial prognoses of the patients been influenced by the therapeutic activities carried out? What differences are there between the effects of the different modes of therapy? What is the connection between the prognosis and the effects of the therapies on it on the one hand and the clinical, psychosocial and psychologic background variables of the patients on the other? What conclusions can be made concerning the effects of the present therapeutic approach on the prognosis in a comparison of the results of the follow-up study and the findings made in other studies on the prognosis of schizophrenic patients?

4. What influences have the therapies had on the family environment of the patients, the state of health of the family members and the mutual relationships between the patients and their family members?
5. What kind of a model for the psychiatric health care system do we arrive at in the treatment of schizophrenia? What therapeutic approaches appear particularly central within this model? What prerequisites do they have in view of the organization as well as the quantitative and qualitative resources? What shortcomings are particularly obvious in the current therapeutic practice, and what should be done to correct them?

The starting-points of our project have been shaped by goals typical of developmental work rather than research in a stricter sense. We develop the therapies along a comprehensive psychotherapeutic approach, taking into account the *individual needs for treatment*. Our project is carried out along *the principles of action research,* and it hence differs from methodologically "controlled" studies of therapeutic outcome.

But the methodologically oriented studies also have their restrictions. As we have already pointed out previously (Alanen et al. 1980), the clinical relevance necessarily remains limited in the investigations where the schizophrenic patients are divided randomly into groups given different therapies without any consideration given to the case-specific indications. Carpenter et al. (1981) also maintained that the meaningfulness of research has been underestimated in comparison with methodologic correctness in the recent works on the outcome of psychotherapeutic treatment of schizophrenia. What they mean by "meaningfulness" is that research should provide significant new information for the development and application of therapeutic methods. The goals of our own work lie in this direction.

The effects of the developmental level of the therapeutic activities on the prognosis of the patients can be analyzed more widely at the future stages of the Turku "schizophrenia project". We have obtained three samples of the same basic population of schizophrenic patients, representing the different stages of the development of our therapeutic approach. The times of their admission and follow-up studies are shown in the following summary.

Table 2. The overall design of the Turku Community Psychiatric Schizophrenia Project

Admission	Number of patients	Stage of development of the psychotherapeutic approach	Follow-up studies	Follow-up studies
1965–67	100	single cases	1973–74	7½ yr.
1969	75	scattered,	1971	2 yr.
		hospital-oriented	1976–77	8 yr.
1976–77	100	more comprehensive	1978–79	2 yr.
		and purposive,	1981–82	5 yr.
		open care included	(1983–85)	8 yr.
(1983–84)	36	especially family therapeutic activities further developed	(1985–86	2 yr.)

The results of the psychiatric follow-up study carried out after 7½ years on the first patient series are included in the monographs by Salokangas (1977, 1978). The second series included the 68 patients admitted into the Clinic of Psychiatry whose basic examination was carried out by Räkköläinen and reported by him 1977. Alanen and Laine (1973) have published some results from the 2-year follow-up study of this series, while Räkköläinen et al. (1979) and Salokangas (1985) have published some findings based on the 8-year follow-up. The latter follow-up study was made on a series of 75 patients, which also included the schizophrenic patients admitted for their first period of therapy into the Kupittaa Hospital in that same year. Results of the 2-year follow-up on the current series have been previously published by Alanen et al. (1982a, 1983) and of the 5-year follow-up preliminary in Alanen et al. (1985 a, b).

The 8-year follow-up on this series is being carried out. The fourth series is a part of a more extensive nation-wide project in which the diagnostic criteria were more narrow, based on the DSM III.

2 Prognosis of Schizophrenia and the Research on Psychosocial Modes of Therapy

2.1 General View of the Prognosis and Factors Contributing to It

An assessment or mutual comparison of studies dealing with the prognosis of schizophrenia is made difficult by the inconsistency of the diagnostic delineations suggested by different authors. It is, however, possible to acquire a relatively unambiguous overall view.

One of the most significant and comprehensive works undertaken in this field is the follow-up study published by Manfred Bleuler in 1972: "The Schizophrenic Disorders: Long-Term Patient and Family Studies" (English translation 1978). The work reports the results of a 23-year follow-up of 208 consecutive schizophrenic patients admitted into hospital in 1942–43. Prior to the last follow-up examination or death, 152 of these patients had reached a status that had remained stable for 5 years of more. 20 % of the patients had recovered, 33 % were only slightly ill, 24 % were moderately ill and another 24 % severely ill. The corresponding figures for those patients who had originally been first admissions were 23 %, 43 %, 19 % and 15 %. A good social adjustment outcome was found in about 30 % of the whole group, and in 40 % in the first admissions group. Bleuler also compared these patients with his follow-up of an earlier series published previously (1941). He pointed out that the relative proportion of mild illness was greater in the later series, while the proportion of serious schizophrenias had diminished. He invited particular attention to the fact that the group with the most severe prognosis – the patients whose acute onset psychosis immediately resulted in grave chronicity – had disappeared. But the number of patients with complete and permanent remissions had remained more or less unchanged.

Another Swiss study covering a large series and a long period, which was made by Ciompi and Müller (1976); (Ciompi 1980), yielded largely similar findings. These authors also found a favourable prognosis (complete remissions or only slightly ill "end states") for half, i.e. 49 %, of the patients in their series. Again, a third of the patients were found to have a relatively good social outcome. The results indicated that the prognosis of schizophrenia has been more or less the same for decades. Nevertheless, Ciompi also says (1980): "For everyone who does not link the concept of schizophrenia to an obligatory bad outcome, the enormous variety of possible evolutions shows that there is no such thing as a specific course of schizophrenia".

One interesting observation was mentioned by Müller as early as 1959 and repeated by these Swiss studies, namely that late remissions are seen in schizophrenia: there are patients who recover after years of illness – often following a life event (e.g. somatic illness, the death of a close relative or a change of environment), or as a response to the introduction of a new kind of therapy. The results obtained from the integrated rehabilitation system run by Sopimusvuori r.y. in Finland – which will be discussed in more detail in chapter 2.3.4. – strongly support this notion (Anttinen 1983, 1985).

Findings in good agreement with those reported by Bleuler and Ciompi and Müller have also been obtained in two other comprehensive works on the long-term prognosis of schizophrenia. Huber et al. (1979) found a favourable prognosis for 22 % of the 500 schizophrenic patients followed up for about 20 years in Bonn, West Germany (these patients showed permanent remission of their psychotic symptoms), while 26 % had a relatively favourable prognosis, 24 % a relatively unfavourable one and 28 % an unfavourable one. Tsuang et al. (1979) considered the 30- to 40-year prognosis of schizophrenics admitted into hospital in Iowa, U.S.A. during 1934 – 44 to be good in 20 % of the cases, relatively good in 26 % and poor in 54 %.

Several earlier studies showed that the prognosis of schizophrenia depended on the original clinical description of the illness. Norwegian Langfeldt (1939) made a distinction between schizophrenia proper and schizophreniform psychoses, which were characterized by the presence of heterogenous precipitating factors. He found the prognosis of such psychoses to be crucially better than that of typical or nuclear schizophrenia : after 7 – 10 years, 62 % of the patients with schizophreniform psychosis in his series had recovered completely, while remissions had only taken place in 5 % of the typical or nuclear schizophrenias (Langfeldt 1956).

Some other Nordic authors (Johanson 1958, Astrup et al. 1962, Astrup and Noreik 1966, Achté 1961, 1967) have confirmed a parallel prognostic difference. A corresponding distinction between "process schizophrenia" and "non-process schizophrenia" or "reactive schizophrenia" was made in the USA (e.g. Garmezy and Rodnick 1959, Stephens 1970). The prognostic difference is emphatically revealed by the extensive survey of prognostic studies with more than 5-year follow-up published by Stephens in 1978. In his own series of 349 patients, 7 % of the "process cases" showed complete remission, 39 % had a relatively good prognosis, and 54 % developed more serious chronicity, the corresponding figures for the "non-process patients" being 36 %, 57 % and 7 %.

In the 1970's Strauss and Carpenter (1972, 1974, 1977), among others, invited attention to the restrictions involved in the fact that most prognostic studies were excessively based to the follow-up of the patients' clinical symptoms. Strauss and Carpenter differentiate between 4 prognostic categories: working capacity, symptoms, social relations and the durations of necessary hospital care, which are naturally interrelated, but each of which is further influenced by specific background variables. The number of social relations, the working capacity and the duration of previous hospitalizations turned out to have the greatest influence on the subsequent prognosis. The most significant negative symptomatic feature was the decrease of affect (Strauss and Carpenter 1977, Carpenter et al. 1978).

The prospective prognostic study by this American team showed the diagnostic categorization on the basis of the primary symptoms by Langfeldt and Schneider (1959) to be of more questionable value than previously estimated (Hawk et al. 1975, Strauss and Carpenter 1977). A similar notion based on a prognostic investigation was also presented by Bland et al. (1978, 1980), in Canada.

Simon and Wirt (1961), among others, have pointed out that certain features of the prepsychotic personality development are associated with favourable prognosis, the most notable of them being a good ability to make contacts, a good working anamnesis, and a presence of peer as well as heterosexual relations. Vaillant (1964) developed a prognostic scale where the first three items correlating with a good prognosis of schizophrenia were a presence of precipitating factors at the onset of psychosis, depressive psychotic symptoms, and development of psychosis within less than 6 months. Salokangas (1977, 1978) particularly underlines the connection between the psychic and social development in schizophrenic patients. Prepsychotic psychosocial development, which is reflected by the psychosocial situation and socioeconomic competence of the patients at the onset of the illness turned out the best predictive factor for clinical and psychosocial development in his series. He also emphasized the negative prognostic significance of asocial tendencies observed especially among the male patients.

The effect of the family environment on the prognosis of schizophrenic patients has been discussed in a row of interesting studies carried out in the Institute of Psychiatry in London. Brown et al. (1972) interviewed the relatives of schizophrenic patients, measuring the number of emotionally coloured comments made by the relatives on the patient within a given period. Vaughn and Leff (1976) replicated these studies and made scales of critical comments and hostility on the hand and comments reflecting excessive emotional involvement on the other. These were called (maybe somewhat imprecisely) "high expressed emotion", EE. They saw that a high EE clearly correlated with the probability of a discharged patient to be rehospitalized within the subsequent 9-month period. Later, clinical studies followed (cf. 2.3.2.).

An international survey carried out by the World Health Organization (The International Pilot Study of Schizophrenia, WHO, 1973, 1979), which consisted of nine centres located in different social and cultural environments, showed that schizophrenic syndromes similar in principle were seen in all these areas. The results of a follow-up study conducted two years later were surprising: both the psychosocial prognosis of schizophrenia and the clinical prognosis associated with the remission of symptoms were regularly better in the developing countries than in the better developed parts of the world (Sartorius et al. 1978, WHO 1979). While in the centres located in the industrialized countries (Denmark, England, USA, USSR and Czechoslovakia) the best two of the five prognostic categories included 35–50 % of the patients, the corresponding figure was 86 % for Ibadan, Nigeria, 66 % for Agra, India and 53 % for Cali, Colombia. The significance of the finding is emphasized by the fact that the diagnoses were made on the basis of a standardized psychiatric interview (PSE, the Present State Examination). A five year follow-up study confirmed these prognostic findings (Sartorius 1984).

Although this investigation has also been criticized, the aforesaid prognostic differences can probably be considered indicative. The tentative explanations of these differences have suggested possible regional differences in the biologic nature of schizophrenia – either constitutionally or following differences in child mortality – on the one hand and factors associated with the social environment on the other. The latter include the greater cohesion of the supportive extended kinship networks in the developing countries (Mosher and Keith 1979, British Medical Journal 1980; cf. also the description of "familism" in rural Nigeria by Abasiekong 1981). A related explanation refers to the generally less complicated social systems making the return to the work and other activities easier for the patients. The present authors also consider the lack of differentiation in the sociocultural development and the consequently more symbiotic nature of the human relations – which has also been described e.g. by a Finnish child psychiatrist Forssen (1979) working in Tanzania – a highly probable explanation for the difference. – The good prognosis of schizophrenia was also confirmed by Waxler's study (1979) in Sri Lanka. She underlines particularly the significance of the cultural beliefs and social labelling as factors influencing the prognosis.

The indicators of a good prognosis which have already become classic in our own culture, such as acute onset of the psychosis, confusion, depressive features and the minor extent of affective blunting, were of less significance in the developing countries compared with the Western countries in the WHO study. Raman and Murphy (1972) had already made a similar finding in an earlier study made on the island of Mauritius in the Indian Ocean. The different population groups differed with regard to the prognosis of schizophrenia. The differences were considered even by these authors to be best explained by the social conditions, particularly the support given by the family to the schizophrenic family member.

Results of some more recent follow-up sudies on schizophrenia will be discussed in connection of the discussion of our own results in Chapter 6.

2.2 Effect of Neuroleptic Medication on the Prognosis

Has the development of neuroleptic medication affected favourably the prognosis of schizophrenia? As early as 1969, Cole and Davis reviewed a hundred studies where the effect of phenothiazines on schizophrenia was compared with placebo groups, using the double blind method. In 86 of these studies the medication alleviated the psychotic symptoms more effectively than the placebo. In another survey of a great number of investigations published about ten years later, Davis et al. (1980) report the mean of rehospitalization to be 19 % for patients on neuroleptic medication and 55 % for control groups.The follow-up periods were short in most of the studies.

The long-term effect of medication on prognosis has been subject to less study. A few conclusions can be made, however, on e.g. the follow-up studies made in England and Finland before and after the advent of neuroleptic medication.

Harris et al. (1956) followed up for 5 years the patients given insulin coma treatment in London, establishing 45 % of them as socially recovered; in addition to these, 21 % lived outside hospital, though socially incapacitated. In another 5-year follow-up study carried out by Brown et al. (1966) on schizophrenic patients first admitted into three English mental hospitals in 1956, 56 % turned out socially recovered and 34 % lived outside hospital as social invalids. Wing (1978), who was himself a member of the latter team, interprets the differences as showing that medication has affected favourably even the long-term prognosis of the patients. It can be pointed out, however, that also the facilities for outpatient therapy and social rehabilitation were better at the time of the latter study.

A similar notion of a relative improvement of the prognosis of schizophrenia was also expressed by Bland et al. (1978) in their Canadian study, which was already referred to earlier on. In a group of schizophrenics followed up from 1963 till 1974–75, they found the prognosis to be good in 53 % of the cases; 33 % of the patients showed no deterioration compared with the prepsychotic level.

In Finland, Achté and his co-workers (Achté 1967, Niskanen and Achté 1972, Achté et al. 1980) conducted a five-year follow-up study on all the patients with psychoses of the schizophrenia group or paranoid psychosis first admitted into hospital in Helsinki in 1950, 1960, 1965 and 1970. The results of this follow-up, which indicate social improvement, are shown in the Table below.

Table 3.

Series	social recovery %	social incapacity %	dead %
1950 (–55)	59	37	4
1960 (–65)	68	27	5
1965 (–70)	64	30	6
1970 (–75)	54	41	4

In the light of these figures it seems that the favourable development of the prognosis from the 1950's to the 1960's – coinciding with the introduction of neuroleptic medication – has come to a standstill or even turned unfavourable in the 1970's, probably influenced by the worsened employment situation.

The most notable changes had taken place in the duration of the first hospitalization, which was 148 days in 1960, but only 38 days in 1970. A parallel change can be seen in the proportion of patients in hospital at the end of the follow-up period, which was 21 % in the first series, 14 % in the second and merely 6 % in the last.

The effects of neuroleptic medication on the prognosis of schizophrenic patients hence appear more clearly as a lesser need for hospital treatments, even in the long run. Together with the development of outpatient care and rehabilitation facilities and partly supporting them – the development of pharmacal therapies has exerted a clearly favourable influence on the social prognosis of schizophrenic patients. Still, the most recent retrospective studies made in Finland, for example, also demonstrate the limits of this influence. We think that the need for developing new modes of therapy is hence apparent even on these grounds.

2.3 Studies on the Effect of Psychotherapy and Other Psychosocial Modes of Treatment

The research on the effect of psychotherapeutic treatment given to schizophrenic patients involves numerous problems. One weakness particularly typical of works made in the Anglo-Saxon area is shortness of the follow-up periods. Although prognostic studies have indicated that reliable data on the course of illness can only be obtained 5 years after the onset – for example, the survey published by Stephens in 1978 only included the works where the follow-up was 5 years or more – the follow-up periods in several works on the effects of psychotherapy are no more than a few months, at best one or two years.

The criteria used in assessing the prognosis are highly variable. Some authors have been content merely to report the duration of hospitalization or the number of readmissions, although these criteria are grossly inadequate, particularly when dealing with the effects of psychotherapy. When assessing the effects of psychodynamic psychotherapy, we should consider, apart from the patient's clinical status, working capacity, hospitalizations and other similar more or less hard facts, even the patient's increased insight into his symptoms as well as his psychological personality development and the reflection of this in the quantity and quality of his interpersonal relations.

Quite justifiably, it has also been suggested that the nature – as well as the description – of the modes of psychotherapy applied in the different works are highly variable in quality, and the therapists also differ in their competence and experience of therapeutic work (Mosher and Keith 1979, 1980).

We might here repeat the points made above (in Chapter 1.2.) on the restricting effects of the excessively method-oriented design of therapy studies on the possibilities of measuring the potentialities of psychotherapeutic treatment. A research design based directly on the natural scientific model still is considered a measure of scientific worth by several researchers and reviewers.[1]

One further addition to the problems is the influence of the therapist's personal characteristics, on which Whitehorn and Betz (1954, 1960) already made important observations. One consequence of this is that the results obtained in one study are not so readily reproducible in another as are the results of pharmacotherapy.

2.3.1 Individual Psychotherapy

In the history of individual psychotherapy of schizophrenic patients, a significant role is played by numerous case reports demonstrating that even patients with severe, and frequently long-standing, schizophrenic disorders have been successfully cured through a long-term empathic dyadic relationship (e.g. Kempf 1919, Knight 1939, Sechehaye 1947, Müller 1955, Johansson 1956, Will 1961). Benedetti (1975) summarizes therapies conducted under his guidance by a talented psychotherapist, Bertha Neumann. Of the 30 patients classifiable as schizophrenics, most of them with quite severe symptoms, who were treated by Neumann, more than half, i.e. 17, had recovered sufficiently to be able to work, to be free of psychotic symptoms and to show no relapse in a follow-up study made several years later. The period of therapy varied from 3 months to 5 years, with 3 hours of psychotherapy weekly in most cases. Of the remaining 13 patients, 7 showed definite improvement and good social adjustment.

Sjöström(1982), in Sweden, recently presented an interesting prognostic study of the schizophrenic patients also treated by one and the same psychotherapist (Barbro

[1]One recent example of this is the review of the pharmacotherapies of schizophrenia by Davis et al. (1982), which also includes a survey of psychotherapies. In addition to their absolute requirement for randomization, the authors also suggest that control groups receiving "psychological placebo treatment" be used in studies of psychotherapy.

Sandin) in the Säter Hospital. There were 14 patients, all of them under 30 years old and classifiable as typically schizophrenic on the basis of the Research Diagnostic Criteria. The control series consisted of 12 other male schizophrenic inpatients of the Säter Hospital matched to the therapy series for age, diagnosis and the most central background variables contributing to the prognosis. The follow-up period was 6 years from 1974 to 1980.

Two of the psychotherapy patients had committed suicide. According to the multidimensional prognostic criteria of Strauss and Carpenter (1977), the other patients undergoing psychotherapy were in a clearly better condition than the control group. Two central prognostic areas, working capacity and the need for hospital treatment during the last year of follow-up, as well as the combined measure of global prognosis showed statistically significant differences ($p < 0.01$), and the difference for the presence of symptoms was also almost significant ($p < 0.05$). At the time of the follow-up, 7 of the therapy patients were without any medication and the mean drug dose of the group corresponded to 25 mg chlorpromazine per day, while only one of the control patients managed without pharmacotherapy and the mean drug dose of the group corresponded to 400 mg chlorpromazine per day.

An average of 200 hours of psychotherapy per patient had been given in this series. All of the therapies had been commenced at the inpatient stage in close cooperation with the ward staff; in almost every case the therapeutic contact was continued at the outpatient stage. Four of the patients were still receiving psychotherapy at the time of the follow-up.

Follow-up studies covering more extensive series consisting of patients of several therapists have failed to give parallel findings clearly more favourable than the conventional prognosis of schizophrenics. These include the retrospective study made by Christian Müller (1961) on the schizophrenic patients treated psychotherapeutically in the famous Burghölzli Hospital in Zürich during 1950–58 as well as Schulz's (1963) and McGlashan's (1984) follow-up reports from the well-known psychotherapeutic centre of Chestnut Lodge in Maryland, USA. These studies hence serve to caution against excessively optimistic generalization of the single reports of favourable outcomes of psychotherapy.

Since the 1960's, at least 7 research projects have been carried out on the individual psychotherapy of schizophrenia, which have been designed more systematically than previously, including a comparison of the results with patient groups treated by other methods. Of these studies, the one made in the Camarillo State Hospital in California under the guidance of Philip R. A. May (1968, 1969) has attracted most attention partly probably because of the findings favourable for pharmacotherapy and unfavourable for psychotherapy. The series consisted of 288 schizophrenics first admitted into hospital (the subjects with the best and poorest predicted prognosis were excluded). The series was divided in a random fashion into five groups receiving different therapies: 1) individual therapy, 2) pharmacotherapy (trifluoroperazine), 3) individual therapy combined with pharmacotherapy, 4) electroshock treatment, and 5) milieu therapy. The psychotherapeutic treatment was given by resident physicians (including recently graduated ones) under the guidance of their seniors. The patients were followed up until they were able to leave the hospital or had been there for 6–10 months and both the therapist and the counsellor considered the therapy as having failed. The "successful" therapies, which here simply mean discharge from hospital, were distributed as follows: psychotherapy 65 %, pharmacotherapy 95 %, psychotherapy + pharmacotherapy 96 %, electroshock treatment 79 %, and milieu therapy (which here does not refer to any specific community therapy, but merely to a control group not receiving any of he abovementioned therapies) 58 %.

Karon and VandenBos (1972, 1975) criticized May's project on the grounds that most of the therapists were inexperienced and the trial was carried out in an atmosphere where the counsellors were even primarily dubious of the chances of psychotherapy applied to psychoses. Further criticism has been directed at the shortness of the therapies – an average of 46 hours per patient – and their restriction to the inpatient stage. May even points out himself that these findings cannot be used for making conclusions on the effects of pharmacotherapy and psychotherapy on outpatients. Together with his team (May et al. 1976, 1981) he subsequently made follow-up studies on his series, trying to prove the permanence of the original prognostic findings (though he was obliged to report a statistical "attenuation" of the effects of pharmacotherapy after a 3-year follow-up). A notable loss of patients detracts from the value of these follow-up studies.

Grinspoon, Ewalt and Shader (1972) examined the results of psychoanalytically oriented psychotherapy in a group of 20 male patients with chronic schizophrenia, who had been inpatients of the Boston State Hospital for at least 3 years without interruption and had "no hope of being discharged in the near future". The patients were transferred from there to a research institute functioning under the auspices of the Harvard University Department of Psychiatry. Half of the patients were given combined psychotherapy and medication (thioridazine), while the other half received psychotherapy and placebo.

The authors maintain that psychotherapy alone – even when given by experienced psychotherapists – helped these patients "little or not at all" during the two years. Psychotherapy combined with medication, on the other hand, alleviated their symptoms, though to a limited extent only. Grinspoon and his co-workers conclude that their findings speak strongly in favour of pharmacotherapy in the treatment of patients with chronic schizophrenia.

Two other American research teams obtained more favourable results. Of these, Karon and VandenBos' (1972, 1975, 1981) project was carried out in the Michigan State University. The project included three groups of patients, the first of which was given psychoanalytic psychotherapy with "direct" interpretations and without medication, while the second received "ego-analytically" oriented psychotherapy (accordant with the psychoanalytic frame of reference) in combination with small or moderate doses of chlorpromazine and the third group of controls was given merely moderate or large doses of chlorpromazine. The psychotherapy groups comprised altogether 21 patients and the control group 12. Most of them belonged to the lowest social group. 2/3 of the patients were being hospitalized for the first time, and the others were also regarded as relatively recent cases of the schizophrenia group.

The psychotherapy of the patients was started quite intensively (3–5 sessions weekly) and continued thereafter with longer intervals (1 session weekly) for altogether 20 months even at the outpatient stage. A careful psychiatric and psychological assessment of the condition of each patient was made at several stages of the therapy, and a follow-up examination was carried out 2 years after the termination of therapy. The results on both the duration of hospitalization and the patients' clinical status reveal a statistically significant difference in favour of the patients given psychotherapy. A particularly significant difference emerged in the psychological testing for thought disorders ($p < .005$), but no differences were noted in the results of projective tests.

This project showed psychotherapy to have better effects on the prognosis of the patients than had pharmacotherapy. Comparing their findings with those reported by May, Karon and VandenBos stress, among other things, that the results achieved by experienced therapists were more permanent in their study than the results reached by less experienced therapists working under guidance.

Rogers et al. (1967) published a study on "client-centered" individual therapy of inpatients diagnosed as schizophrenic, where the clinical status and interactional relations of 24 patients on therapy were found to be clearly better than those of a large group of patients receiving "conventional hospital treatment" only. The therapists in this trial were experienced psychologists, and therapy sessions were held twice a week.

Norwegian Endre Ugelstad (1978) studied 30 chronic male schizophrenics aged 25–40 years, who had all been in hospital for at least 3 years, and had now been treated for at least 1 year without a break in the Gaustad Hospital in Oslo. He divided these patients into a group of 12 receiving intensive psychoanalytically oriented individual therapy at least twice a week for one year or more, a group of 6 given active milieu therapy on a special ward established for this purpose, and a control group of 12, which consisted of patients having jobs or doing sheltered work outside the hospital despite the fact of being still inpatients. According to a quantitative assessment of the psychic status developed by Rockland – Pollin (1965), the therapy groups were initially more seriously disturbed than the control group.

According to a follow-up made two years later, the outcome in the group given individual therapy was clearly better than that in the control group. This was also shown by the discharge figures: 7 patients had been discharged from the psychotherapy group, 4 from the control group and 1 from the milieu therapy group. Another survey conducted 4 years after the beginning of the project demonstrated a levelling of this difference between the psychotherapy and control groups. A psychiatric assessment using the Rockland – Pollin scale supported the results favourable for psychotherapy, as did also an independent psychologic test carried out on the patients of the psychotherapy group. Ugelstad emphasizes the significance of social factors (work and dwelling) as well as the relations outside the hospital for the achievement and permanence of therapeutic results.

Beck et al. (1981) examined the results of the one-year psychotherapy of 27 schizophrenic patients in a community-psychiatric unit operating under the auspices of a university in Cambridge, Massachusetts. Most of the therapists (94 %) and patients (85 %) described the therapy in favourable terms. In 12 cases (44 %) definite improvement in the work and/or social relations was observable. The more experienced therapists achieved better results than the less experienced ones. The authors invite attention to the fact that the descriptions by the therapists and the patients of the therapeutic relationship were well accordant in the cases where the outcome was good, but often highly divergent in the cases where no progress had taken place. They take this as evidence of a connection between the therapeutic process and progress.

A remarkable research project for the study of individual psychotherapy of schizophrenia was designed in 1970's at the MacLean Hospital, Belmont,

Massachusetts, under the leadership of Alfred H. Stanton. Afterwards the project has been led by John G. Gunderson. The results of this project were published in the Schizophrenia Bulletin magazine (Stanton et al. 1984, Gunderson et al. 1984).

The project's aim was to measure the results and relative benefits of exploratory, insight-oriented (EIO) psychotherapy and reality-oriented, supportive (RAS) psychotherapy comparing them with one another. The project was realized with utmost thoroughness and care. The treatments were provided by experienced therapists independently of the research group. The follow-up examinations encompassed all the most important instruments used in previous American studies.

The sample included 186 patients; the diagnoses were confirmed by the Discriminating Criteria for Schizophrenia used in the WHO research. Like in the May (1968) study, the most severely and mildly disturbed patients were left out of the sample.

EIO therapists were psychoanalytically oriented, RAS therapists had a supportive, more biologically oriented approach. The frequency of treatments in the EIO groups was clearly greater (more than 2 sessions a week on the average, in the RAS therapy it was less than 1). The researchers conclude that the therapies differed from each other as expected regarding the direction of discussions (in the EIO therapies the stress lay on the interpersonal relationships including clarification of unconscious motivation and transference; the RAS therapies were more directive). The difference still remained small; also the EIO therapies had supportive qualities. The pharmacotherapy for the patients was planned in a "controlled" manner by experts of psychopharmacology, and a time limit was set for the group and family therapies the patients could receive in addition to the individual therapy.

The dropout rate presented a big problem in this study. Only 72 patients (44 %) could be studied after 12 months and 51 patients (31%) after 24 months, when the most essential results were being evaluated. The differences in the prognosis of the groups proved to be small. Regarding cognitive functioning (disorganization of thoughts, insight-ability) positive development was seen in both groups in comparison. In the development of the ego functioning a moderate-sized effect favoring the EIO therapy was found.

There were no verifiable differences in the development of interpersonal relationships; in both groups about one third of the patients were able to form meaningful relationships during the follow-up time. In both groups the symptoms were relieved alike. As to the social abilities the result was clearly better in the RAS group concerning the occupational functioning; whereas there was no difference in the self-sufficiency and social functioning of the patients. Both groups received a considerable amount of pharmacotherapy throughout the study period and so did not differ from each other here.

Again, the hospitalization time was longer for the EIO patients than the RAS patients, which was largely accounted for by the longer initial hospitalization of the EIO patients; the RAS patients were rehospitalized somewhat more often.

It should be noticed, that in this study the comparison was not drawn between psychotherapy patients and those left out, but it was made between two psychotherapeutic approaches, which in the end differed from each other partly diffusely. As a whole the study did not prove that the EIO therapy would have had any remarkable benefits compared as against the RAS therapy. The reseachers debate in their discussion whether the result had been different had the patient sample remained bigger during the follow-up or the time of the follow-up longer. In their view the latter factor might have had a certain effect. In the light of our own experiences, we also would regard this as probable.

2.3.2 Family Therapy

Family therapy is a more recent mode of treatment than individual therapy. It is, however, interesting to note that even Federn and Sullivan, the pioneers of individual therapy in schizophrenia, were aware of the importance of the family environment for the prognosis of their patients.

Hence Federn (1943) points out that each schizophrenic psychosis "is related, consciously or unconsciously, to conflicts or frustrations of family life", and says that the treatment of psychotic patients is a Sisyphean task, unless the unfavourable aspects of family life can be altered. Several individual therapists have seen it to be useful to have a favourable contact with the members of their patients' families, or have included the family in their therapeutic work at some stage. As an example we can mention the pioneering work carried out by Kauko Kaila and Allan Johansson in Finland as early as the 1950's (Johansson 1956, 1985, Kaila 1954).

Experiences on the family therapy of schizophrenics and its outcome have been published by e.g. Bowen et al. (1961), Jackson and Weakland (1961), Gralnick (1963), Shellow et al. (1963), Esterson et al. (1962), Scott and Ashwoth (1967), Scott and Montanez (1972), Scott and Alwyn (1978), Alanen (1973, 1976), and Kaufmann (1976). What these papers have in common is a notion of family therapy as an expedient method of treating schizophrenia which also has a favourable outcome in many cases. The therapeutic technique (which was generally based on the psychodynamic concept) as well as the criteria used for evaluating the outcome vary in the different works. Hence Bowen's work is based on a very thorough examination and treatment of 15 families – where the symptomatic member was a very ill young schizophrenic – and his criteria of the outcome include both a remission of the symptoms and an improvement of the family system: according to him, a "definite" change was only achieved in one case, while moderate or slight improvement took place in 7 other families, no change occurred in 4 cases, and 3 families discontinued the therapy so early that no assessment could be made. Jackson and Weakland, in turn, evaluate the improvement of both the patient's symptoms and social adaptation and the interfamily communication, considering the outcome good in 15 of their 18 families and poor in only 3 families.

Alanen as well as Kaufmann emphasize the significance of a sufficietly long family-therapeutic contact. According to Alanen, it is possible for the family therapist in a long-term therapeutic relationship to promote the psychologic individuation of a young patient both by activating the patient's capacity of expression and by allowing the parents to transfer to the therapist their needs for dependence previously applied to the patient. In such a case the parents may gradually identify with the attitudes of the therapist, while the relationship thereby created lessens the ties previously existing between the parents and the patient.

Kaufmann also emphasizes the significance of this therapeutic principle, which he calls the "Trojan horse strategy", but also points out the associated risk of getting stuck in continuous pseudo-mutuality (Wynne et al. 1958) with the family and the need for more active interventions.

The investigations by Scott and his co-workers are interesting, particularly from the viewpoint of identifying the factors which contribute to the social prognosis of the patients. Scott and Ashworth (1967) described the psychologic event they called "closure". This essentially consists of the rejection of a schizophrenic patient previously bound to his parents in hospital as assumably incurable, while his care is delegated to the hospital staff. Scott et al. (1972, 1978) then examined the schizophrenic patients who easily became chronic hospital inmates and compared them with ones who did not suffer this fate. They found significant differences between the "hospital-oriented" group and the "home-oriented" group, when they applied an interpersonal test method (the Family Relationship Test) to illustrate the notions of the patient on the one hand and the patients on the other of themselves and each other. In the hospital-oriented group the parent's image of themselves and the patient's image of them differed greatly, while in the home-oriented group the images were parallel, which meant in practice that the patients had identified themselves with their parent's "good" notion of themselves as parents. According to Scott et al., family therapy should be particularly applied to the patients of the hospital-oriented group. Otherwise, Scott and his co-workers considered the treatment of this group – including about 35 % of the schizophrenic patients living with their parents – both useless and doomed to failure.

Over the past few years, the development of family therapy has been notably influenced by the therapeutic technique based strategically on the systems theory. The therapists using this technique work as a team and make active efforts to find out the role played by the symptoms of the identified patient in the maintenance of the psychological state of the family. When successful, the interpretation by the therapists of their views in accordance with the carefully designed strategies has a marked altering effect on the family's internal feedback cycles. The therapists applying this technique to the treatment of schizophrenics report favourable results, which, so far, have been mostly casuistic (Selvini Palazzoli et al. 1977, Sluzki 1981, Stierlin 1983). Systematic investigation of the effects of strategic family therapy on the prognosis of schizophrenia still awaits to be undertaken.

Another current line of development is the combination of short active and directive family-therapeutic intervention – often called the psycho-educational approach (e.g. Anderson et al. 1980) – and pharmacotherapy. An important stimulus for this line of therapeutic practice was provided by the EE studies of Leff and Vaughn described in chapter 2.1. The disturbances of family communication are here seen as affecting the course of the illness, but not necessarily its etiology.

Goldstein et al. (1978) reported interesting results in their carefully planned study of 104 acute young schizophrenic patients first hospitalized for a short period and then given crisis-oriented family therapy. The series was randomly divided into 4 groups, of which 2 were given family therapy and 2 were not; the groups further differed in that 2 were given a higher and 2 a lower dose of injected fluphenazine enantate at 2-week intervals. The family therapy was restricted to six sessions given at one-week intervals with clearly defined objectives: 1) to make the patient and his family accept that the patient has had a psychosis; 2) to make them identify some stress factors of their life probably precipitating the psychosis; 3) to make them develop strategies for identifying possible future stresses; 4) to make them plan ways to alleviate or prevent these stresses. Goldstein et al. point out that they thus tried to help the patient and his family utilize the event of the psychosis psychologically rather than seal it over and externalize it.

A follow-up study carried out 6 months after the discontinuation of therapy showed that 75 % of the patients had not been rehospitalized, while the corresponding figure for previous series treated in the same therapeutic unit in Los Angeles had been 55 %. The outcome was clearly the best in the groups given family therapy: no rehospitalizations took place in the group that received both family therapy and more intensive drug therapy, while 22 % of the patients given family therapy and less intensive drug therapy were rehospitalized, the corresponding figures for the groups without family therapy being 14 % and 48 %.

Another follow-up study undertaken 3 years later showed, however, that the differences between the groups had levelled off (Goldstein and Kopeikin 1981, ref. Gunderson & Carroll 1983).

Leff et al. (1982) carried out a therapy investigation on the families of schizophrenic patients with high EE values of the family members. This study also dealt with patients on continuous neuroleptic medication administered as long-acting injections. In the study group (12 families), this medication was supplemented with three-part social intervention, including lectures on the nature and prognosis of schizophrenia given to the relatives, relatives' groups and family therapy sessions (1 to 25 sessions per family, mean 5.6.) The control group consisted of 12 families also with high EE values, whose patient member was given similar pharmacotherapy, but otherwise conventional treatment.

The study was begun at the time of discharging the patients from hospital. During the following 9 months, half of the control patients, but only one of the patients in the study group were rehospitalized. In the light of the follow-up results, the goal of bringing down the high EE values was reached well in the case of critical comments, but less well in the case of expressions showing emotional involvement. The authors consider their results to demonstrate the causal significance of the relatives' attitudes for the rehospitalization of schizophrenic patients, concluding that these attitudes can be therapeutically corrected. –There is a two-year follow-up study being carried out on the series, for which no results have been published yet.

American Falloon et al. (1982) also report the results of a 9-month follow-up survey on schizophrenic patients on continuous neuroleptic medication, who were given family therapy on home visits, to diminish stress factors through increased understanding of the illness and learning-therapeutic methods. The goal of this work, too, was to avoid rehospitalization, which was successfully accomplished for all but one (6 %) of the experimental patients compared with 8 patients (44 %) in a control group of the same size given similar drug doses and supportive individual therapy.

Good results of family therapy with largely similar goals have also been reported by the team of Liberman et al. (1981), which also included Falloon and Vaughn.

As early as the 1960's Laquer et al. (1964) described the results they got in treating jointly the families of several schizophrenic patients, which were relatively good in their series of 80 patients: considerable improvement took place in about half of the cases, and only 10–20 % of the patients showed no response to the therapy. Lansky et al. (1978) also reported moderately favourable experiences with a similar therapeutic method. Schindler (1980) recently reported the results obtained with "bifocal therapy" (the patients as one group, the relatives as another ; Schindler 1957, 1959) as early as 1949–59 in Vienna, which were exceptionally good even in the light of 20-year follow-up: of the 116 patients, 90 % were able to work. 76 % had found a dwelling partner,

16 % lived in their original families, only 3 % were "isolated" and 5 % were in hospital. A more detailed account on these follow-up data would be useful.

Seeing to the fact that the spouse relations of married schizophrenic patients have long been an object of scientific interest (e.g. Lichtenberg & Pao 1960, Towne et al. 1961, Dupont et al. 1971, Alanen and Kinnunen 1975, Buddeberg and Kesselring 1978), there are relatively few written reports on spouse therapy. Apart from Becker's (1963) small series of 7 patients, the only other report to be found in the literature is a study by Alanen and Kinunen (1975) on the marital relations of patients collected from Finland, with spouse therapy given in 18 ot the total of 30 cases. The marital relations in this work were divided, mainly on the basis of the Spouse Rorschach tests, into three groups, which also correlated to the identified chances of successful spouse therapy. The results were best in the groups where either both of the spouses were helpless or the patient was more dominant and his or her spouse an empathic "follower". Poorer results were obtained in the group where the spouse dominated the patient in an unempathic way and the patient was submissively dependent on the spouse.

2.3.3 Group Therapy

In the treatment of schizophrenic patients, group therapy has a longer tradition than family therapy. Papers on group therapy were written as early as the 1920's and 1930's (Lazell 1921, Marsh 1933, Schilder 1936). The increase of outpatient therapies over the past 15–20 years has contributed to the development of group activities for the aftercare of schizophrenic patients. Group therapy has often been considered both a cost-saving method and an expedient mode of therapy for increasing the interpersonal contacts and social skills that are so important for long-term schizophrenic patients. On hospital wards and rehabilitation homes, group therapy and other, less specific group functions and meetings have become an important part of the activities of the therapeutic communities.

Reviews of works on the group therapy of psychotic patients have been published by e.g. Bednar and Lawlis (1971), Parloff and Dies (1977) as well as Mosher and Keith (1979, 1980) in a more extensive survey on psychosocial treatment of schizophrenia. The general conclusion made in these reviews and the papers discussing them is that group therapy really is most consequential for the expansion of the patient's interpersonal field and the associated activation of social skills. From the viewpoint of clinical recovery, however, the results do not seem particularly good.

Parloff and Dies discuss the results of group therapy reported in 1966–1975. In 5 out of 7 studies of schizophrenic patients, the patients given group therapy on a hospital ward did not benefit from it crucially in comparison with the patients without therapy. Nevertheless, 5 of the 6 other studies where group therapy was combined with other forms of treatment showed it to have a favourable effect on the outcome. The forms of treatment with which group therapy was combined in these works included neuroleptic medication, video tape feedback, conventional ward activities and "dyadic social interaction". Mosher and Keith point out that the results were generally better in settings where the therapeutic programs were relatively well structured (e.g. Robinson 1970, Corder et al. 1971, Olson and Greenberg 1972), and that this agrees well with the notion that structured programs are particularly practicable in the treatment of chronic patients.

The use of group therapy in the after-care of outpatients has also been discussed by many authors. O'Brien and his co-workers (1972) divided 100 discharged patients randomly into groups receiving either individual therapy or group therapy; in both groups the therapy consisted of supportive sessions given at relatively long intervals by relatively inexperienced therapists. Follow-up studies 12 and 24 months later showed that the patients given group therapy were able to manage better socially and also had a slightly better clinical status than the patients given individual therapy. The rate of rehospitalization was the same in the two groups. Herz et al. (1974) also studied the difference between group and individual therapy in a series of 108 chronic schizophrenics, who were treated for 11 months by residents. The results revealed no differences in the prognoses of the two patient groups, although the authors mention that the therapists felt group therapy to be a more favourable mode of treatment. Levene et al. (1970) saw no differences between patients on group and individual therapy. Claghorn et al. (1974) investigated the effects of group therapy compared with a group of patients given merely pharmacotherapy, stating that group therapy improves the social coping and interpersonal skills of the patients, but does not alleviate the clinical symptoms. In a more long-term study, Lindberg (1981), of Sweden, combined injected fluphenazine medication with both individual and group psychotherapy in the treatment of 14 chronic schizophrenic male patients. There was a control group of 13 patients receiving only drug treatment. The psychotherapy program was more intensive for three first years of investigation and less intensive for 2 further years. Variables measuring intellectual capacity and thought disorders (The Holtzman Inkblot Technique) indicated a favourable development in the psychotherapy group during three years but a slight decrease after that. The psychotherapy group also stayed more days outside the hospital than the control group. However, only during the fifth year was the difference statistically almost significant ($p < .05$) and when the patients were followed further three years there was a levelling between the groups in this respect.

2.3.4 Other Studies

Among the studies on the *milieu therapy* of schizophrenic patients, two interesting projects opposite to each other in many respects were undertaken in the 1970's. In 1973, Gordon Paul and his co-workers (also Paul & Lentz 1977) reported the results of a carefully planned study of chronic schizophrenic patients. They divided their series into three groups, of which the first underwent a precisely structured behaviour-therapeutic program of therapeutic community (token economy program), the second was treated in accordance with the conventional therapeutic community principles, and the third served as a control group receiving conventional mental hospital treatment. Within three years, 96 % of the patients in the first group could be discharged, the corresponding figure being 68 % in the second group and 46 % in the control group. The rehospitalization percentage in the first group was less than 5 %. Although only a few of these patients (10 %) were able to live independently, they managed to live as outpatients with the help of extramural supportive arrangements. Paul et al. also pointed out that the patients whose pharmacotherapy was discontinued benefited more from the active therapeutic program than those on continuous medication, who were less able to learn new and socially more adaptive modes of activity. Liberman (1980) also demonstrated the utility of structured therapeutic programs accordant with the "training and education model" in the rehabilitation of chronic patients in particular.

Loren R. Mosher and his co-workers (Mosher et al. 1975, Mosher and Menn 1978, 1983) approached the treatment of acutely psychotic patients with the objective of supporting particularly the patients's own efforts towards integration that are included in psychotic regression. The team founded in California the small Soteria home staffed by laymen without psychiatric training or therapeutic identity, but enthusiastic about their task. The patients accepted were unmarried first admission schizophrenics 15–30 years of age, who were treated by the staff in conversation contacts under guidance. The periods in Soteria home were generally long, lasting for 5–6 months; pharmacotherapy was only given if no observable recovery had taken place within 6 weeks. The control group consisted of similar patients admitted for "short and effective" (average 21 days) mental hospital treatment. A follow-up carried out 2 years after the termination of the treatment showed that the chances of the Soteria patients to manage without readmissions were greater by about 20 % than those of the control patients despite the fact that 50 % of the controls had been on neuroleptic medication until rehospitalization or the end of the follow-up period, while only 19 % of the Soteria patients had been given corresponding pharmacotherapy. The Soteria patients had also been more successful occupationally and more effective and lived independently or with their friends more often.

Mosher and his team emphasized, among other things, the importance of the relatively long duration of the community therapy for the separation from home and the significance of the peer group thereby created for the psychosocial development of their patients. It is partly on the basis of these results that Mosher and Keith (1979), discussing the milieu therapy of acute schizophrenic patients, underline the small size of the therapeutic unit, the positive expectations and active involvement of the staff in the therapeutic process as well as practicable, down-to-earth and problem-oriented therapeutic principles.

Hogarty et al. (1973, 1974a, b, Goldberg et al. 1977) carried out a large project in the USA, studying the contribution of pharmacotherapy on the one hand and *sociotherapy* consisting of social casework and occupational rehabilitation (Major Role Therapy) on the other on the prognosis of schizophrenic patients discharged from hospital. The contribution of pharmacotherapy was unambiguous: 48 % of the patients given chlorpromazine and 80 % of those receiving placebo were rehospitalized within the following two years. Sociotherapy promoted significantly the patient's social adjustment, particularly in the pharmacotherapy group. What is significant, however, is that this effect emerged relatively slowly: it was not yet discernible in the one-year follow-up, but was statistically significant at 18 months and even more pronounced at 24 months. In a later report the authors conclude that sociotherapy was most beneficial for patients in a relatively good condition, but occasionally even precipitated the rehospitalization of patients with severe symptoms. They hence recommend that sociotherapy be started at the time when the patients no longer have any manifest psychotic symptoms (Goldberg et al. 1977). In an another project, where the sociotherapy consisted of intensive social casework on both the individual and the family, the results were essentially the same (Hogarty et al. 1979).

The *rehabilitation* of long-term psychiatric patients became an important mode of action and object of study in the 1960's. It was particularly pursued in England and

Holland, where units of industrial therapy were established in hospitals (pioneered by Early 1960, and Wing 1960) and sheltered workshops outside them (e.g. Speijer 1961).

It has become evident that successful rehabilitation cannot be based exclusively on efforts to make the patient capable of working through work experiments, but requires the support of a more extensive therapeutically oriented community outside the hospital. Over the past few years, increasing numbers of rehabilitating dwelling communities, "halfway homes", have been founded for this purpose. As a pioneer in this field emerged the Fountain House established in New York as early as the 1950's, where more than 300 people had been staying by the mid-1970's. This therapeutic community, which was established on an outpatient basis and emphasized the dweller's own activity, has served to diminish the rehospitalizations of many previous inmates (Beard et al. 1978).

In 1970, a system of rehabilitation homes called the Sopimusvuori programme was established at Tampere, in Finland, upon the initiative of Erik E. Anttinen, Ritva Jokinen and Leena Salmijärvi. It now incorporates rehabilitation units of various levels that accommodate more than 200 patients. The ideology is based on community and group activity which involves both clients and staff and is as far as possible based on equality (Anttinen 1983). Altogether 500 clients, most of them schizophrenic chronics hospitalized for long periods, have been discharged from hospital through this integrated rehabilitation system. The preliminary follow-up data on the first 201 patients rehabilitated – 52 % of them had been hospitalized for altogether more than 10 years and 2/3 for more than 5 years – revealed that 3/5 of them had been able to start living in supported dwellings or dormitories, apartments owned or rented by themselves or together with their families. For 1/5 the rehabilitation home came to be permanently the highest level of living milieu, and for the remaining 1/5 the rehabilitation turned out unsuccessful, and the clients had to be returned to hospital (Anttinen 1983; 1985).

Good results of the rehabilitation of chronic patients in dwelling units have also been reported by e.g. Engelke and Haselbeck (1980), Gomez (1981) and Mezquita (1982).

The effects of *psychiatric home care* on schizophrenic patients have also been studied. In the project carried out by Anttinen and his co-workers (1971, 1974) in Finland in the 1960's, 264 schizophrenic patients discharged from hospital were followed up for two years. Of these patients, 97 belonged to the home care group, while the control group received conventional outpatient therapy. The results of the study provided unambiguous proof of the superiority of home care for the social coping of these patients, most of whom were chronically ill. The home care patients were working for 52 % of the follow-up period, while the control patients had a working time percentage of 38.5 %, and an opposite ratio prevailed for rehospitalizations: 42 % of the home care patients and 56 % of the control patients were rehospitalized. Anttinen et al. emphasize particularly the attention given to the family milieus. According to their estimate, the relatives of the patients in the home care group were in need of therapeutic support in 87 % of the cases, and actual family therapy would have been indicated in 65% of these families. The authors also pointed out that for about 30 % of the home care patients the best solution would have been a dwelling unit or a rehabilitation home.

Equally favourable results were reported by Davis et al. (1972), who conducted a study on the preventive effects of home care on rehospitalization in Louisville, Kentucky. Along with the development of home care – and often in association with it different modes of supportive cooperation with the relatives of schizophrenic patients often on a group basis have been developed over the past few years (e.g. Kanter and Lin 1980, Thornton et al. 1981, Fink 1981, Bernheim 1982, Katschnig & Konieczna 1985).

Many of the studies described above have stressed the significance of pharmacotherapy for the social management of schizophrenic patients. It is therefore justifiable also to comment on a couple of reports on the opportunities of *treating schizophrenic patients without medication*. These studies are partially stimulated by the observation on the adverse sideeffects of long-term neuroleptic medication (for this, also cf. Wilson et al. 1983).

Carpenter et al. (1977) conducted a therapeutic trial on 49 patients with acute schizophrenia in the research centre of the National Institutes of Health, strictly limiting the share of pharmacotherapy. The therapy took place in a psychotherapeutically oriented milieu, where the patients were given psychoanalytically oriented individual therapy 2–3 times a week, group therapy once a week and most also family therapy once a week. No pharmacotherapy was given during the first 3 weeks; later on, 22 patients were also given neuroleptic treatment, which was, however, discontinued at least 3 weeks prior to the discharge. The average duration of hospital therapy was 4 months. This series was compared with 73 patients treated elsewhere with medication. The follow-up was made one year later in the research series and 2 years later in the control series. Attention was given to the working capacity of the patients, their social abilities, the duration of hospitalizations and the clinical symptoms observable during the month preceding the follow-up. The results indicated a small but significant difference in favour of the patients treated in the NIH. No differences were seen between the NIH patients with and without medication.

Rapaport et al. (1978) studied a Californian series of 80 young male schizophrenics, half of whom were treated with chlorpromazine administered in daily doses of 300–900 mg and the other half with placebo. The study consisted of as many as 8 follow-up assessments, the last being made 36 months after the termination of the hospital treatment. As it was to be expected, the results indicated that pharmacotherapy alleviated the patient's symptoms at the initial stages of the treatment. The follow-up examinations, however, revealed a group which had not received medication either in hospital or afterward, and which had a better prognosis than any other of the groups. These patients belonged to the category with a "good premorbid prognosis", and their clinical picture was predominantly paranoid. According to Rapaport et al., one should not resort to pharmacotherapy in the treatment of these patients, but rather endeavour to promote the reintegration of their personality without medication.

Mosher and Keith (1979, 1980) concluded their reviews of the studies on the psychosocial therapies of schizophrenia by pointing out that by now there are more data available on the effects of these therapies than is generally realized, and that most of the results obtained are favourable. They particularly emphasize the good outcome of family therapy and milieu therapy as well as the other modes of therapy influencing the social environment of the patients. It is easy to agree with these opinions yet by adding that, besides the environmentally oriented approach some studies demonstrate that long-term individual therapy also may have importance in the development of the treatment of schizophrenic patients.

On the whole, we can interpret the findings of the research on the effects of psychotherapy as lending definite support to the need for therapeutic development accordant with the integrated model of illness presented above in chapter 1.

We have not found any studies where this model of treatment would have been applied with the purpose of meeting both holistically and individually the therapeutic needs of all the new schizophrenic patients in a given area.

3 Study Project, Material and Methods

3.1 Beginning of the Project and the Patient Series

3.1.1 The Research Team and the Planning of the Project

The economic possibilities of carrying out the project were based on a research contract made with the Academy of Finland for the period April 1, 1976 – March 31, 1980. It permitted the formation of a four-member team with Professor Yrjö O. Alanen as the head and psychiatrist Viljo Räkköläinen, psychologist Juhani Laakso and specialized psychiatric nurse Riitta Rasimus as the members. Below they will be called the head of the project, the psychiatrist of the team, the psychologist of the team and the specialized nurse of the team. Alanen, Räkköläinen and Rasimus were members of the staff of the Clinic of Psychiatry – the first of them being the head of the Clinic of Psychiatry as well as of the Psychiatric Outpatient Department of the University Central Hospital of Turku – while Laakso was a staff member of the Turku Mental Health Office.

One important goal of our approach is to provide psychotherapeutic treatment to as many as possible of the patients for whom it is considered indicated. This presupposes a wide assortment of activities, which can only be ensured by using a multiprofessional staff as therapists.

The basis for this was the on-the-job training and supervision system already established at the Clinic of Psychiatry and extended during the project. The team members were engaged in this together with other members of the staff. Our explicit goal was that the research project should not remain a separate entity but intertwine organically with the activities of the Mental Health District. In that way it's effects would become permanent and have a continuous influence upon the development of the every-day treatment practices.

Riitta Rasimus was the only member of the team who was employed in research and the associated therapeutic work on a full-time basis during the period covered by the research contract, whereas the others participated along with their regular employment.

The team planned the project in their meetings prior to the collection of data. At the same time, a 163-item form was designed for the psychiatric basic study. This form was developed on the basis of the forms used at the earlier stages of the schizophrenia-project conducted in Turku (Räkköläinen 1977, Salokangas 1977, 1978). The renewal of the form was made in such a way as to permit comparison with the previous patient series. Another objective was to include clinically innovating items for applying the knowledge obtained from psychodynamic and family dynamic studies to the planning and follow-up of the treatment of schizophrenic patients. We assumed the function of the form not to be restricted to its use as an instrument of research, but hoped it would also be of use in the orientation and organization of clinical and therapeutic work both in this project and later on.

As early as 1971 and 1972, the head of the project and the psychiatrist of the team had conducted a reliability test of the earlier edition of the form. When further developing the form, the team members weighted the items with inter-rater reliabilities of more than 60 %. No reliability test was carried out during the present psychiatric basic study. Each form was jointly filled in by the same team members (the psychiatrist and psychiatric nurse of the team).

The contents of the form can be seen from the findings described in Chapter 4.

At the planning stage, the team negotiated with Christer Sourander, M.D, the chief psychiatrist of the Kupittaa Hospital, who also acted as the Medical Director of the Turku Mental Hospital District, and with Lyyli Hyry, assistant chief psychiatrist of the Turku Mental Health Office (cf. Alanen et al. 1978a). Representatives of the city administration of Turku and the hospital board were also informed of the project in a common meeting. The meetings and the consequent planning of cooperation in the different working units served to increase the coherence of the study and to facilitate the action research by the team.

3.1.2 Diagnostic Criteria for Inclusion in the Series

The diagnostic criterion for inclusion in the series was the presence of distinct psychotic symptoms of the schizophrenic type and indicative of disintegration of the previous functional level of the personality in the patient. When defined in this way, the schizophrenia group turns out to be relatively large, but it is quite consistent with the essential signs proposed by Eugen Bleuler (1911), who developed the term schizophrenia: at least partial loss of the integration of associative functions and/or affects. The definition also agrees with the classic psychoanalytic notion of the regressive development characteristic of psychotic conditions, which include disintegration or at least serious "splitting" of the higher-level psychic functions emerging along with age-appropriate psychologic development, and a simultaneous breakthrough of psychic functions of the primary process area previously controlled by the ego (e.g. Fenichel 1945, Räkköläinen 1977).

This diagnostic delineation was justified by our wish to keep the criteria of inclusion the same they were in the previous series of the Turku schizophrenia project. In those cases, too, the head of the project had made the ultimate decision concerning inclusion. But we also considered a relatively wide patient sample most appropriate considering the developmental goals of the project.

At the time of the basic study made upon inclusion in the series, we divided our patients into five sub-groups as follows:

nuclear schizophrenia	44
severe paranoia	4
acute schizophreniform psychosis	18
schizo-affective psychosis	13
borderline psychosis	21

This division was also used in our first reports based on the findings of the basic study (Alanen et al. 1979, 1980).

At the time of the first follow-up made two years after inclusion in the series, some changes were made in this division. They were due to a longer experience of the patient's clinical features. The patient labelled as nuclear schizophrenia were reclassified as a group of typical schizophrenias, which was also made to include the four severe paranoias; they can also be defined as paranoid schizophrenias, where the disintegration of ego functions is less extensive, but the psychotic thought disorders based on schizophreniform ideas of reference and other delusions are the more persistent.

The group of schizophreniform psychoses was simultaneously reduced, because many of the patients classified as belonging to it were later diagnosed for features characteristic of typical schizophrenias. Some other diagnostic specifications in individual cases were also made.

We also decided to replace the term "borderline psychosis" with "borderline schizophrenia", to emphasize the difference of this group from the "borderline personalities" as defined e.g. in the DSM-III system (American Psychiatric Association 1980).

After that, the diagnostic categorization of our series turned out as follows:

typical schizophrenia	56
schizophreniform psychosis	10
schizo-affective psychosis	14
borderline schizophrenia	20

Parallel diagnostic shifts of relatively equal magnitude from initially diagnosed schizophreniform psychosis to typical schizophrenia have also been noted in other Finnish follow-up studies (Achté 1961, 1967, Salokangas 1977). It might also be pointed out here that the DSM-III system, which has emerged as an important diagnostic system in the 1980's, only differentiates between schizophrenia's and schizophreniform psychoses on the basis of the duration of the symptoms, which means that the final diagnostic line can be drawn when the symptoms (including the symptoms of the prodromal and residual stages) have lasted for 6 months.

Nevertheless, our conscious goal in our final diagnostic categorization was that the major determinant would be the clinical picture, not the prognosis established through follow-up. In this we were aided by the notion suggesting that the prognosis of an individual patient suffering from typical schizophrenia need not necessarily be less favourable than the prognoses in the other diagnostic categories of our system.

We can best *define our diagnostic categories* on the basis of the following *clinical signs:*

The group of *typical schizophrenia* included the patients who, besides a schizophrenic-type thought disorder (in practice, the criterion for inclusion in the whole series), had some other characteristic and distinct schizophrenic symptoms which had set about without any toxic or organic precipitating factors and indicated a tendency to persistence. We paid particular attention to the presence of eight nuclear symptoms of schizophrenia: autism, schizophrenic thought disorder, hebephrenic affective disorder ("blunting" of affect), schizophrenic auditory hallucinosis, physical delusions of being influenced, massive psychologic delusions of being influenced, typical catatonic symptoms (stupor or excitement), and sensations of depersonalization and/or derealization when the patient's consciousness is clear.

We here slightly modified the comprehension of "process schizophrenia" prevalent in the Nordic tradition created by Langfeldt (1937, 1953, 1956) and followed, e.g. by Achté (1961, 1967). Compared with the ten symptoms selected by Achté as the criteria of typical schizophrenia, we left out an alteration of character prior to the onset of the psychosis (because it is not a psychotic symptom and difficult to differentiate from a schizoid adolescence crisis or heightened opposition to parents), and linked together the experiences of derealization and depersonalization.

It was further required that the patients classified as having typical schizophrenia lacked any manic or depressive symptoms occurring parallel to the schizophrenic symptoms and notably colouring the clinical picture.

The group of *schizophreniform psychoses* included short or recurrent psychotic states, where the onset of schizophrenic symptoms had regularly been sudden and the symptoms had been of short duration. In four cases the patient had serious problems of alcohol abuse or drug addiction, which had reached a culmination at the onset of the psychosis, without the psychosis resembling delirium tremens or alcoholic hallucinosis. Psychologic precipitating factors clearly different from the regular course of life of the patients were also common in this group. They were not, however, included among the diagnostic criteria, because the onset of typical schizophrenias also is associated with the patient's life course and the changes taking place in it, even if most frequently not very acute but rather characterized by developmental crises of longer duration (cf. e.g. Alanen et al. 1966, Räkköläinen 1977).

Schizo-affective psychoses were characterized by a simultaneous occurrence of schizophrenic symptoms and a clearly manic or depressive mental stage. The group hence did not include the cases where the depressive mood only became manifest after the termination of the schizophrenic symptoms of psychosis. The psychoses belonging to this group regularly had a sudden onset, but often lasted longer than the schizophreniform psychoses.

The group of *borderline schizophrenia* included the patients whose schizophrenic symptoms were mild, less characteristic and usually short in duration, although they tended to recur in most cases, occasionally even become chronic. The patients typically had character pathology of the kind called borderline personality (Kernberg 1967, 1975, Gunderson and Kolb 1978), a tendency to intense anxiety and various neurotic symptoms, mostly "splitting" of the ego functions, along with psychotic symptoms. A borderline personality pathology as such did not lead to inclusion in our series, unless the patients also had psychotic symptoms.

Fenton, Mosher and Matthews (1981) point out in a critical review of the current diagnostic systems dealing with schizophrenia that they all – despite their endeavours towards objectivity and reliability – are arbitrary and depend on mutual agreements between the raters. We cannot claim that our own classification would be strict; it probably could not be without being untrue to reality. Some of the statistical correlations between these groups and the observations made on the patients at the time of the basic study are of certain illuminating interest.

We observed – in agreement with Hawk et al. (1975) and Salokangas (1977) – that the nuclear schizophrenic symptoms enumerated above also occurred in many cases defined as schizophreniform psychoses, although transiently. The only exception was the hebephrenic affective disorder, which was not diagnosed in any of the patients in the group of schizophreniform psychoses. Another symptom infrequent in this group was autism, which was only seen in one schizophreniform patient at the time of the basic study, though three patients were autistic in the groups of schizoaffective psychoses and borderline schizophrenias and as many as 33, i.e. more than half of the patients, in the group of typical schizophrenia.

When we combined these eight symptoms to make a measuring instrument, which was classified according to the number of symptoms diagnosed (cf. Appendix 4, item 2), *the number of schizophrenic symptoms* noted at the time of the psychiatric basic study turned out to have a significant statistical correlation ($p = .003$) with the group of typical schizophrenia, an equally significant negative correlation with the group of borderline schizophrenia ($p = .008$), and further an almost significant negative correlation with the group of schizo-affective psychoses ($p = < .05$). This scale did not, however, differentiate between the group of schizophreniform psychoses and the rest of the series.[1]

The duration of psychotic symptoms prior to admission (Appendix 1, item 12), on the other hand, made a significant distinction between the group of schizophreniform psychoses and the rest of the series ($p = .0012$): The symptoms were of shortest duration in this group. Only one patient had had symptoms for more than a month. A parallel, though only marginally significant finding was made in the group of schizo-affective psychoses, while the borderline schizophrenic patients differed from the rest of the series into the opposite direction at an almost significant level ($p = .017$). The group of typical schizophrenias had no correlation with this clinical background variable.

We did not divide our patients into the classical sub-groups of schizophrenia, hebephrenic, catatonic and paranoid subgroups. This was replaced by studying prognostic variables in relation to the occurrence of the nuclear schizophrenic symptoms enumerated above. Instead of this we supplemented our diagnostic categorization with another clinical classification based on the quality of the disturbance of ego functions. This classification is described in more detail in Chapter 4.2.3.

We did not consider it possible to diagnose our patients in retrospect with the DSM-III system adopted into use since the time of the beginning of our study (American Psychiatric Association 1980). As far as we can see, the diagnostic limits of our group of typical schizophrenia largely coincide with the criteria of "schizophrenic disorder" as defined in the DSM-III, though they remain slightly wider because of the absence of the criterium based on the duration of symptoms.

In our later analyses, *we will take a special notice of the findings related to our whole series, on the one hand, and of the findings related to the group of typical schizophrenia, on the other.*

---

[1] In the statistical analysis of our results, the significances have been calculated with the Khi square (X^2) method, unless otherwise mentioned. They are divided as follows.

highly significant: $p < .001$, in some tables***
significant: $.001 \leq p < .01$, in tables**
almost significant: $.01 \leq p < .05$, in tables*
marginally significant: $.05 \leq p < .10$, in tables (*)
nonsignificant: $p \leq .10$

3.1.3 Inclusion of the Patients in the Series

The series consisted of 100 successive residents of Turku aged 16–45 years, who were admitted for the first time into one of the units of the community psychiatric system of the Turku district for psychosis of the schizophrenia group, i.e. meeting the aforesaid diagnostic criteria. If the patient had been earlier admitted for other than psychosis diagnosis, he was considered to be a first admission schizophrenic and included in the series. The patients who had been earlier admitted into a community-psychiatric unit of some other district, were not considered first-admission schizophrenics and were excluded from the series (unless the treatment was a direct continuation of an acute treatment set about elsewhere).

The new cases possibly to be included in the series were reported to the team, whose psychiatrist interviewed the patients and made preliminary diagnostic classifications. The cases were thereafter discussed by the team. In a majority of the cases, there was no disagreement as to the inclusion or exclusion of the patients; in the few ambiguous cases the decision was made by the head of the project after a discussion on the matter by the team.

Epidemiologically speaking, it is notable that our sample is greater than the incidence of psychoses of the schizophrenia group among the original population of Turku, because the resident population also included the approximately 15000 students of the colleges and schools resident in the town area. Most of these students had been registered in the census lists of Turku; only three were registered elsewhere. Of the patients admitted into the Psychiatric Out-patient Department of the University Central Hospital of Turku, too, only those resident in Turku were included.

The collection of patients was started on April 1, 1976, and the sample of 100 successive patients was completed by October 31, 1977. There were 52 male and 48 female patients. The age group of 16–25 years consisted of 34 patients, the age group of 26–35 years of 45 patients and the age group of 36–45 years of 21 patients. The distribution of these patients into the diagnostic sub-groups is shown by the table below:

Table 4. The age groups and diagnostic distribution of the patients

Age	Typical schizophrenia	Schizophreni-form psychosis	Schizo-affective psychosis	Borderline schizophrenia	Total
16–25	24	1	3	6	34
26–35	22	5	8	10	45
36–56	10	4	3	4	21
Total	56	10	14	20	100

The typical schizophrenic patients included 32 males and 24 females. The sex-bound difference was most marked in the group of schizophreniform psychoses (7 males, and 3 females) on the one hand and in the group of borderline schizophrenia (7 males and 13 females) on the other; the difference in the latter group emerged as marginally significant compared with the rest of the series ($p = .089$). As it was to be expected, typical schizophrenias were more frequent in the younger age groups and

Table 5. Admission of patients into the different working units

Unit	Number of patients
Clinic of Psychiatry	47
Kupittaa Hospital	27
Day Hospital of the Clinic Psychiatry	5
Mental health offices of Turku	8
Out-patient activity of the Clinic of Psychiatry	2
Psychiatric Out-patient Department of the University Central Hospital of Turku	11
Total	100

schizophreniform psychoses in the older groups, although these differences – again in comparison with the remaining series – were not even marginally significant.

The findings correspond to other studies (e.g. Bland et al. 1978, Schwartz et al. 1978) according to which there is a greater amount of men than female patients among first admission schizophrenics. In the Schwartz et al. material from Mannheim, W. Germany, where the diagnoses had been defined on the basis of the PSE-interviews at the initial assessment, the sex distribution was 41 males (58.6 %) and 29 females (41.4 %) which is almost exactly the same as in our group of typical schizophrenia. The age distribution also was close to ours, although the eldest group was slightly smaller in the Mannheim material.

Table 5 shows the numbers of patients admitted into the different working units.

Hence 74 or three fourths of the patients were taken into our series as hospital patients, 5 as day hospital patients and only 21 from the out-patient units.

At the initial stages of the treatment, four of the out-patients included in the series were admitted into hospital. Patients were also transferred from one hospital into another at the early stages of the treatment. The reason for transferring a patient from the Kupittaa Hospital to the Clinic of Psychiatry was generally the need for psychotherapy by the patient included in the research series, while the reason for transferring a patient from the Clinic of Psychiatry into the Kupittaa Hospital was the patient's violent behavior, which could not be controlled by the psychosis ward of the clinic, as it was weaker in external structure and had fewer male nurses.

Considering the very early transfers from one treatment unit to another, *the first therapeutic units for our patients were divided as shown by Table 6.*

Table 6. The distribution of the first treatment unit of the patients

Unit	Number of patients
The Clinic of Psychiatry, in-patient	54
The Clinic of Psychiatry, day-patient	5
Kupittaa Hospital, in-patient	24
Out-patient units	17

3.2 Course of the Project

3.2.1 Psychiatric Basic Examination

The psychiatrist of the team carried out a psychiatric interview on all the patients included in the series as soon as possible after their admission. The two exceptions to this practice were the patients admitted into the Psychiatric Out-patient Department of the University Central Hospital of Turku, who refused any interviews that were part of our study apart from a telephone conversation, and for whom the information elicited in the interviews made in the therapeutic unit had to suffice.

The specialized nurse of our team also met the same patients and further interviewed their relatives. She met the mothers of 56 patients, the step-mother of one, the fathers of 40 and the step-father of one, the spouses of all the 28 married patients and the spouses of 9 patients living in legal separation, siblings of 29 patients, children of 4 patients, and another relative of 3 patients. In addition, she met a friend of 1 patient. A relative of altogether 90 patients were seen. In addition to the two patients who refused interviews for purposes of research, 6 patients did not permit us to see their relatives, and in one case the parents of the patient refused to be interviewed, and in yet another case the patient had no relatives alive.

The goal in all of these interviews was to understand the patient, his life history and developmental situation. This was considered of essential importance for elucidating the therapeutic needs and making the therapeutic plan. According to our experience, this approach in general makes it easier to collect patient data than is possible with strictly structured interview methods. The data thus obtained were recorded in detailed notes made after the interviews.

Care was also taken to collect during the interviews as accurately as possible the information needed for the aforesaid 163 item psychiatric basic study form. The form was divided into five main sections: data on the family background, the patient's development and life course, description of the situation upon admission, specification of the clinical status and symptoms, and the design of the therapeutic plan. The whole team participated in the discussion and design of the therapeutic plans in their regular meetings. The goal in making the therapeutic plans was to make them meet optimally the therapeutic needs of the patients and their family environments within the resources that were realistically available.

The basic study form was re-structured, to facilitate statistical processing, but there was also room for clarifying notes and arguments. On the basis of the form we constructed the clinical and psychosocial background variables for the patient series (cf. Appendix 1).

3.2.2 Psychologic Basic Examination

The psychologist of the team conducted the *psychologic basic examination* of the patients. This regularly took place slightly later than the psychiatric basic examination; in the case of patients in a severely psychotic condition it was necessary to wait until the most serious stage of the psychosis was passed. The psychologic basic examination was therefore not connected directly to the planning of therapy, but rather constituted a parallel tool for the psychiatric variables measuring the clinical status, which was especially utilized for elucidating the individual-psychologic factors influencing the treatment, the prognosis and the intrapsychic condition of the patients. The study could be carried out with 88 patients.

The psychologic basic examination consisted of patient interviews and the following tests:

1. Wechsler Adult Intelligence Scale (WAIS)
2. The Kahn Test of Symbol Arrangement (KTSA)
3. Rorschach test (RO)
4. Object Relations Technique (ORT)

At the first stage, the data obtained from the tests were processed psychometrically, calculating the numeric scores of the sub-tests. At the second stage, the psychologist made global assessments of the patients he had met, forming the central variables reflecting the patient's intrapsychic condition. The starting-point in forming the variables (cf. Appendix 2) consisted of the test protocols and the single scores, which were modified with the data obtained in the psychologist's interviews on the basis of clinical experience (the method used as a supplementary tool to psychotherapy research has been described by e.g. Appelbaum 1977).

The psychologic basic study covered 88 patients.

3.2.3 Action Research by the Team

The therapeutic plans made by the team for the different patients were reported to the different therapeutic units, and the team members often participated in the planning meetings discussing the therapy of the patients in most of the units (the out-patient units and the Clinic of Psychiatry). The members of the team also personally participated in the therapeutic activities and the supervision given for them and also tried in other ways to stimulate the implementation of the psychotherapeutic treatments. All in all, the team members made the following contributions to the therapeutic activities concerning the different patients:

psychotherapeutic responsibility	16
other therapeutic responsibility	4
responsibility of supporting the relatives	15
responsibility for supervision	23
other consultations on therapy	24
administrative responsibility	60

The figures were obtained for the first two years of follow-up. Several patients continued their individual or family therapy even beyond those two years; in 2 cases a member of the team initiated psychotherapy belonging to the project only during the latter follow-up period. The greatest personal responsibility for the therapeutic work and the work on supporting the relatives was taken by the full-time specialized nurse of the team. The responsibility for supervision was divided more or less equally between the four members, and administrative responsibility refers to the administrative and therapeutic decisions concerning the patients treated in those units of the Clinic of Psychiatry and the Psychiatric Out-patient department of the University Central Hospital ofTurku which were directly administered by us.

It should be emphasized, however, that – despite the working contribution of the team – the *responsibility for the treatment of the patients always belonged to the therapeutic unit in charge of this treatment.* Most of the psychotherapies were carried out by therapists other than the team members. Nor did the team members try to influence any more profoundly the activities taking place in the different therapeutic units. This was also considered to serve best the developmental goals of the project. Our action research was not intended merely to increase transiently the quantitatively scant resources of the mental health district – although this increase did take place – but to promote permanently the development of the therapeutic activities in the different units.

3.2.4 Two-Year Psychiatric Follow-up

The first *psychiatric follow-up study* of the patients and their family members was undertaken two years after the patient's admission for treatment. It consisted of *two different parts.* The first part consisted of a follow-up of the patients and their family members by the *psychiatrist and the specialized nurse of the team,* using the same division of tasks as in the basic examination. Their acquaintance with the patients and their families had become quite considerable during the course of the project, although the different cases differed notably in this respect. This acquaintance provided a good basis for making assessments on the development of the patients. There was, however, the risk of there being subjective factors involved for the same reason, especially concerning the patients whose psychotherapies were conducted by the team members themselves.

For this reason, a *parallel psychiatric follow-up study* was planned, which was carried out by a psychiatrist not a member of our team. This *independent psychiatric investigator* was Dr. Ritva Järvi, a specialized psychiatrist and then working at the mental health office of Parainen, near Turku. She had familiarized herself with the therapeutic orientation of our team while trained at the Turku Clinic of Psychiatry and possessed several years' experience of in-patient and out-patient work in community psychiatry. Owing to her post in another mental hospital district, she was completely unfamiliar with our patients. Her assessments were hence believed to be independent of the possible expectations coloured by the examiner's previous acquaintance with the patients.

The follow-up studies were methodologically similar to the basic study. Structured follow-up forms were made. The form used by the team had 114 items and the form used by the independent investigator 84 items. The most central assessment of the patient's condition were included in both of the follow-up forms, so as to allow mutual comparison. The same also applied to the most important assessments of the therapeutic outcome.

The follow-up study illuminated the patient's clinical status and their psychosocial and psychodynamic life situation as well as the changes that had taken place in them during the follow-up. The investigators also collected information on the therapies accomplished and tried to estimate their significance as well as their relation to what would have been the actual need for therapies. Moreover, the team determined the need for therapy and rehabilitation in the patient series at the time of the follow-up study.

Information on the patients and of their treatments was obtained from the patient files of the therapeutic units. In addition to this, the *therapists* in charge of the patients in the different therapeutic units, including those working in private offices, were mailed a *questionnaire* for elucidating the nature of the psychotherapies accomplished, their duration and the supervision connected with them. Nearly all of the therapists replied; in a couple of cases the most essential data regarding the mode of therapy were obtained on the telephone.

The *National Pensions Institute* gave a permission to collect information on the sickness allowances granted to the patients during the follow-up period and the disability pensions granted on the basis of the illness. The information was collected via the Turku office of the National Pensions Institute.

The follow-up studies were undertaken as soon as possible after the termination of the follow-up period of each patient, and they were completed by the end of 1979. This stage also involved action research: in altogether 14 cases, the follow-up study gave rise to a stimulation of new therapeutic measures or a revision of the therapies being carried out.

Three patients had died during the follow-up period. The psychiatrist of the team personally interviewed 87 patients in the follow-up study. There were 7 patients who refused to be interviewed, including the 2 who also refused the basic study. 3 of the patients refusing the interview had a long conversation on the telephone with the psychiatrist. It turned out otherwise impossible to reach 3 patients. With the exception of 2 patients, it was possible in the follow-up study to meet relatives of the patients who either refused the interview or were otherwise out of reach. When we further take into account the information acquired from the patient files of the different therapeutic units, it can be said that the follow-up by the team covered at least the most essential aspects of the development of all the patient's condition in quite a satisfactory manner.

Of the relatives of the patients, the specialized nurse of the team met during the follow-up 47 mothers (in addition to which she had telephone conversations with three more) and one step-mother, 31 fathers, 27 spouses and 7 divorced spouses, siblings of 19 patients and children of 8 patients as well as 3 other relatives. In 3 cases furthermore a friend of the patients was seen. Altogether 8 patients refused to give a permission for us to meet their relatives, and one had no relatives. All in all, relatives of 88 patients were seen during the follow-up study, which number is nearly equal to that in the basic study.

The independent psychiatrist met 80 of our patients. Some of the patients who had consented to be interviewed by members of the team refused absolutely the interview by the new psychiatric investigator.

3.2.5 Two-Year Psychologic Follow-up

The psychologic follow-up study carried out by the psychologist of the team consisted of an interview and the same tests that were used in the psychologic basic study, with the exception that abbreviated versions of the WAIS and KTSA were used. On the basis of the data material obtained from the results of the tests, the changes that had taken place in the patients during the follow-up period were assessed using 14 4-class variables. The assessment was congruent with the assessment made by the rest of the team and the independent investigator, but was made independently of these.

At the time of the follow-up study, the patients' experiences of their illness and the treatment given for it were analyzed with two attitude tests. The form for the experience of illness was originally based on the attitude-measuring instrument developed by Soskis and Bowers (1969), which has previously been applied in the Finnish circumstances by Alanen and Laine (1973). The form concerning the experiences of therapy was particularly designed for purposes of this study. The results of these studies will be published separately.

The psychologic follow-up covered 71 patients. The loss of patients was hence 27 %, consisting mainly of those unable to endure the interpersonal closeness of the interview and the testing situation. The group of loss was compared with the study group with regard to several background variables and the therapeutic outcome. Discrimination analysis indicated that the groups as a whole did not essentially differ from each other. The differences between single variables, which were analyzed with t-tests, indicated that the patients participating in the follow-up study had more conscious motivation for the therapies and had more conspicuous depressive symptoms.

3.2.6 Five-Year Psychiatric Follow-up

The second psychiatric follow-up study of the patients and their family members was carried out five years after admission for treatment. This follow-up study was no longer part of the research contract made with the Academy of Finland, but the Academy supported it financially with a research grant.

The follow-up study was carried out by the team in such a way that the head of the project, the psychiatrist of the team and the psychologist of the team divided between them the psychiatric patient interviews in such a way that each got one third of the patients. Thereby none of the investigators interviewed any patients who were, or had been, in his own psychotherapy. The specialized nurse of the team, in turn, interviewed relatives of the patients, as in the previous follow-up study.

The 5-year follow-up was more restricted than the 2-year follow-up, as it did not include patient interviews by an independent investigator or a psychologic follow-up of the patients. This was partly due to practical reasons. It should also be emphasized, however, that the experiences of the use of an independent investigator in the previous follow-up study had indicated that the independent assessments were otherwise quite parallel to those made by the team (see Chapter 6.1.), but – particularly as regards the assessments of the patient's clinical condition – more "favourable" than those made by the team. The independent investigator, for example, saw clearly fewer psychotic symptoms in the patients than the team, who based their statements not only on the patient interviews, but also on the information obtained from relatives and the different therapeutic units. Moreover, the team was better able to estimate particularly the changes taking place in the psychodynamic status of the patients than was the independent psychiatrist, who only met the patients once.

The 5-year follow-up proved to include *the most important assessments concerning the prognosis of the patients and the effect of the therapies on it,* one reason for it being that the 2-year follow-up period appeared too short particularly for estimating the effects of therapy. 44 patients continued their psychotherapy beyond the 2-year follow-up period; they accounted for more than 3/4 of the group we subsequently labelled as "psychotherapy cases". Although our series included several patients whose therapy still continued after the 5-year follow-up period, it was, however, possible in these cases to obtain a sufficiently long-term and reliable idea of the suitability of the therapy to the patient and the therapeutic outcome.

The framework of the 5-year follow-up study again consisted of a structured form comprising 95 items. Most of the assessments concerning the condition of the patients were identical to those used in the previous forms, which facilitated the assessment of the changes that had taken place. This form also included some new assessments, the most important of them being the four-dimensional system of determining the prognosis developed by Strauss and Carpenter (1972).

Data on the therapies were again obtained from the *patient files* of the different therapeutic units. Similarly, the *therapists* in charge of the patients in the different units were again mailed a questionnaire, and replies were got from all of them. The information on the sickness allowances received by the patients during the follow-up period and the *disability pensions* granted on the basis of the illness was again collected via the Turku office of the National Pensions Institute.

The follow-up studies were, in a majority of cases, made immediately after the termination of the follow-up period in this case, too. In the cases where the patient interview was delayed, the interviews were made with the purpose of illuminating, as far as possible, the situation that prevailed at the time of the termination of the patient's follow-up period. The project was completed in February 1983, when 4 months had passed since the termination of the follow-up period of the last patient.

We did not hear of the deaths of any patients during the new follow-up period. We obtained no data on one patient, because we were unable to get hold of either her or her relatives.

We interviewed personally 79 patients. 8 patients refused to be interviewed and 10 patients could not be met for other reasons. Of these patients not interviewed personally, 5 had a telephone conversation on their condition with the investigator.

The specialized nurse of the team met personally the mothers of 44 patients and the fathers of 26 patients, 18 spouses and 9 previous spouses, 22 siblings, 8 children, 3 other relatives and 1 friend of a patient. She further had telephone conversations with 8 mother, 5 father, 2 siblings and 3 previous spouses. The purpose of these interviews and conversations was to elucidate the development of the condition of the members of the patients, families and to acquire information concerning the patients who were not seen personally.

In addition to the patient who had disappeared completely, the data on only 2 patients remained clearly inadequate. One of these 2 refused interviews of both himself and his relatives, but the team was provided information by the therapeutic unit in charge of him. In the case of the other patient it was possible to meet relatives, but they knew little of the patient, who had moved abroad.

3.3 Data Analysis and Statistical Methods

The statistical analysis of our material was carried out on the DEC – 2060 computer of the University of Turku, using BMDP programs. Since most of our variables were categorical, the material was mainly analyzed using statistical methods for describing the mutual relations between categorical variables: the X^2-test, Fisher's exact test, kappa coefficient (K), stepwise linear logistic regression analysis, and log-linear models. The statistical analyses were executed by Anne Kaljonen.

Since the number of variables was high and the number of cases low in our series, each problem was generally approached by means of *cross-tabulation* and the *X^2-test*. This provided an idea of which factors seemed to be connected with the matter under study. If the cross-tabulation did not meet the criteria set for its application (the cell frequencies too small), the dependence was analyzed by means of *Fisher's exact test,* which is only suited to analyzing the dependence of two dichotomous variables. The statistical significances given in the text (p) are hence mostly based on the X^2-test. The corresponding basic analytic method for the numerical variables (in-patient days and episodes, Strauss-Carpenter total scores) was the t-test, which was applied as either one- or two-sided test, depending on what were the preliminary hypotheses pertaining to the matter. The *kappa coefficient* was used as a measure of agreement e.g. when comparing the assessments by the team and the independent examiner in the two-year follow-up. Since many of the assessments under comparison were categorical, the analysis of agreement was usually better carried out by means of the weighted kappa coefficient than by the conventional kappa coefficient (Cohen 1968); when certain assumptions are valid, the weighted kappa receives the same value as Pearsons's product moment correlation coefficient.

The multivariate analyses consisted of *stepwise logistic regression analysis and log-linear models.* Logistic regression analysis (Breslow & Day, 1980) is a statistical multivariate method suited to the analysis of the mutual relations between categorical variables when one of the variables is a dichotomous response and the others are factors or explaining variables, which may be categorical and/or numerical. The purpose of the logistic regression analysis is to bring out the most essential part of the information obtained from the numerous cross-tabulations of two variables. The results of the analysis are interpreted by observing the statistical significance of the connection between the response and each factor, when the connections of the other factors to the response have been taken into account. If the connection between the response and the factor is not genuine, but is explained by another factor, the factor which originally appeared significant is dropped out of the model. Since the logistic regression analysis is based on a contingency table, it is obvious that the number of factors that can be included as explaining factors depends on not only the selection, but also the size of the material. The weak point of the logistic regression analysis is that it does not take into account the interaction of more than two variables; the connection between a factor and the response may be different at the different levels of another factor (and statistically significant), although the connection obtained as a result of the analysis may not be significant. Even for this reason, the connections between e.g. the therapies and the prognosis or this changes had to be analyzed in more detail by means of the log-linear models.

When the basic analysis of the material had first been carried out with the X^2-, Fisher's or t-test, the analysis was then continued by grouping the variables explaining each response according to which sub-area of the patient's life situation it was considered to measure. This had to be done owing to the large number of variables and the small number of cases. Each group of variables was subjected to stepwise logistic regression analysis, whose purpose was hence to select the variable(s) that explained most strongly the response in question. Finally, on the basis of these sub-analyses the best explaining variable of each group of variables were selected for the play-off analysis, which was performed with the method of maximum likelihood ratio (MLR). In addition to the response, the explaining variables were also mostly constructed as two-class yes/no variables. The actual procedure of dichotomizing the variable depended on the results of the X^2-test it was thus possible that several different dichotomies may have been obtained of one original variable. When examining the change that took place in the prognosis during the five year follow-up period, we made the analysis separately on the group of patients considered to have progressed in this prognostic area from the time of the basic examination and the group which had regressed respectively.

Of the results of the logistic regression analysis, the statistical significance of the connection between each explaining factor and the response (p) is given, when the connections between the other explaining factors and the response have been taken into account. Some tables also include the relative risk (R), which reflects the ratio between the percentages obtained from a cross-tabulation of two variables, but does not take into account the connections between the other factors and the response.

It was further desirable to apply the theory of log-linear models (Bishop et al. 1975), to analyze separately the connections between certain therapies and the prognosis or certain favourable changes in the prognosis. Since the size of our series, 100 patients and 56 typical schizophrenic patients, restricted the number of explaining variables in the logistic regression analysis to 3–5 possible factors, it was deemed necessary to analyze separately the connections between the therapies and the prognosis regardless of how significant they appeared on the basis of the cross-tabulations. When interpreting the results, the main attention was given to the statistical significance of the connection between the therapy and the prognosis, when the connections between the other factors and the prognosis had been kept constant (partial association).

We also analyzed the interaction of more than two variables. Hardly any interaction of this kind were found in our models, which means that the logistic regression analysis we applied previously turned out a highly suitable method for eliminating explaining factors. Since the log-linear models are based on the X^2-test the small cell frequencies were increased by adding a constant 0.5 to each cell frequency.

4 Findings of Psychiatric Basic Examination. Indications of Therapeutic Plans

We will here describe the findings of the psychiatric basic examination. The main emphasis will be laid on those included in the psychosocial and clinical background variables constructed for statistical analysis in subsequent accounts of therapeutic practice and prognosis (Appendix 1). At the same time, the definitions connected with these variables and their categorization are clarified. In later chapters, the connections of these variables with the implementation of different modes of treatment as well as with prognostic findings will become the focus of our interest.

In addition to numerical findings, the statistical connections between these background variables and the diagnostic subgrouping of our series will be presented.

4.1 Psychosocial Background of Patients

4.1.1 Sex and Age

The psychosocial background variables also included the sex and age distributions of the patients, which were described above in Chapter 3.1.3.

4.1.2 Family Background

4.1.2.1 Mental Health of Members of Primary Family

Of the *parents* of our patients, 6 mothers and 7 fathers had been *in hospital or institutional care* because of mental disorders, in addition to which 6 mothers and 3 fathers had been given outpatient treatment. Siblings of 14 patients had been given hospital or institutional treatment, and siblings of 3 patients had been psychiatric outpatients. In the families of altogether 34 patients, i.e. 1/3 of the entire series, a family member other than the patient had been given psychiatric treatment.

While conducting the interviews, we also assessed the *personality disorder of the parents*. The findings are shown in the Table 7.

This assessment is laden with several weaknesses. The data on 27 mothers and 27 fathers were inadequate to allow assessment. The diagnosis of the disorder of the psychotic level was based on observations made at the time of meeting the parents, reliable interview data and, in many cases, on patient files of the treatment units. Most of the psychoses encountered were classified as belonging to the schizophrenia group. "Other severe ego disorder" refers to personalities characterized by borderline states, character disorders, alcohol abuse and

Table 7. Personality disorders of the patient's parents

Degree of disorder	Mother	Father
Is or has been psychotic	9	7
Other severe ego disorder	23	45
Neurotic disorder	38	8
No disorders	3	13
Inadequate data	27	27

addiction as well as exceedingly severe character-neurotic disorders. The high number of fathers in this group is due to alcohol abuse, which is particularly typical of men, and which was frequently identified on the basis of information proffered by the mother and/or the patient, even without meeting the father. It is probable that more extensive individual examinations would have increased the number of women belonging to this disorder class. We can therefore hardly conclude that the fathers of our patients would have been more seriously disturbed than the mothers; this is also supported by the fact that the "normal" personalities were estimated to be more frequent among the fathers than among the mothers.

We applied a binary classification to the background variable of maternal or paternal personality disorder, drawing a line between "other severe ego disorder" and "neurotic disorder". What makes this expedient is the fact that *subjects with definite ego pathology are often characterized by an obscurity of the boundary between the personalities of oneself and others* – particularly one's children. They tend to use relatively primitive defences, which have been described by Kernberg (1967, 1975) as typical of the borderline personality organization: denial, splitting, early forms of projective mechanisms (including projective identification), primitive idealization as well as omnipotence and devaluation. These defensive operations often lead to excessively possessive attitudes towards the children. Stierlin (1974, 1976) has described such relationships with transactional models of binding and delegation. We have developed the term "transactional defence mechanisms" (Alanen 1978, 1980; Räkköläinen and Alanen 1982). This refers to the way in which e.g. the notions and fantasies of the parents pertaining to their relationships with and images of their children are significant for the maintenance of their own equilibrium. A successful warding-off of anxiety is then dependent on whether the child behaves in the manner expected of him, or whether at least such a fantasy can be sustained. Such transactional defences often bring the two parties of an interrelationship into mutual entanglements, which must necessarily be treated by family-therapeutic means.

There were no statistical differences between the diagnostic subgroups with regard to these findings.

4.1.2.2 Atmosphere and External Structure of Primary Family

When assessing the *parent-patient relationship* in childhood, we found that mothers with possessive features were more frequent in our series than mothers who were hostile or indifferent to the patients: the former numbered 61, the latter 25. The corresponding figures for fathers were 30 and 30. Only in the case of 2 mothers and 12 fathers met by us were these features completely absent.

The only significant difference between the diagnostic groups regarding the parent-patient relationships in childhood was that of the 9 cases where the father had been lacking 4 were included in the small group of schizophreniform psychoses.

The finding on the overall *atmosphere of the primary families* of our patients showed that both "chaotic" and "rigid" atmospheres (Alanen et al. 1966) were common. A predominantly chaotic atmosphere, which is characterized by inconsistency, unreliability and unpredictability of attitudes, often defective interpersonal boundaries and disturbances of reality testing owing to the mental disturbances of a parent or another influential adult of the family, prevailed in the primary families of 18 patients. A predominantly rigid atmosphere, which typically involves "impervious", often projective attitudes of the patients or other influential adults towards the children, emotional poverty and heightened intrafamilial role expectations, were found in 32 families. Almost all of the other families displayed minor chaotic and/or rigid features. The atmosphere of 12 families could not be estimated.

Both the chaotic and the rigid atmospheres were somewhat less common in the group of borderline schizophrenics. The difference was not statistically significant.

Deviations in the external family structure when the patient was less than 16 years old – including parental separation and divorce and long-term presence of people not members of the nuclear family in the family – were seen in 54 cases, while 45 patients had not experienced any such deviations in their family conditions. The background variable constructed on the basis of this finding was statistically nearly significantly related to the group of schizophreniform psychoses ($p = .018$), where 9 out of the 10 patients had experienced such external deviations.

23 of our patients had been *away from home for long periods* prior to the age of 15.

4.1.2.3 Social Background of Primary Family

The social group of the primary family was assessed in accordance with the four-class system applied by the Statistical Office of the Town of Helsinki, which has also been used in some other social-psychiatric investigations carried out in Finland (Achté 1967, Väisänen 1975, Salokangas 1977).

The criteria for the social grouping applied by the Statistical Office of The Town Helsinki are presented briefly below:

Social group I: Persons with a college or university degree, a major part of the self-employed professionals, commissioned officers from captain upward, teachers, persons in leading positions etc.

Social group II: Small-scale entrepreneurs, supervisors and higher office personnel (e.g. technician, printing press overseer, nurse, office clerks, transport contractor) shopkeepers, farmers.

Social group III: Skilled labour and lower office personnel (e.g. assembler, assistant nurse, telephone operator, non-commissioned officer, shop assistant, small farm owners).

Social group IV: Unskilled workers, auxiliary personnel, farm hands etc.

When the classification was made according to the social group of the parent or other guardian of the patient who was in a better position during the patient's childhood and adolescence, 11 families were included in the social group I, 11 in group II, 51 in group III and 27 in group IV.

We also constructed a background variable according to whether the patient's *primary family* had experienced some of the following *deviations of the normal life course* during his or her childhood: more than one move to another locality (these cases numbered 23 in our series), inclusion of the family in a local minority group on the basis of linguistic, national or racial characteristics (5), shortage of financial resources (long-term in 4 families and short-term in 7), asocial or antisocial behaviours of family members (14), or their participation in the activities of political or religious extremist movements (11). Some of these "deviations" had occurred in altogether 48 families. A comparison of these families with the remaining 52 families provided no statistical connections with the diagnostic categorization.

4.1.3 Prepsychotic Development of Patients

4.1.3.1 Physical and Psychologic Development

Three of our patients suffered from permanent disability due to a *physical illness or injury.* One of these was on a disability pension because of a physical illness (rheumatoid arthritis). Other kinds of permanent or recurrent physical illness were seen in the anamnesis of 23 patients.

The data on the potential injuries of the central nervous system at the perinatal stage remained inadequate. But a more comprehensive view was obtained on the *psychic symptoms* of our patients *in childhood,* i.e. prior to the age of 16. 19 patients had exhibited tendencies to withdrawal at that early age already, and one of these 19 had had psychotic symptoms. Behavioural disorders were reported for 6 patients, use of alcohol or drugs for 3, and a suicidal attempt for one. Neurotic or psychosomatic symptoms turned out more frequent than more serious symptoms in the childhood of our patients: neurotic or psychosomatic symptoms were seen in the anamnesis of 54 patients.

When these data were combined to make a background variable, where the first group consisted of the patients with a withdrawal tendency in childhood, the second consisted of those with some other symptom formation and the third included subjects with no data on psychic symptoms, an almost significant statistical connection emerged with the group of patients suffering from borderline schizophrenia. They differed from the rest of the series in that they were known to have suffered more often from mild psychic symptoms in childhood ($p = .033$).

The psychodynamic development of our patients was examined in the light of data pertaining to their sexual development and their habit of coping with aggressions on the one hand and the quality of their interactions with their parents and outside their primary families on the other.

The prepsychotic stage of sexual development was approached from the viewpoint of information on the concrete *sexual relationships* of our patients on the one hand, and assessments of their *psychosexual development level* on the other.

Of our patients, 64 or nearly 2/3 had had a heterosexual relationship on a long-term basis, 9 had had several transient relationships, and 2 had had only one transient relationship, while 23 patients had lacked any such relationships. For 2 patients this assessment could not be made. As it was to be expected, sexual relationships were fewest in the group of patients with typical schizophrenia, where 18 had lacked any, 5 had had transient relationships and 32 long-term ones. The group differed from the remaining series at an almost significant level. All in all, a surprisingly large portion of the patients had had sexual relationships, which is, however, accordant with the relatively wide diagnostic spectrum and age structure of our series.

The following assessments were made concerning the psychosexual development of the patients:

Table 8. Overall assessment of the psychosexual development level of the patients

Situation of development	Number of patients
Delayed	17
Chaotic or characterized by identity crisis	20
Established homosexual	—
Established heterosexual	61
Inadequate data	2

Delayed development here refers to mainly heterosexual development which is clearly retarded relative to the age of the subject. There occur marked inhibitions and repressions, occasionally also excessive guilt feelings, and drive satisfaction is concentrated, to an abnormal degree, to masturbation or fantasy.

The sexual development is *chaotic* or characterized by *identity crisis* when its orientation is clearly ambivalent. There may occur various perverse tendencies, such as homosexual fantasies, though not exclusively these, anxiety-provoking fears of homosexuality and/or tendencies to incest. Some other cases involve ostensible hypersexuality and uncontrolled sexual impulses reflected in a predisposition to numerous short-term detached heterosexual and/or possibly homosexual relationships.

Established *homosexual* development means that the subject has adopted a definitely homosexual identity. Established *heterosexual* development refers to "normal" age-appropriate heterosexual identity. This does not necessarily exclude masturbation or deviating tendencies, though the latter do not markedly interfere with the patient's age-appropriate heterosexual behaviour. Established heterosexual or established homosexual psychosocial development does not necessarily imply that the subject has or has had a sexual partner, although they do imply that he or she has had at least one long-term "dating" relationship.

Quite understandably, there was a highly significant statistical connection between the data on concrete relationships and the assessments of the level of psychosexual development ($X^2 = 74.0$, $p < .001$). This is also suggested by the roughly equal sizes of the healthiest groups in both assessments. Contrary to the date on concrete relationships, however, the two-class variable of the psychosexual development level did not correlate even marginally with the diagnostic groups.

There were no established homosexual patients in our series, although the homosexual panic associated with the identity crisis seems to have contributed to the onset of the illness of some patients.

Overtly violent behaviour had occurred in the case of 26 patients, while 73 patients were known not to have behaved violently. The patient's *characteristic ways of coping with aggression* were assessed on accordance with the table below.

Table 9. Overall assessment of the patient's way of coping with aggressions.

Way of coping with aggressions	Number of patients
Avoiding aggressive behaviour	63
Impulsive	32
"Normal"	2
Inadequate data	3

We know that schizophrenia often involves a difficulty to control in an integrated manner the aggressive feelings towards other people. The way of coping with aggressions here refers to the most characteristic attitude of the subject in coping with and expressing his or her aggressions.

Avoidance of aggressive behaviour means that the individual tends to avoid showing outward aggressiveness through a general tendency to withdrawal and by evading situations where aggressions easily arise; if aggressions occur, after all, there is an effort to conceal them and keep them to the fantasy level.

Impulsive aggressiveness refers to an inclination to repeated uncontrolled and impulsive outbursts of aggressiveness, which take the form ot either physical violence or (more often) verbal explosions, which results in continuous conflict situations with the environment.

"*Normal*" control of aggressions means that the individual does not avoid situations provoking aggression, both excessive submission and uncontrolled aggressiveness are rare, and the personality contains an ability to deal with the arising conflicts at the level of realistic conversation.

An effort to avoid aggressive behaviour turned out typical of about 2/3 of the patients, while the others had a tendency to impulsive aggressiveness; "normal" ways of coping with aggressions were seen in no more than a couple of patients.

A highly significant mutual connection also prevailed between these two assessments of aggressiveness ($X^2 = 64.1$, $p < .001$). As regards overtly violent behaviour, only the borderline schizophrenics differed from the rest of the series: they lacked the feature of overtly violent behaviour with a frequency of marginal significance. In the assessment of the ways of coping with aggressions, this group differed from the remainder of the series almost significantly, being characterized by notable avoidance of aggressive behaviour. Impulsive aggressiveness, in turn, was marginally significantly more frequent in the group of patients with schizophreniform psychosis. The distribution of typical schizophrenic patients in this respect was quite precisely parallel to the distribution of the total series.

The relations of our patients to their parents were assessed according to our notion of the parental relation in early adulthood or upon entering this stage. Apart from a couple of cases where a parent had died when the patient was already at an adult age, this assessment corresponded to a notable extent to the patient's relation with the parents prior to the psychosis. The relationship with the mother was clearly more often (41) close and dependent than the relationship with the father (16), while the father the relationship was clearly more often distant or broken (23) than the mother relationship (11).

The overall assessment of the patient's *relative differentation from his or her primary family* was considered quite important for the planning of therapies. This assessment was also primarily one of psychological development, although the patients *notably entangled with their primary families* were regularly also incapable of external separation – they continued to live with their parents (or one of them). We encountered relatively frequently the actual process of *separation struggle*, which was reflected by unsuccessful attempts at independence.

These attempts were manifested now as concrete, but unsuccessful, efforts to move away from home, now as plans to do so, though not yet realized. Conflicts in heterosexual relationships, field of study or occupation, when they simultaneously involved the problem of gaining independence from the parents, were also interpreted as a process of separation struggle. Some married patients were also undergoing a separation struggle in an ambivalent situation between their primary family and spouse.

For about half of our patients the separation from the primary family had come about in a way that also shifted the focus of the interpersonal relations outside the family. Since, however, ambivalent relationships with the parents were common – and the dependence had frequently been transferred to new relationships – we have grouped these cases under the heading *"at least ostensibly successful separation"*.

Our findings are shown in the table below:

Table 10. Assessment of the level of the patient's psychologic separation from their primary families

Relation with primary family	Number of patients
Notable entanglement	16
Characterized by separation struggle	35
At least ostensibly successful separation	49

Patients who were entangled with their primary family or were undergoing the separation struggle were relatively the most numerous in the group of typical schizophrenias on the one hand and in the group of borderline schizophrenias on the other, but the differences between the diagnostic groups were not significant.

The quantity and quality of the patients' *interpersonal relationships outside their primary families* were also elucidated.

The following finding was made on the *quantity* of interpersonal relationships.

Table 11. Assessment of the quantity of the patient's significant interpersonal relationships outside their primary families

Quantity of significant relationships	Number of patients
No significant relationships	21
One significant relationship	36
Several significant relationships	42
Inadequate data	1

The relations that were classified as significant were concrete current relationships which the patient had clearly experienced as personally involving. Since we were dealing with relationships outside the primary family, we also included the marital relationships of the married patients.

Only one fifth of the patients seemed to have been lacking any such relationships; 3/4 of these had typical schizophrenia. It was relatively common that the patient only had one significant relationship.

Table 12. Quality of the patient's interpersonal relationships outside their primary families

Quality of relationships	Number of patients
Labile and brief	29
Characterized by recurring conflicts	35
Deeply involving and fairly permanent	31
Not assessable	5

For assessing the *quality* of the interpersonal relationships, the classification shown in Table 12 was used. Most of even those patients who were above classified as having no significant relationships had had short-term relationships outside their primary families.

Of the different diagnostic groups, the group of schizophreniform psychoses emerged at the level of statistically marginal significance, being characterized by labile and brief relationships on the one hand and by relationships disturbed by repeated conflicts on the other, while these patients lacked any deeply involving and constant relationships without conflicts.

4.1.3.2 Social Development

The *basic education* of our patients is shown in Table 13.

Table 13. Basic education of the patients

Basic education	Number of patients
Primary school not finished	—
Primary school finished	61
Secondary school finished	11
Graduation from senior secondary school	28

The data on the *occupational education* of our patients are shown compiled in Table 14.

Table 14. Occupational education of the patients

Occupational education	Number of patients
No occupational education	35
Trade school or training sufficient for occupational competence	49
Technical, commercial or other corresponding school	4
Technical, commercial or other corresponding college	6
Academic degree or corresponding education	6

The level of basic education in our series is high. The number of senior secondary graduates is somewhat increased by the fact that Turku is a university town: the series includes students who have moved to Turku from elsewhere.

More than one third of the series, however, lacked occupational education, and less than one fourth of the senior secondary graduates had an academic degree. The onset of illness had often taken place halfway through the occupational education.

The background variable composed of basic education did not correlate with the diagnostic groups. The lack of occupational education was somewhat more pronounced among the typical schizophrenic patients, but the difference was not significant. On the other hand, those with schizo-affective psychosis had marginally significantly more often completed occupational education than the others.

The *social group* of each patient was determined in accordance with the classificatory system of the Statistical Office of the Town of Helsinki (see 4.1.2.3.). The students were classified as belonging to a social group one step lower than that resulting from the degree they were studying for, and the housewives working at home were classified in the social groups of their husbands.

The social group distribution of our patients then turned out the following (Table 15).

Table 15. Social groups of the patients

Patient's social group	Number of patients
I	4
II	27
III	56
IV	13

When we defined the *social role* of each patient at the time of the admission we ended up with the following classification.

Table 16. Social roles of the patients at the time of admission to treatment

Social role	Number of patients
School pupil	1
Student	19
Working	45
Spouse at home or working at home	12
Unemployed	22
In army or civil service	—
In prison	—
On pension	1

Table 17. Degree of occupational identity at the onset of the illness

Degree of occupational identity	Number of patients
Occupational identity lacking	24
Occupational identity developing	15
Ostensibly stable identity	61

Of the 20 school pupils or students, 18 belonged to the diagnostic nuclear group ($p < .01$). The number of unemployed subjects in the class of typical schizophrenia did not differ from that seen in the total series.

Another statistical connection emerged between the patient's social role and group of schizo-affective psychoses ($p = .032$): there were no students in that group, while the proportion of working subjects including patients working at home was relatively greater than in the rest of the series.

In addition to the social role, we also made an effort to define the *occupational identity* achieved by the patients in the manner shown in Table 17.

The assessment of the occupational identity achieved was based primarily on the manner in which the patient felt he had found his occupational position in the working life of society. In order that a patient was classified as possessing a stable occupational identity, it was required that he had moderate experience of working in an occupation and that he considered this occupation suitable for himself. Most of those lacking an occupational identity were students, but some of the students were at the phase of developing an occupational identity through temporary jobs etc.

An at least ostensibly stable occupational identity had been achieved by nearly 2/3 of our patients. The patients with typical schizophrenia lacked stable occupational identity at an almost significant level compared with the rest of the series ($p = .033$), while an opposite situation prevailed in the group of schizophreniform psychoses ($p = .048$).

4.1.3.3 Data on the Patients' Secondary Families

Secondary family here refers to the family of procreation that comes about through marriage.

On the basis of the data on marital status, the patients in our series were divided as follows:

Table 18. Distribution of the patients on the basis of sex and marital status

Marital status group	Number of patients		
	female	male	total
Unmarried	22	35	57
Married for the first time	16	9	25
Separated	2	7	9
Divorced	3	1	4
Widowed	1	—	1
Married for the second time	3	—	3
Divorced or separated for the second time	1	—	1

There were 57 unmarried patients, 28 married ones, 14 separated or divorced and 1 widow. The group of unmarried subjects was the largest, as it was to be expected, and the number of separated or divorced subjects was precisely half of the number of married ones. The figures hence reflect clearly the problems of the patients with schizophrenia group psychoses in getting married and maintaining their marriage.

The number of "separated" patients in Table 20 is greater than that of "divorced". This indicates that many patients had fallen ill soon after the breakdown of their marriage and the following separation. These problems clearly precipitated the onset of psychosis in many of our patients, especially male patients, who had fallen ill with schizophreniform psychosis.

When we combined our data on marital status into a variable with unmarried patients as one group, married ones as another and separated, divorced or widowed ones as a third, the group of typical schizophrenics did not – perhaps surprisingly – differ from the rest of the series at all, though the other diagnostic subgroups did. The group of schizo-affective psychoses contained the relatively highest proportion of married patients, 8 out of 14 ($p = .046$; the group also included 2 of the 3 patients married for the second time). The group of schizophreniform psychoses differed from the others with marginal significance on the basis of the relatively greater number of separated or divorced subjects and widows, the group of borderline schizophrenia with the same significance on the basis of the greater number of unmarried and the lower number of married subjects.

Table 18 indicates that a clearly larger portion of the female patients were married than of the male patients, while a clearly larger portion of the men were unmarried than of the women. The sex-bound difference in marital status was almost significant.

25 female patients and 14 male patients had *children*. Only three patients had had a child die (one of them her only one, so as to remain childless). 25 patients had 1 child,

9 had 2, 4 had 3 and one had 4, which brings the number of surviving children of the patients in our series to a total of 59. In addition to these, 4 patients had altogether 6 children of the previous marriages of their spouses in their families. Of the patients with children of their own, 26 were married, which means that only 2 of our 28 married patients were childless. Of the other patients with children, 7 were separated from their spouses, 4 were divorced, 1 was a widow, and 1 was unmarried.

Both the married patients and those who had recently divorced had numerous different problems in their marital relationship and family life. This is also reflected by the *psychologic data of the secondary families* acquired in the basic investigation.

Our series includes one married couple where both of the *spouses* became psychotic and were therefore admitted for treatment during our sampling period. Of the other spouses or divorced spouses – who numbered altogether 41 – 9 turned out to have other serious ego disturbances and 18 neurotic disorders. One divorced spouse had been in psychiatric hospital treatment, while 3 married spouses and 1 separated spouse had been given psychiatric outpatient treatment. Examining the distinctly observable disturbances of the patients' spouses that had begun during the marriage, we found one psychosis, 4 cases of alcohol abuse or other addiction, one suicidal attempt and one severe neurosis.

Fowler and Tsuang (1975) found that 28 % of the spouses of 50 schizophrenics had personality disorders (including 5 alcoholics). Our findings correspond nearly to those of their study.

The *psychodynamic atmosphere* of the existent secondary family was assessable for 26 patients out of 28. The atmosphere was assessed as chaotic in 5 cases, rigid in 9 cases and a combination of both chaotic and rigid features was found in 10 cases; in only 2 cases were these features lacking. The *relationship between the spouses* was schismatic and laden with serious and persistent mutual conflicts in 15 marriages and skewed, that is, disproportionately dominated by one spouse, in 5 cases. In another 5 cases the relationship was estimated to be predominantly balanced and integrated.

Of the children of the patients, psychic disorders had been present in at least 4, of whom 2 had been in psychiatric outpatient care. Our team did not meet children systematically.

One of the spouses of our patients and one of their children had a long-term illness resulting in physical disability.

4.1.3.4 Relatives' Attitudes Towards the Patient

The *relatives' attitudes towards the patient* were observed during their interviews and the other contacts with them. The findings on the attitudes of the spouses and parents are presented in Table 19.

Table 19. Attitude of the closest relatives towards the patient at the basic investigation

Attitude towards patient	Spouse[a]	Mother	Father
Empathic, willing to understand	15 (19)	20	16
Helpless, anxious	10 (11)	24	13
Poorly understanding or hostile	2 (5)	18	17
Indifferent	1 (4)	2	5

[a] The figures in parentheses also include the 11 spouses divorced or separated who continued to have a close contact with the patient.

Although the marital relationships were so often schismatic, the group of spouses contained a relatively larger proportion of empathic relatives willing to understand the patient than the parental groups. They also often had a helpless and anxious attitude. The parents were divided more or less equally between an effort at empathy, helplessness and anxiety, and poorly understanding or hostile attitudes. Of these features, helplessness and anxiety were particularly common among the mothers.

We are aware of the subjective nature of this kind of assessment of attitudes. Even so, we tried to elucidate the significance of the relatives' attitudes for the treatment and the factors involved in the therapeutic plans by constructing two background variables of them. One was made according to *whether the patient had an empathic parent and/or spouse*. These patients numbered 43, while the patients without an empathic close relative numbered 44. 13 patients remained outside this background variable because of lack of sufficient information. The other variable was constructed according to *whether the parents and spouses included some who understood the patient poorly or were hostile towards him*. There were 42 such patients in the series, while in the case of 45 patients no such features were noted in the closest relatives. 13 patients were also excluded from this variable.

The group of schizo-affective psychoses contained slightly more patients with empathic parents or spouses than the other groups ($p < .072$). The other background variable, the presence of hostile or poorly understanding close relatives, in turn, distinguished the group of borderline schizophrenia from the remaining series by indicating that the patients of this group had significantly ($p = .007$) more often relatives with such attitudes.

4.2 Admission for Treatment and the Clinical Background Variables

4.2.1 Previous Treatments. Admission for Present Treatments

Despite the fact that the patients had been admitted for the first time into units of the community psychiatric health care system because of psychotic disorders of the schizophrenia group, an unexpectedly large proportion of the patients in our series had already been *treated previously* for psychic disturbances. There were altogether 36 patients of this kind. Four of them had been treated for a psychotic disorder, 32 for milder disturbances. The former group consisted of patients who had received out-patient care for their psychosis outside the system of community psychiatry, but now entered the public system. The reason for this in all cases was that the patient's condition had been aggravated so as to require hospital treatment.

The previous treatments were divided between the different therapeutic units as follows:

child-psychiatric hospital or institution	–
child guidance center or some other child-psychiatric out-patient unit	2
psychiatric hospital treatment (for reasons other than psychosis)	2
other hospital or institutional therapy for a psychic disturbance	1

out-patient care within the public psychiatric health care system (for reasons other than psychosis)	5
other psychiatric out-patient care (e.g. the mental health services of the students' health care foundation, private psychiatrist or psychologist)	21
general practitioner or a specialist other than psychiatrist	7

Some of the patients had been treated in several therapeutic units. The group of patients with previous treatment did not correlate with any of the diagnostic subgroups.

The *initiative for the present admission* was made by the patient in 20 cases, by parents or siblings in 21 cases, by the spouse or children in 20 cases and by another relative in 3 cases, by a friend or an acquaintance in 8 cases, by an official or health care worker of the patient's employer or school in 11 cases, by another doctor or health care worker in 13 cases, and by the police in 14 cases. 26 patients *first arrived in the therapeutic unit* alone, while 26 were accompanied by parents or siblings, 24 by the spouse or children and 2 by another relative, 5 by a friend or an acquaintance, 1 by a doctor or health care worker, and 16 by a policeman. These findings clearly indicate the family and environmental orientation of the initial situation in the treatment of a schizophrenic patient.

57 patients in our series were brought for treatment – into hospital in these cases – by *judicial sanctions*. These patients were relatively the most numerous in the diagnostic group of schizophreniform psychoses, which differed from the rest of the series almost significantly. The patients with typical schizophrenia admitted on the basis of judicial sanctions were also marginally significantly more numerous than those in the other series, while the group of borderline schizophrenia only included 2 patients with judicial sanctions for treatment ($p < .001$).

We also tried to find out how many of the patients, regardless of the judicial sanctions, were really admitted against their will, and how many attended the therapy willingly. The results of this assessment of the *patients' own attitude* towards admission is shown in Table 20.

In the light of these figures, it seems that judicial sanctions were used unnecessarily often for bringing the patients into hospital. The reluctance to attend treatment was particularly notable among the typical schizophrenic patients, which differed from the remaining series at an almost significant level ($p = 0.29$). The willingness to receive treatment was greatest in the group of borderline schizophrenia, which differed clearly significantly ($p = .005$) from the others. The patients with schizophreniform psychoses, on the other hand, who had been admitted for treatment on the basis of judicial sanctions with one exception, were not significantly correlated with this attitude assessment.

Table 20. Patient's attitude towards admission for treatment

Was the patient admitted for treatment	Number of patients
willingly	38
passively conforming	37
clearly unwillingly	25

During the course of the basic study, we also examined the *attitudes of the patients towards the therapeutic plans* presented to them. 59 of the patients refused no form of therapy, while 41 took a negative stand to at least one of the modes of treatment suggested. The negative attitudes were most numerous concerning the necessity of hospital treatment (27 patients), and next came the contacts with the family (14 patients) and drug treatment (7 patients). The binary variable constructed of attitudes did not correlate with any diagnostic category.

Of the families, 60 considered hospital treatment most suited to the patients, taking a favourable attitude towards it. 16 families preferred out-patient therapy, and 15 seemed willing to withdraw completely from the problems of therapeutic responsibility.

4.2.2 Clinical Pictures

The first background variable of the clinical picture was the *time* that had elapsed between the *manifestation of psychotic symptoms* and the admission for treatment.

Table 21. Time between the manifestation of the first psychotic symptoms and the admission for treatment

Time between manifestation of psychotic symptoms and admission for treatment	Number of patients
less than 2 weeks	25
less than a month	17
less than 3 months	19
less than 6 months	15
less than a year	9
less than 2 years	4
2–5 years	5
more than 5 years	6

The psychotic symptoms of 42 patients had appeared during the month preceding admission, while the symptoms of 34 patients had become manifest during the preceding six months and those of 24 patients even prior to that. Attention is attracted by the fact that about one tenth of the patients had had psychotic symptoms for at least two years prior to admission for treatment. These patients consisted of two groups: a few paranoid schizophrenics and similarly a few borderline schizophrenic patients, both of whom typically had had transient rather than persistent psychotic symptoms, which were relatively well controlled by the ego. Only one of the patients in our series could be considered a clearly chronic schizophrenic upon admission.

The correlations between this background variable and the diagnostic categories were examined in Chapter 3.1.2.

The *nuclear symptoms of schizophrenia* were found to occur with the following frequencies in our series:

Table 22. Frequency of the nuclear symptoms of schizophrenia in our series

Symptom	Number of patients
Autism	40
Schizophrenic thought disorder	99
Hebephrenic affective disorder (blunting of affect)	11
Schizophrenic auditory hallucinosis	25
Somatic delusions of being influenced	20
Psychic delusions of being influenced	19
Catatonic symptoms (stupor and/or excitement)	8
Sensations of depersonalization and derealization	28

The schizophrenic thought disorder, defined according to Bleuler (1911), was a criterion for inclusion in the series in nearly all cases (cf. 3.1.2.). A majority of the autistic patients, 32, suffered from typical schizophrenia ($p = .000$). The groups of schizophreniform psychoses and borderline schizophrenia included an almost significantly lower-than-average number of autistic patients. A hebephrenic affective disorder was noted in 9 typical schizophrenics and in 2 patients classified as having schizo-affective psychosis. The presence of schizophrenic auditory hallucinosis was significantly higher than average ($p = .0011$) in the group of typical schizophrenias, while the group of borderline schizophrenias had an almost significantly and the group of schizo-affective psychoses a marginally significantly lower than average number of patients with this symptom.

The delusions of being influenced based on somatic sensations as well as the sensations of depersonalization and derealization were relatively most frequent in the category of schizophreniform psychoses, where both symptoms were seen in 5 patients. The group of typical schizophrenias did not differ statistically from the remaining series with regard to either these symptoms or the psychic delusions of being influenced. The latter symptom had a marginally significant connection with the group of schizo-affective psychoses. Of the patients with typical catatonic symptoms, 6 had typical schizophrenia, 1 schizophreniform psychosis and 1 schizo-affective psychosis.

Our findings confirmed the assumption that the presence of a psychosis of the schizophrenic type certainly does not exclude the possibility of there being also *other psychic symptoms*. 25 of our patients had conspicuous *neurotic* symptoms and as many as 54 had *depressive* symptoms. 27 patients were diagnosed for *acting-out behaviour,* which is common in character disorders, and 35 patients had a tendency to *alcohol abuse* or other addiction.

We also examined the statistical connections between these symptoms and our clinical-diagnostic categories. It appeared that the group of typical schizophrenias did lack neurotic symptoms at a highly significant level: they were only noted in 5 of the 56 patients in this category ($p = .000$). They were, however, highly significantly frequent in the group of borderline schizophrenia (14 patients, $p = .000$).

Depressive symptoms were also correlated with the diagnostic categories, although less manifestly. The patients with borderline schizophrenia also had a significantly higher frequency ($p = .007$) of depressive symptoms, while the group of typical schizophrenics had a lower relative frequency than the other series, though only approaching marginal significance ($p = .11$). The finding of there being no relation between the group of schizo-affective psychoses and depressive symptoms can probably be considered unexpected. This is explained by the fact that several of these psychoses (8 out of 14) were maniform.

The occurrence of acting-out behaviour had no statistical connections with our clinical-diagnostic categories. The same was also true of the tendency to alcohol abuse or other addictions.

The degree of the *regressive need for help* among our patients is shown by the fact that our team considered 50 of them to be clearly in need of outside support to be able to manage in their environment at the time of admission. 97 were regarded as suffering from intensive *anxiety* or fears, 2 as slightly anxiety-ridden, and only one as showing no signs of anxiety.

During the course of their illness, 17 patients had attempted suicide or other physical self-mutilation, and 10 others had had serious thoughts of self-destruction. In addition to this, 40 patients had had less serious tendencies to self-destruction or delusional fears of destruction. 33 patients appeared to have no tendencies to self-destruction. The suicidal tendencies thus identified had no significant correlations with the clinical-diagnostic categories.

Violent behaviour prior to admission was reported for 15 patients and violent behaviour had been seriously threatened by 7 others. Lesser aggressive features or delusional ideas of surrounding destruction were further noted in 15 patients. 63 patients lacked any aggressive tendencies classifiable into these categories. Violent behaviour had a marginally significant correlation with two of our diagnostic subgroups: patients with borderline schizophrenia had a lower-than-average frequency of violent behaviour, while the schizo-affective group was characterized by more violent behaviour than was the average.

The *patient's ability to make contacts* was divided as follows:

Table 23. Quality of the contact between the patient and the interviewer

Quality of patient's contacts	Number of patients
No contact established	—
Suspicious or reserved contact	37
Symbiotic need for reliance	55
"Normal" contact	8

There were no patients unable to enter into contact, but 37 patients had a suspicious and reserved contact with the interviewer. On the other hand, there were 55 patients who made a reliant contact with symbiotic features in the interview. This is accordant with the notion presented in several psychodynamic investigations suggesting that schizophrenic patients actually have marked need for reliance and dependence directed at their environment: autistic withdrawal is partially interpretable as a reaction to the inability of the surrounding people to respond to these heightened needs and the wish of the patient to shield himself against frustrations through withdrawal.

Burnham et al. (1969) described the need-fear dilemma as the basic problem of the schizophrenic patients: on the one hand they have an intense need for contact, while on the other they have a fear of the risks involved in it – not only frustration, but also excessive dependence on someone else, i.e. being "swallowed" by the other. On a hospital ward functioning as a therapeutic community, it often turns out that a patient initially inclined to autistic behaviour becomes symbiotically reliant having experienced an empathic attitude to himself on the part of the environment; this frequently takes place in an excessively "unprotected" way, which easily results in frustrations in a normal environment. Our own estimate was based on the experience obtained during the first few interviews. The patients who openly express their symbiotic needs also find it easier to establish a psychotherapeutic relationship than do the suspicious or reserved subjects, although they are often also exposed to disappointments and frustrations even during brief separations, e.g. cancellation of therapeutic sessions or the therapist's vacations.

The relatively serious disturbance of the personalities of our typical schizophrenic patients in comparison with the other diagnostic groups is indicated by the frequency of suspicious and reserved contacts amongst them: of the 37 reserved or suspicious patients, 28 belonged to this group ($p < .01$). The number of symbiotically reliant patients in the group of typical schizophrenics was nearly equal to that of suspicious or reserved patients, 25, which is, however, almost significantly less than in the other diagnostic sub-groups. The group of borderline schizophrenias included a marginally significantly smaller number of suspicious or reserved patients. The highest relative frequencies of symbiotically reliant patients occurred in the groups of borderline schizophrenia – 14 out of 20 patients – and schizo-affective psychoses – 10 out of 14 patients –, which figures, however, lack any statistical significance.

Our patients' *insight into their own problems* was divided into the following categories in the basic examination:

Table 24. Patient's insight into their own problems and their connection to the onset of schizophrenia

Patient's insight	Number of patients
Denies completely his illness and his problems in general	20
Admits there are problems, but thinks they are caused by other people	29
Has some insight into his own role in the coming about of his problems and/or symptoms	48
Sees his problems and symptoms as part of himself and endeavours to solve them	3

As shown by the above Table, about half of our patients showed at least some insight into their problems, while the other half either denied their illness or regarded their problems as being caused by others. When the patients were divided into these two groups of approximately equal size, no statistical correlations with our diagnostic sub-groups emerged. The patients partially capable of insight were relatively the most numerous in the group of borderline schizophrenia (13 out of 20).

4.2.3 Categories Constructed on the Basis of the Quality of Ego Dysfunctions (Ego-Dynamic Sub-Grouping)

We decided to deepen our clinical approach psychodynamically by classifying our patients, apart from the diagnostic categorization, also according to an overall assessment of the disturbance of their ego function, i.e. the severity, duration and dynamic meaningfulness of its disintegration. One reason for the new classification was the expectation that it might also be of significance for the determination of the weight placed on the different therapeutic procedures. In principle, the classification is independent of the diagnostic classification, although these two categorizations are partly interrelated.

The term "ego" is here used in the psychoanalytic sense. "Ego" refers to the group of psychologic functions responsible for the integrated and logical control of the personality functions both internally and in relation to the external world. The presence of psychotic symptoms always means that the ego functions are disintegrated to some extent and for some time.

We call our new classification *ego-dynamic sub-grouping of psychoses of the schizophrenic type*. We divided our patients into the appropriate groups in the basic study already. Similarly to the diagnostic categorization, this grouping was also revised somewhat during the course of the first follow-up study.

The following four ego-dynamic groups were established:

1. The patients whose psychotic status is characterized by sinister imminent disintegration of the ego functions. These patients have relatively slight – or at least short-term – though often recurrent, psychotic symptoms, particularly ideas of reference and other paranoid delusions or delusions pertaining to one's own ego image, but no massive psychotic condition which would result in clearly observable and extensive psychotic behaviour in the social environment. The patients usually also have neurotic symptom formation. Both the neurotic and the psychotic symptoms are of clearly defensive significance in the protection against internal anxiety and more profound disintegration of the personality. The symptoms are hence clearly related to the long-term adaptive dynamics of the personality, which is mostly relatively easy to verify by empathic investigation.

   We call this sub-group the *group of imminent disintegration*.

2. The patients in whom the onset of the psychotic condition is relatively sudden and so massive that the patient is clearly not able to control his psychotic behaviour or cope in his social environment at his previous functional level. In a typical case, the onset of psychosis is triggered by a precipitating factor, either somatic, psychic or social, which differs from the patient's normal course of life. The symptoms are rather characterized by a decompensation of the previous psychic balance – often resulting in at least ostensibly good adaptation – than by a defensive significance. Adequate treatment usually brings about relatively rapid compensation of the psychotic symptoms, although this improvement also depends on the patient's life situation and the development of his closest interpersonal relationships.

   We call this sub-group the *group of acute disintegration*.

3. The patients in whom the onset of psychosis is most clearly related to persistent and serious problems of interpersonal relations and difficulties in adjustment through social coping. This is often reflected in isolation, gradual deterioration of social functions and special behavioural features. Psychotic symptoms usually appear gradually and slowly; in some cases they may be sudden, but even then there are clearly observable difficulties in the prepsychotic adaptive development. The psychotic symptoms are clearly more profound than in the group of imminent disintegration. The dominant features include long-term thought and affective disorders and an autistic, often hallucinatory mental world where projective and introjective elements vary. The symptoms are of internal defensive significance for the patient at the psychotic level. They tend to be established as part of the patient's means of adaptation as a whole, but they generally do not promote his social adjustment.

We call this sub-group the *group of regressive disintegration.*

4. The patients whose psychotic development is generally dominated by rigid, typically paranoid symptom formations, which, psychodynamically speaking, signify a projective way of solving psychologic problems. The patients have schizophrenic delusions which may be accompanied by hallucinations, but the disintegration of the ego as a whole is less comprehensive than in the previous group and the patient is better able to cope socially. This group differs from the group of imminent disintegration on the basis of the persistence, and often also the systematic nature, of the paranoid symptoms; they are of increasingly permanent defensive significance for the patient, who is usually convinced of their ultimate reality.

We call this sub-group the *group of paranoid disintegration.*

The classification turned out to be clinically appropriate: the grouping of patients according to this principle involved no great problems.

The sizes of the groups were more equal than in the diagnostic classification. The group of regressive disintegration was the largest, consisting of 31 patients. The patients with acute disintegration numbered 28, those with imminent disintegration 21 and those with paranoid disintegration 20. The connections between the ego-dynamic groups and the diagnostic groups are shown in table 25.

Table 25. Connections between psychodynamic groups and diagnostic

Ego-dynamic group	**Diagnostic group**				
	Typical schizo-phrenia	Schizo-phreniform psychosis	Schizo-affective psychosis	Border-line schizo-phrenia	Total
Imminent disintegration	0***(−)	2	1	18***(+)	21
Acute disintegration	9** (−)	6*(+)	11***(+)	2*(−)	28
Regressive disintegration	29***(+)	0*(−)	2	0***(−)	31
Paranoid disintegration	18***(+)	2	0*(−)	0*(−)	20
Total	56	10	14	20	100

The asterisks indicate the statistical significances between the psychodynamic and diagnostic groups, (+) = a connection going in the same direction, (−) = a connection going in the opposite direction.

Nearly all of the borderline schizophrenia patients were classified as belonging to the group of imminent disintegration, which further included 2 schizophreniform psychoses with mild symptoms and one mildly symptomatic schizo-affective psychosis. There were no typically schizophrenic patients in this group. The group of acute disintegration comprised patients from all the diagnostic sub-categories. This group had a highly significant connection with schizo-affective psychoses, and it also included a majority of the schizophreniform psychoses. The number of typical schizophrenic patients in this group was, however, of the same order – despite the fact that there was a significant negative connection between the groups of typical schizophrenia and acute disintegration.

Most of the typical schizophrenic patients belonged to either the group of regressive disintegration or the group of paranoid disintegration. The former group further included 2 schizo-affective psychoses and the latter 2 schizophreniform psychoses. Schizophreniform psychoses were completely lacking in the group of regressive disintegration, schizo-affective psychosis in the group of paranoid disintegration and borderline schizophrenic patients in both of these groups.

The connections between the ego-dynamic groups and the other clinical and psychosocial background variables were analyzed specifically for each group.

The *group of imminent disintegration* was highly significantly connected with the presence of neurotic symptoms ($p = .001$) while the positive connection with depressive symptoms ($p = .020$) and the negative connection with schizophrenic symptoms ($p = .042$) were almost significant. Other highly significant connections were found with the exclusion of judicial sanctions as well as with a willing attitude to treatment. Neurotic or psychosomatic symptoms in childhood were almost significantly more frequent than in the anamneses of other patients, and the same finding was seen in the longer-than-average duration of the psychotic illness. As in the diagnostic group of borderline schizophrenia, hostile or poorly understanding relatives were common ($p = .004$), while the tendency to avoid aggressions was less pronounced ($p = .083$) than in the borderline group.

The group had a better insight ability than our sample in the average, but the difference was not even marginally significant ($p = .106$).

The only highly statistical connection of the *group of acute disintegration* was found present with a shorter-than-average duration with psychotic symptoms ($p = .0004$). A relatively good social and psychosocial adjustment was illuminated by almost significant connections with an established heterosexual identity ($p = .025$) and the occupational role (fewer students, more people with jobs or working at home; $p = .024$). As opposed to avoidance of aggression, there were more individuals with a tendency to impulsive aggressiveness in this group as compared with the other patients ($p = .031$).

The *group of regressive disintegration* quite clearly consisted of the patients with the most seriously retarded social and interactional development, especially as regards the working life (more students, fewer people with jobs or working at home; $p = .000$); fewer subjects with established occupational identity ($p = .009$), separation from home ($p = .002$) and sexual relationships ($p = .037$). The youngest age group was notably numerous ($p = .002$). As it can be expected, nuclear schizophrenic symptoms were also more frequent in this group than in the rest of the series ($p = .022$). If we compare these findings with all the patients diagnosed as typically schizophrenic, we can see that the serious problems of psychologic and social development are particularly frequent in the group of regressive disintegration: the group of typical schizophrenias as a whole lacked most of these statistical connections. As regards the clinical features, however, the group does not differ from the group of typical schizophrenias in the same way: the connection with the numerical incidence of nuclear schizophrenic symptoms was even more marked in the latter group.

An unexpected finding was the marginally significantly better insight ability found in this patient group compared with the remaining series.

The connections between the *group of paranoid disintegration* and the background variables were quite different from those emerging in the regressive group despite the fact that a majority of this group also consisted of patients diagnosed as typically schizophrenic: Compared with the rest of the series, the paranoid group was characterized by a reluctant attitude towards therapy and a conspicuous lack of insight ability (both, $p = .002$). Suspicious or reserved contact mode and negative attitudes to treatment were also visible, although only at a marginally significant level, as was also an overtly violent behaviour. A majority of the paranoid patients had accomplished separation from the primary family ($p = .036$). With regard to nuclear schizophrenic symptoms, the group did not differ from the rest of the series either way.

The correlations with the background variables definitely suggest that the therapeutic challenge is weighted quite differently for the patients diagnosed as typical schizophrenics belonging to the group of regressive disintegration on the one hand and the group of paranoid disintegration on the other.

In comparison with the diagnostic categorization, the ego-dynamic sub-grouping led to somewhat clearer connections with background variables based on clearly psychodynamic assessments. These include assessments concerning psychologic separation from the primary family, psychosexual identity, coping with aggressions as well as insight ability, and the patient's willing attitude to treatment. The connections with background variables based on clinical symptoms are, on the other hand, somewhat weaker than in the diagnostic categorization.

4.3 Case-Specific Therapeutic Plans

The last part of the form used in the psychiatric basic examination consisted of the plans for case-specific therapy. The therapeutic plans were designed in team meetings, and the goal was to create a therapeutic plan which

a) seemed to meet most appropriately the therapeutic need of the patient and/or his family, and
b) seemed to be realistic from the viewpoint of both the therapeutic resources available and the therapeutic motivation that could probably be created.

A *summary of the team's indications for the different modes of psychotherapy* is shown in Table 26.

We considered *neuroleptic medication* indicated for 97 patients. There were, however, only 5 patients whose need for medication was defined so as to alleviate rapidly the psychotic symptoms with relatively massive pharmacotherapy. For the

Table 26. The numbers of patients with indications for the different modes of psychotherapy in the therapeutic plans designed at the time of the basic study

Modes of therapy	Number of patients	
1. **Intervention in crisis**		
On an out-patient basis	16	
On an in-patient basis	10	26
2. **Individual therapies**		
Intensive individual therapy	25	
Infrequent individual therapy	44	69
Other individual contacts	27	96
3. **Family therapies**		
Conjoint therapy of primary family, intensive	6	
Conjoint therapy of primary family, supportive	10	16
Spouse or couple therapy, intensive	13	
Spouse or couple therapy, supportive	13	26
Separate support for member(s) of family		36
Contact with patient's family established		19
Families with one or several of the above modes		92
4. **Group therapy of out-patients**		10
5. **Psychotherapeutic community on a hospital ward**		
Primarily indicated	59	
Upon failure of out-patient-therapy	4	63

remaining 92 patients, the medication with individual dosage was regarded as part of an overall therapeutic plan, where it primarily served the purpose of treatment designed on psychotherapeutic premises.

Electroshock treatment at the initial stage was considered possibly indicated for two patients. Both were suffering from catatonic psychosis.

The need of our patients for *rehabilitation and/or socially helpful measures* turned out to be great at the time of the basic study already. We considered 60 of these first admission patients to be in need of such measures. The need was divided between various activities as follows:

Occupational guidance	17 patients
Assistance in getting employment	37 "
Other job-related arrangements	10 "
Need for financial assistance	15 "
Residential arrangements	22 "
Social arrangements relating to the family situation	6 "
Total for need of rehabilitative measures	60 patients

Below, we will describe our thoughts of the indications for the most important modes of psychotherapy (cf. Alanen et al. 1979).

4.3.1 Intervention in Crisis

This mode of therapy consists of help provided in an acute psychosis or an otherwise critical condition by means of rapid and frequently repeated measures. It may take place entirely on an out-patient basis, or it may include a short period of hospital or day-hospital treatment. Sometimes crisis intervention concentrates on the patient as an individual, but more often it is family- or environmentally oriented, which means that, apart from helping the patient, contacts are flexibly made with the family members or other individuals close to the patient (seen either separately or together with the patient). Contacts with the working milieu and other social support are also possible.

Intervention in the crisis of acute psychosis was regarded as particularly indicated when the goal was to protect the patient from more serious injuries or being branded in his interpersonal relationships and social environment. Most of these patients had fallen ill rather suddenly, in connection with conflicting life situations.

4.3.2 Individual Therapies

By *intensive individual therapy* we did not mean a strictly analytic insight-oriented therapy, but an empathic and prolonged therapeutic relationship in which a conscious attempt to enhance the patient's own insight into his problems was included.

The most important determinant in the case of this treatment was the investigator's view as to whether the patient would be able to benefit from a therapeutic process that would deal with deep-rooted developmental problems, and whether such a process could be motivated in his particular case. It was also assumed that the patient's life situation did not include problems which made his possibilities for a long-term individual psychotherapy questionable – no such entanglement of intrafamilial relationship which would necessarily indicate a conjoint family therapy as the primary treatment, or such life situation which would not permit a commitment to a long-term psychotherapeutic relationship.

The indication for *infrequent individual therapy* occurred most typically when it was considered beneficial for the patient to have an opportunity for a fairly long-continued, supportive treatment contact. This was combined with the control of drug therapy, which constituted a more important part in the treatment of many of these patients than in the group indicated for intensive individual therapy. Still, the infrequent setting was also assumed to prepare the way for a more intensive therapy for some patients.

4.3.3 Family Therapies

Conjoint family therapy of the primary family was considered indicated "when the basic disturbance of the patient and the onset of the illness appeared to be so closely related to intrafamilial relationships, and the mutual dependency of the family members so intensive, that it was felt impossible for the patient to emancipate himself without an active psychotherapeutic intervention directed into these actual intrafamilial interactional processes". It was also assumed that the interviews with the patient and his parents had given some grounds for concluding that conjoint family therapy would be possible and useful, and that motivation for it could be aroused.

Family therapy of the secondary family, which in our plans most often consisted of *couple therapy* of the patient and his or her spouse, was indicated notably more often than conjoint therapy of the primary family at the basic study stage.

This was associated with the fact that our previous experiences of couple therapy had proved favourable even in cases where the therapist had little experience of family therapy. The most important indication for couple therapy was the relation of the patient's illness to the marital relationship (or other partner relationship) involving shared problems. The other indication was that the therapy of some patients was considered to be particularly promoted by the support given by the spouse: shared therapy is often safer for the patient and alleviates his fears of being rejected by the spouse.

The possibility of including the patient's children in the therapy was not excluded, either, but this inclusion was rare within the implemented therapeutic practice. It was considered important, however, that the discussions of couple therapy also touched upon children and problems related to them.

Indication for a *separate support for member(s) of the families* was present in the following situations:

- when a family member appeared to need help as an individual
- when the relatives appeared to need support in order to prevent the patient's illness or its treatment from becoming too heavy a burden for them
- when it was thought that the patient's individual treatment would possibly fail without such contact with the family
- when the patient's lack of treatment motivation actually led to a situation in which the contact with a family member constituted the only possibility for providing care
- when these contacts were seen to serve as possible preliminary work for the subsequent family(or individual) therapy

4.3.4 Group Therapy of Out-Patients

Within the framework of our therapeutic principles, group therapy has been mostly given in the psychotherapeutic communities set up on wards of the Psychiatry Clinic. Some group therapy had been conducted among out-patients in the Mental Health Office of Turku.

A conscious indication for this mode of therapy was, above all, the effort to improve the social contacts of relatively lonely patients, but there were also other, mainly supportive objectives.

4.3.5 Psychotherapeutic Community on a Hospital Ward

We call the in-patient wards of the Clinic of Psychiatry *psychotherapeutic communities,* underlining their therapeutic orientation (Alanen 1975). In accordance with the therapeutic community ideology developed by Jones (1953), our effort has been to minimize the hospital hierarchy inexpedient for psychiatric work. Therapeutic measures have been considered of primary significance, however, and the difference in position between the patients and the staff has remained clear-cut.

We have underlined the following three features as being particularly characteristic of the psychotherapeutic community treating psychotic patients (Alanen 1975):

1. shared empathic basic attitude towards the patients,
2. open mutual communication,
3. development of individual therapeutic relationships within the therapeutic community.

Along with the progress of the work, family-oriented therapeutic work has emerged as a fourth central starting-point. Art therapy and creative physical activity have served as important additional modes of therapy for many patients.

Within our therapeutic system, psychotherapeutic communities signify a maximal use of the resources, which is particularly useful for the most seriously disturbed, regressive patients. But even in less profound or more persistent disturbances, the psychotherapeutic community may provide a pivotal system for clarifying the patients' topical problems and planning the necessary therapeutic interventions on a more long-term basis. To make this possible, we have made intentional efforts to promote the contact between our psychotherapeutic communities and the units for out-patient therapy, particularly the mental health office.

4.4 Summary and Discussion

When evaluating these findings on the basic examination, we must bear in mind that our *goals* even here were *clinical*. The findings were primarily used to ascertain the background factors affecting the prerequisites for the implementation of psychotherapies as well as the indications and outcome of these therapies. In the two next chapters we will resume the topic of which the initial background variables turned out most relevant for these purposes.

The psychiatric basic examination in our project always also included therapeutic viewpoints, particularly the creation of contact with the patient and the other individuals interviewed. The basic examination hence served as a preparation for therapy. The technique of inquiry then requires an empathic attitude towards the individual being interviewed and his problems. Unstandardized interview is better suited to this endeavour than standardized inquiry, which technique has been used in several works with a purely scientific emphasis.

These viewpoints should be especially emphasized as regards the questions pertaining to the patient's manner of contact and his own attitude towards therapy, but they are important also concerning several other psychodynamically weighted assessments. These include the patients' insight into their own problems, which, quite understandably, is clearly related to the prospects of psychotherapy. It is obvious that if the interviewer has an attitude that makes it possible to approach the patient in a genuinely empathic way – possibly even pointing out preliminary connections between the patients's problems and the events of his life or the emotional reactions he shows in the interview – he is able simultaneously to stimulate the patient's insightfulness and also to describe it in terms more relevant to the psychotherapeutic situation than a more distant "objective" inquiry conforming to a given standardized formula.

This finding was further emphasized in the investigation of schizophrenic patients first admitted in 1983–84 in Turku, where both individual interviews of the patients and a family-centered initial investigation in joint meetings of the patient and his family members were accomplished. According to the findings thereby made, even two thirds of the patients had at least some insight into their problems and symptoms. The investigators concluded that the research approach – aiming both at individual- and system-oriented understanding – itself clearly increased the patient's insightfulness at this early stage already, thereby possibly also lessening their tendency to passive chronicity (Aaltonen et al. 1984).

The findings of our basic examination confirmed the notion of *disorders frequently present in the primary family milieus of schizophrenic patients.* Slightly less than 10 % of the parents had had disorders of the psychotic level, which corresponds to the previous findings. Other disorders graver than the neurotic level, especially serious personality disorders, were clearly more numerous. Despite the relatively high number of parents not examined individually, we can take our results as supporting the previous findings (Lidz et al. 1957, 1965; Alanen et al. 1966) on the prevalence of serious personality disorders among the parents of schizophrenic patients.

The differences in family background between the diagnostic subgroups of the present series might be described as unexpectedly small. What attracts attention, however, is the finding that disorders of the external structure of the patient's childhood family were clearly most frequent in the group of schizophreniform psychoses, a finding also made by Salokangas (1977) in an earlier series collected in Turku.

We also explored the *attitudes of the closest relatives* – parents and spouses – towards the patients in the interviews made in the basic examination. About half of the patients appeared to have at least one relative with an empathic attitude. There was a group of the same size with a relative classified as "poorly understanding" or "hostile". What may be unexpected was that the latter group of relatives – in these cases regularly parents – were significantly more frequent in the group of borderline schizophrenias than in the rest of the series. As regards the parents with an empathic attitude, the group of borderline schizophrenias did not differ from the others, while the patients with schizo-affective psychosis had an empathic parent or spouse slightly more often than the other patients.

The problems of the *psychosocial development of our patients* are most clearly reflected in the fact that the significant interpersonal relationships outside the primary family numbered one at the most in slightly more than half of our series – one fifth of the patients had no such relationships at all – and that two thirds of the patients only had relationships which were labile and short in duration or characterized by repeated conflicts. The lack of occupational identity was prominent in the group of typical schizophrenias. 50 % of our patients continued to be psychologically – and often even concretely – bound with their primary families, although separation struggle was more common than complete enmeshment with the primary family.

There were 28 married patients, but when we also include the divorced and widowed subjects in this category, the number of patients with a marriage anamnesis comes up to 43. Unmarried patients numbered 57, respectively. The percentage of unmarried subjects was 46 % among the female patients and 68 % among the males, the corresponding ratio for divorced patients being opposite (10 % and 15 %).

The characteristic way of *coping with one's aggressive feelings* was avoidance in two thirds of the series, while one third of the patients typically had impulsive outbursts of aggression. The former group was associated with the borderline schizophrenias and the latter with schizophreniform psychoses, while the group of typical schizophrenias did not differ from the average. There was, however, a difference in *sexual relations*. At least short sexual relations were reported by all but 23 of our patients; 18 of these 23 belonged to our nuclear schizophrenic group. 61 of our patients had an *established heterosexual identity*, the others being divided more or less evenly between delayed sexual development on the one hand and chaotic development with identity crises on the other. None of the patients had an established homosexual identity.

As to the *social status* and the *educational level*, our series included a notably high number of senior secondary school graduates, i.e. 28. This, together with the high proportion of students in our series, is due to there being a large amount of university students in Turku. A conspicuous finding pertaining to education was that many of the patients had become psychotic halfway through the occupational education following the stage of basic schooling.

Slightly more than half of our patients had been admitted for therapy on the basis of *judicial sanctions*, their number being almost significantly higher in the group of schizophreniform psychoses than in the rest of the series. The group of borderline schizophrenias, on the other hand, included hardly any patients admitted with judicial sanctions. Only 25 patients came to treatment clearly against their own will, which suggests that the use of judicial sanctions upon admission was relatively often unnecessary. 41 patients had a negative attitude towards one of the modes of therapy recommended for them.

It was already pointed out in Chapter 3 that the number of *schizophrenic nuclear symptoms*, as defined in accordance with the Nordic psychiatric tradition established by Langfeldt (1937, 1952), was significantly higher in the group of typical schizophrenias, whereas a negative correlation emerged between the number of nuclear symptoms and borderline schizophrenias at a significant level and between the symptoms and schizo-affective psychoses at an almost significant level. Schizophreniform psychoses did not differ from the remaining series in this respect, but the symptoms had been of significantly shorter duration in this group than in the others. The longest average duration of psychotic symptoms before the admission was reported by the patients with borderline schizophrenia. Autism, hebephrenic affective disorder and schizophrenic auditory hallucinosis were particularly typical of patients of the nuclear group. Exploration of *other than psychotic symptoms* indicated that neurotic symptoms were highly significantly more frequent and depressive symptoms significantly more frequent in the group of borderline schizophrenias than in the rest of the series. The typical schizophrenic patients, however, lacked neurotic symptoms at a highly significant level.

The findings on the *nature of the contact between the patients and the team members* were considered important for the establishment of psychotherapeutic relationships. 55 of our patients were clearly symbiotically reliant, while 37 patients had a suspicious or reserved attitude towards the interviewer. The latter type of contact was significantly more common among the typical schizophrenic patients than among the other patients despite the fact that this group also included 25 patients with a symbiotic contact.

About half of our patients had at least some *insight* into their own role in the development of their own problems and/or symptoms. Preliminary insightfulness of this kind was most common in the group of borderline schizophrenias, but no significant differences emerged between the diagnostic categories – unexpected as it was.

All in all, our basic examination revealed quite clearly the characteristic problems of our patients. Their internal dynamics, their connections with the family background, and their contribution to the onset of the disease were perceived illustratively by the interviewers in most of the cases. In this way *the findings also confirmed our own notions of the contribution of psychologic factors to the onset of schizophrenia.* But they simultaneously demonstrated the *heterogeneity* of our series. The life situations of the patients, their family and other social backgrounds as well as the severity of their problems varied from case to case, thereby supporting our suggestion that the therapeutic plans really should be designed specifically for each patient to meet his or her subjective needs. In Chapter 4.3. we shortly presented our ideas for designing therapeutic plans at the time of the basic examination. The indications of different treatment modes will be discussed in more detail in Chapter 7, after our findings on the implementation of the therapies and on the prognostic results have been presented.

We will, however, discuss here the innovative classification presented in Chapter 4.2.3., which we call *ego-dynamic grouping of psychoses of the schizophrenia group.* One starting-point of this classification, too, was the conspicuous heterogeneity of our series, the other motive being the need to find a classificatory principle that would be better suited to the needs of a comprehensive therapeutic approach based on psychodynamic notions than the classical diagnostic sub-categories of schizophrenia. The grouping should simultaneously be so simple as to be applicable to the everyday clinical practice. The fact that we met with no great difficulties while dividing the patients into our ego-dynamic groups seems to suggest that the latter goal was reached.

The term "ego-dynamic" indicates that the classification is based on the findings of the nature of the ego dysfunctions, while it specifically invites attention to the quality and orientation of the dynamically expedient defensive functions.

An ego-psychologic analysis of the schizophrenic syndrome with profiles for the different ego functions has been presented by Bellak et al. (1973). They discuss 12 ego functions, including e.g. reality testing, regulation and control of drives, object relations, thought processes and defensive functions. Their goal seems to have been, however, to demonstrate the intragroup similarities within the schizophrenic population and discrimination between the schizophrenics and patients with other disorders rather than differentation of schizophrenics into subcategories. The ego function profiles are based on ratings of interviews and/or psychological tests, and they are relatively complex to be applied in the everyday clinical practice.

A classification somewhat closer to our own purposes is the one presented by Pao in his book Schizophrenic Disorders (1979), where the groups are called simply schizophrenia I, schizophrenia II, schizophrenia III and schizophrenia IV. The first three are differentiated on the basis of the severity of the disorders seen in the individual developmental histories of the patients, which, according to Pao, is clearly related to the quality of the symptoms and particularly their way of manifestation. According to Pao, the disturbances of these patients' parents also increase in the same order, corresponding to a greater need for family-oriented treatment. By schizophrenia IV

Pao means chronically ill patients who have been in hospital for long periods and lost their hopes for a better future. They may have originally belonged to any group, but the effects of chronicity must be taken into account quite specially in their therapy.

When we compare Pao's description of his patients with our own patient series, we can postulate that his patients were more seriously disturbed on an average than ours. This agrees with the fact that the series consists of patients of the private Chestnut Lodge sanatorium, who need long-term hospital therapy and had often been ill for a long time before this hospitalization. A majority of Pao's patients – particularly those classified as schizophrenia II and III – would probably belong to our group of regressive disintegration.

Of our own ego-dynamic groups, the *group of imminent disintegration* in practice consists of more or less the same patients as the diagnostic category of borderline schizophrenias. These patients struggle at the borderline of ego disintegration, which is shown by the presence of generally mild, but often quite anxiety-provoking psychotic symptoms. The nuclear symptoms of schizophrenia are less frequent than in the other ego-dynamic groups. Neurotic symptoms, however, are highly significantly more common than in the other groups.

This also shows that the defensive ego functions take place, for a notable part, at the neurotic level. The occurrence of psychotic symptoms is often restricted to the psychologically more stressful life situations, though they are frequently recurrent. Depressive symptoms are also common. These patients are clearly better motivated to treatment than the other groups.

The *group of acute disintegration* include the acute psychoses usually associated with distinct reactive, triggering factors regardless of whether their symptom formation is accordant with typical schizophrenia, schizophreniform psychosis or schizo-affective psychosis. The ego dysfunction is characterized by decompensation of the previous functional level (which is often, though not always, easily reversible) rather than by syndromes with regressive defensive significance. The level of prepsychotic personality development is higher among the patients in this group than in the other groups, which was shown by e.g. the high frequency of stable heterosexual identities and marriages and the high number of patients with an established occupational identity and a job. The time that had elapsed since the onset of psychotic symptoms was highly significantly shorter than in the other groups. Many of the patients typically give impulsive expression to their aggressive emotions, which is opposite to the tendency of avoiding aggressive behaviour predominant in the anamneses of the rest of the series.

The patients in our third ego-dynamic group, the *group of regressive disintegration* are characterized by a very severe disturbance of the prepsychotic personality development, which, in the light of our background variables, is manifested as a lack of psychologic separation from the primary family, a lack of stable heterosexual identity (as well as concrete sexual relationships) and a lack of occupational identity. A significant proportion of the patients belongs to the youngest age-groups, and the number of students is high. On the conflict-deficiency continuum described by Pao, the deficiency of the psychologic and psychosocial development of these patients is conspicuous.

Nuclear symptoms of schizophrenia were more frequent in the patients of this group than in the others. What was typical was that they developed gradually during the adolescence. There were also a few patients who became acutely psychotic, but their prepsychotic difficulties were, however, quite as obvious as those of the other patients in this group. The psychotic symptoms were dominated by deeply regressive, but variably both introjective (associated with the subjective and autistic mental world) and projective (associated with an external delusional system) elements. Although such regression of the ego functions does not help the patients to adjust to his social environment, it does seem to involve defensive functions. Will (1967) described the schizophrenic behaviour as an "unsatisfactory, but necessary resolution of long-standing and various attempts to secure a minimal satisfaction of needs" in the environment constituted by other human beings.

Our fourth *group of paranoid disintegration* is characterized at the clinical level by typically paranoid, projective delusions and/or hallucinations, which are often quite rigid. The overall regression of the psychologic functions, however, is less marked than in the aforesaid group, and the patients' ability to cope in the social environment is better. The background variables indicated that the patients of this group – unlike the regressively disintegrated patients – were more often separated from their primary families than the rest of the series. The insightfulness and willingness to therapy in this group were significantly poorer than in the other groups, which was probably also associated with the fact that a greater proportion of these patients than others had been admitted on the basis of judicial sanctions. The patients in this group typically also lacked neurotic symptoms and had a suspicious or reserved contact with the investigator.

Some psychophysiologic and experimental psychologic investigations (e.g. Venables and Wing 1962, Silverman 1964, Venables 1967, McGormick and Broekema 1978) have shown that paranoid and non-paranoid schizophrenics differ with regard to the physiological level of arousal and to the observation of the environment. The behaviour of paranoid patients turned out to resemble more the behaviour of normal individuals, whereas the non-paranoid schizophrenic patients show signs of greater disorders in the control of the level of arousal and narrowness of the field of observation (possibly based on autism interpretable as defensive).

On the basis of our own findings, both the background variables and the clinical features of the patients with paranoid disintegration differ clearly from the corresponding parameters of the regressively disintegrated patients, who make up a major portion of the other patients classified as typically schizophrenic in our series. The clinical features of the regressively disintegrated patients suggest clearly greater severity, which is compatible with the definitely more serious prepsychotic disturbance of their personality development. But particularly as regards the opportunities of giving psychotherapy, the difference is reversed by the clearly poorer motivation of the paranoid patients to attend therapy, which is also reflected by the reserved and distrustful attitudes towards the investigator in the interviews. Although autistic patients were more numerous in the group of regressive disintegration than in the group of paranoid disintegration, the former group also included more patients with a tendency to symbiotic reliance. Insightfulness was also very clearly poorer in the group of paranoid disintegration than in the group of regressive disintegration. This is doubtless associated with the projective defensive system of the paranoid patients, which serves to place the problems outside their own selves.

Some investigators (e.g. Pulkkinen 1982, comparing the clinical picture and prognosis of paranoid and non-paranoid schizophrenic patients) have concluded that paranoid schizophrenia might be a completely different disease from the other forms of schizophrenia. We find it difficult to agree with this notion. Instead, we wish to emphasize the differences between the four ego-dynamic groups found among the schizophrenic psychoses. This also means that the therapy must be planned differently for these groups. As regards the psychodynamically most essential background variables, this grouping appeared clearly more relevant than the diagnostic categorization based on classical clinical features only.

5 Implementation of Therapies and Factors Influencing It

In this chapter, we will *describe our therapeutic activities* and examine *how widely the different treatment modes could be implemented during the study.*

Even before launching our project, we were aware that the greatest obstacle in the implementation of our psychotherapeutic principles was the excessive hospital-centred orientation of our treatment system. One of our goals at the time of introducing the present project was to promote the orientation towards out-patient care. This was not quite easy. There still was no staff appointed to out-patient therapy in the Clinic of Psychiatry. This shortcoming had been compensated for by the arrangement that the residents specializing as psychiatrists and several other members of the ward staff continued to meet some of the patients treated in hospital after their discharge. Since the beginning of our project on April 1, 1976, until March 31, 1980, these after-care activities were assisted by the specialized nurse of the team, who also participated in the therapeutic work. It was hoped that the after-care activity should be especially directed at patients, who had during the hospital treatment formed a long-term psychotherapeutic relationship breaking of which would have been injurious to the patient.

At the same time, we endeavoured to promote cooperation with the main open care unit of our community psychiatric system, the *Mental Health Office* of Turku. This included mutual therapeutic plan meetings and supervision activities described in Chapter 3.2.3. The same also applies to the psychiatric outpatient clinic of the University Central Hospital of Turku, which was not, however, responsible for treating chronic psychotic patients and which therefore played a relatively minor role in our therapeutic activities.

The scant quantitative resources of out-patient care were increased even through cooperation with the *private sector.* The private psychiatric work in Turku is relatively closely related to the public psychiatric health care through e.g. training and supervision activities. Both the Clinic of Psychiatry and, to a lesser extent, the Mental Health Office and the psychiatric out-patient clinic of the Turku University Central Hospital recommend some patients in need of more complex psychotherapeutic treatment for further treatment by private psychiatrists or psychologists. A further special addition to the overall picture of psychiatric activities in Turku in the private sector – though receiving some support from the town Turku – is the small Toivola out-patient psychotherapy clinic, which was set up by a private foundation, and which closely cooperates with the Clinic of Psychiatry both functionally and administratively.

The *two hospitals* of the mental health district (cf. 1.2.) developed no cooperation in the psychotherapeutic activities, the reason for this being their different therapeutic orientations. Even so, the cooperative relationship was moderately good at the time of the basic study of the patients. Difficulties were later increased especially in connection with transfers of the patients from one hospital to another. The psychosis ward of the

Clinic of Psychiatry had fewer male staff and violent behaviour of a patient could not be controlled as well as in the Kupittaa Hospital. If a patient was transferred from the Clinic of Psychiatry to Kupittaa Hospital in the midst of the treatment, this always involved a discontinuation of the therapeutic relation established in the Clinic, for reasons that could not be influenced by the team. Such happened in the case of a few male patients.

The practical implementation of the therapeutic activities was affected by several factors.

Even the units where the team members themselves worked and had central administrative positions did not always put in practice the plans drawn up by us. Contributing to this was the tradition which had emerged on the wards of the Clinic of Psychiatry and which afforded the spontaneity of the therapeutic staff and the patients an important position in the selection of more long-term therapeutic relationships. Our experiences had indicated that this was the best procedure to use the available resources so as to ensure a successful implementation and outcome of the therapeutic relationships, although the administrators and the supervising personnel were to prevent the designing of plans with unrealistic goals (cf. Alanen 1975, Aaku et al. 1980).

Various patient-specific background variables were included in this process of selection in a multifarious manner. As far as we can see, this is what generally takes place in the treatment of schizophrenic patients. *One of the objectives of this chapter is, consequently, to analyze the patient-specific background variables influencing the selection of patients for different modes of therapy* and to discuss the possibilities of extending the therapeutic activities to apply even to the patients now excluded.

During the course of this work, we found out quite concretely that anybody responsible for designing therapeutic plans for schizophrenic patients should *avoid strict formality* and be prepared to *re-assess the plans when the need may be.* The lives of several patients involved changes that had to be taken into account as possible causes for revising the therapeutic plans. This was not always done, however: the therapy occasionally continued parallel to the old routine and got into a standstill. There were also patients and/or families whose motivation for therapy was not at first successful, but who became more and more motivated as the time elapsed. The psychotherapeutic treatment of some of these patients was only started after the two-year follow-up.

5.1 Use of In-Patient and Out-Patient Treatment

5.1.1 In-Patient Treatment

74 of our 100 patients were included in the series as hospital in-patients, most of them, i.e. 66, being either emergency cases or otherwise in need of urgent help. There were additionally 4 patients admitted as out-patients, who were recommended by the out-patient units for hospital therapy almost immediately, in a couple of cases after an unsuccessful attempt at intervention in a crisis. 5 other patients whose therapy was started on an out-patient basis were admitted into hospital during the first follow-up year. The same was true of 2 patients included through day hospital. During the latter follow-up period, 3 patients included as out-patients were first admitted into hospital.

Our series thus contained altogether 12 patients who were not admitted into a psychiatric in-patient ward at any stage of their illness. Three of these patients were in day hospital, while the remaining 9 continued to be actual out-patients throughout the study period. Four of these 9 and two of the day hospital patients were classified as typical schizophrenics. Of the 31 patients in the group of regressive disintegration, 10 began as out-patients, but, with the exception of one, all these patients were admitted into hospital at some stage, and even the remaining one was admitted into day hospital treatment. More urgently than the others, this group of patients had a need for the support provided by the psychotherapeutic community of the ward.

The day hospital ward available for our use was connected to one in-patient ward of the Clinic of Psychiatry, in addition to which the other wards of the clinic were also able to admit a couple of patients for day care. Five patients were initially included in the series from the day hospital, and the day hospital services were used in altogether 24 cases, mostly as a continuation for in-patient therapy.

5.1.1.1 The Length and Number of the In-Patient Periods

A case-specific overall view of the use of in-patient and day hospital services is provided by the following tables. All of them refer to the 5-year follow-up period.

Table 27 pertains to the total series, table 28 to the patients diagnosed as typical schizophrenics.

The average duration of the first hospitalization as an inpatient was 63.23 days for the 85 patients admitted into hospital during their first year of treatment, while the *corresponding figure for the typical schizophrenic patients was 72.68 days.* The figures are relatively high compared with the tendency towards shorter hospital treatments, which has gained ground even in Finland. A follow-up study made in Helsinki indicated that the duration of the first hospitalization of new schizophrenic patients was 148 days in 1960, 72 days in 1965, and only 38 days in 1970 (Niskanen et al. 1973). In the series of

Table 27. In-patient and day hospital treatments during the follow-up. Total series

Days of treatment	Number of patients			
	first in-patient admissions	follow-up in-patient admissions, total	follow-up day-hospital admissions, total	follow-up in-patient and day hospital admissions, total
0	12	12	76	9
1– 30	32	11	8	12
31– 90	38	24	8	23
91–180	13	18	4	17
181–365	5	18	3	17
366–730	—	13	1	17
731–	—	4	—	5
	100	100	100	100

Table 28. In-patient and day hospital treatments during the follow-up. Typical schizophrenic patients

Days of treatment	Number of patients			
	first in-patient admissions	follow-up in-patient admissions, total	follow-up day-hospital admissions, total	follow-up in-patient and day hospital admissions, total
0	6	6	43	4
1–30	17	3	3	3
31–90	22	11	4	11
91–180	7	10	3	10
181–365	4	12	2	10
366–730	—	10	1	13
731–	—	4	—	5

100 schizophrenic patients admitted into hospital in Turku during 1965 – 67, which was investigated by Salokangas (1977), the average duration of the first stay in hospital was also 38 days. The Clinic of Psychiatry did not yet exist at that time, and all of the hospital therapies were given in the Kupittaa Hospital, where also the "university wards" were situated.

The total duration of the hospital periods of the patients during the follow-up years remained relatively small. *The five-year average per patient was 193.16 days, being 265.02 days for the patients diagnosed as typical schizophrenics.* The corresponding figures for day hospital treatment were 27.32 days and 35.18 days. *Only 4 patients had been in hospital for altogether more than 2 years.* Three of them were males and one female. If we take into account even the day hospital patients, the figure goes up to 5, and another female patient is included. All these patients were suffering from typical schizophrenia.

Table 29 shows the annual number of days spent in hospital in the series and the average number of patients per day in hospital during each follow-up year.

We can see that the *need for hospital treatment levels off after the first year, so that the differences between the years from the 2nd to the 5th are small.* From the 3rd year onwards, *the focus of hospital treatment is very clearly on the group of typical schizophrenias.*

Table 29. Annual distribution of the hospital treatment during the follow-up period. The figures in parentheses refer to the group of typical schizophrenias

Follow-up year since admission	Number of days in hospital	Number of patients in hospital per day on an average
1st year	7529 (4678)	20.6 (12.8)
2nd year	2932 (1943)	8.0 (5.3)
3rd year	3145 (2922)	8.6 (8.0)
4th year	2603 (2562)	7.1 (7.0)
5th year	3107 (2736)	8.5 (7.5)

Table 29 also shows that *an average of 7–9 patients per day were in hospital during the 2nd–5th follow-up years.*

The use of day hospital simultaneously decreased to reach a minimum at the latest stages of the follow-up. The total duration of day hospital treatments in our series was 1610 days during the 1st follow-up year, 698 days during the 2nd year, 58 during the 3rd year, 184 days during the 4th year and 61 days during the 5th year. It should be pointed out here that the day hospital treatment was calculated similarly to conventional in-patient therapy, also including the weekends, when the patients were not on the ward.

At the end of the follow-up period, 8 patients were in hospital and none were in day hospital. Only *2 patients could be regarded as chronic hospital inmates,* and even of these 2 only one had been in hospital without interruption for the last follow-up year. *About one fourth of the patients, however, were at least once in hospital for shorter periods anually during the latter follow-up period.*

The graphic diagrams include the average duration of hospital therapy per patient required by the total series and the diagnostic categories as well as the ego dynamic groups each follow-up year (Figures 2 and 3).

The figures for the 1st year was calculated on the basis of the data on all the 100 patients, while the figures for the following years exclude the patients dead by then, and the figures for the 3rd- 5th years further exclude the 2 patients for whom follow-up data could not be obtained. The number of patients is hence 98 on the 2nd follow-up year and 95 on the next three years.

The figures show quite unambiguously that the hospital treatments needed by the whole series decreased after the 1st follow-up year, but remained roughly the same level throughout the 2nd–5th years, being around 30 days per patient. The *group of typical schizophrenic patients clearly differed from the other groups during the follow-up.*

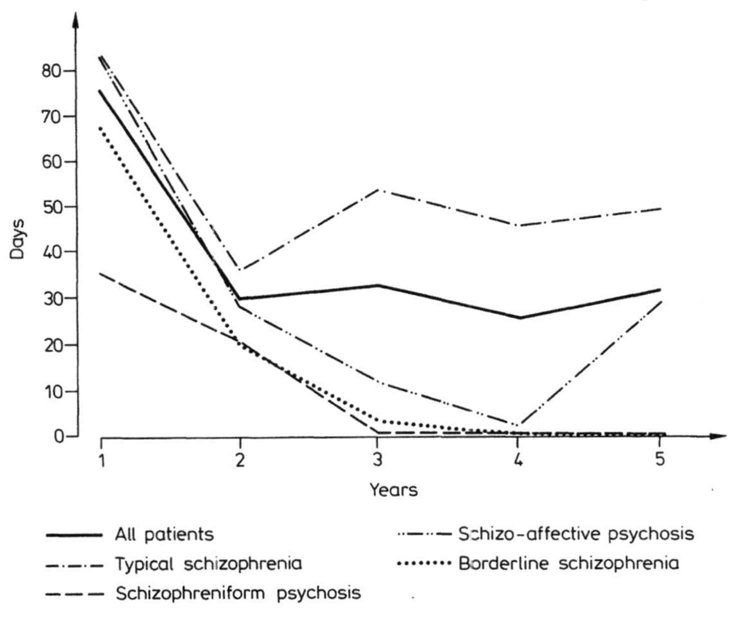

Fig. 2. In-patient days on the average per year in the different diagnostic groups

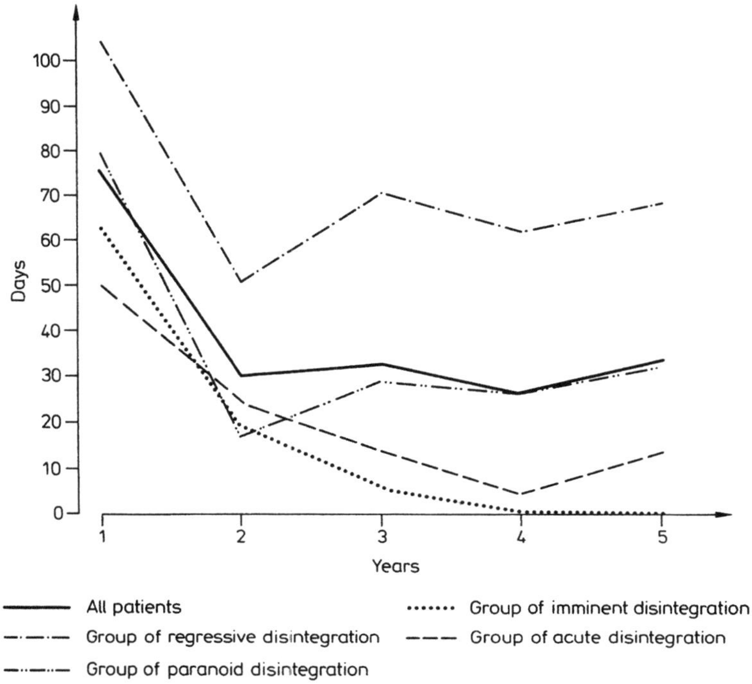

Fig. 3. In-patient days on the average per year in the different ego-dynamic groups

The results on the ego-dynamic groups indicate that *the focus of hospital treatment takes an increasingly firm position in the group of regressive disintegration. But the other groups also differ from each other during the follow-up period:* the need for hospital treatment is second greatest in the group of paranoid disintegration, and some need for hospital treatment is also seen in the group of acute disintegration during the last few follow-up years, while this need disappears almost completely in the group of imminent disintegration.

The number of in-patient admissions of the patients during the follow-up period are presented in Table 30. *32 patients had only been in hospital once and 21 patients twice.* When we include in this group the 12 patients who had not been hospitalized at all, we can see that *about two thirds of the patients had had two or fewer hospital admissions. Six patients, however, had been in hospital 10 or more times during the 5 years.* All these patients belonged to the group of typical schizophrenias. This diagnostic sub-category differed clearly from the other sub-categories as to the number of hospital admissions. However, even this group included more than 50 percent of patients, who had had two hospital admissions at the most and 6 patients with no hospital admissions at all.

Among the ego-dynamic groups, the groups of regressive disintegration (average number 4.10) and paranoid disintegration (average number 3.65) differed clearly from the other two groups, which were close to each other (acute disintegration 2.07, imminent disintegration 1.52). When we remember that the duration of annual hospital treatments in days was clearly longer in the group of regressive disintegration than in

Table 30. Number of hospitalizations of the patients during the follow-up period classified according to the diagnostic sub-categories

Number of hospitalizations	Diagnostic category				
	Typical schizophrenia	Schizophreni-form psychosis	Schizoaffec-tivepsychosis	Borderline schizophrenia	Patients total
0	6	1	1	4	12
1	16	2	5	9	32
2	8	5	3	5	21
3	3	1	2	–	6
4	4	–	3	1	8
5	4	1	–	1	5
6	3	–	–	–	3
7	2	–	–	–	4
8	2	–	–	–	2
9	–	–	–	1	1
10	3	–	–	–	3
11	2	–	–	–	2
18	1	–	–	–	1
Average	3.73	2.00	2.07	1.60	

the group of paranoid disintegration, we can conclude that many patients in the latter group characteristically had repeated, but short hospital treatments, while the in-patient periods in the group of regressive disintegration were longer.

Men had clearly higher number of hospitalizations than women: an average of 3.65 compared with the female average of 2.08 ($p < .01$). Ten or more hospitalizations during the follow-up period were recorded for 5 males and only one female. The annual average of hospital treatments in days during the follow-up period was also greater among the men than among the women, being 50.37 days compared with the 33.26 days of the women. *None of those hospitalized 10 times or more often belonged to the group of psychotherapy cases* (cf. Chapter 5.2.6.).

5.1.1.2 Did a Longer First Hospital Period Lessen the Need for Later Hospital Treatments?

The relatively long average duration of the first period of hospital treatment depended particularly on the therapeutic practice of The Clinic of Psychiatry, whereby the duration of the in-patient therapy of new patients was planned on the basis of the case-specific needs. The patients who were in a poorer clinical condition and were less well motivated to therapy needed, in our opinion, a longer time to establish a therapeutic contact, and their stay in the hospital was occasionally prolonged considerably for this reason. Different factors of the patient's life conditions also contributed to this. *The first in-patient therapies clearly took a longer time in the Clinic of Psychiatry than in the Kupittaa Hospital.* The average duration of the first hospitalization was 73.44 days in the former hospital and 27.0 in the latter ($p < .001$).

We illustrate the therapeutic practices with two examples, which represent the two extremes. The total duration of the first inpatient therapy and the day hospital therapy following it in the case of the first of these patients was the longest in the whole series, while the corresponding time in the case of the latter patients was the shortest in the series.

K, a 29-year-old married trained worker consulted the Mental Health Office because of psychotic disintegration, auditory hallucinations and autism, which had developed over the past few months. For the past couple of years, he had only had temporary jobs, the family – where a second child had been born recently – was poorly off financially, and the patient's self-esteem was very badly depressed. Regressive psychotic disintegration involved omnipotent religious delusions.

The family situtation was characterized, first of all, by mutual helplessness. The wife was 6 years younger than K, frustrated by her husband's illness and the poor life conditions, trying to manage one day at a time without "thinking too much about it".

As the patient's condition persisted unchanged, he was referred for in-patient therapy in the Clinic of Psychiatry 3 months after his first visit at the Mental Health Office. He remained there as an in-patient for 240 days and thereafter in the day hospital for 323 days. The autistic condition soon gave way to a childishly symbiotic and openly trustful attitude towards the ward staff. Even so, K remained disintegrated for a long time, experiencing "continuous dreams".

During the patient's stay in hospital and day hospital, he and his family were supported in various ways; they were, for example, assisted in getting a new dwelling. The day hospital treatment was prolonged, because the wife continued to feel that K's being at home was difficult – K was the "third child" of the family.

After-care sessions at relatively long intervals took place in the out-patient care of the Clinic of Psychiatry. More than a year after his discharge from the day hospital, K was re-admitted into hospital, because he had "got a fit of rage at home". He continued to have delusions. He was only re-admitted for a week, but was admitted again 2 months later, this time for more than a month. At that time the chief ward nurse started couple therapy of K and his wife, which was continued within the out-patient system for altogether 30 sessions.

At the time of the 5-year follow-up, K was at home and practically free from psychotic symptoms, but on a disability pension. His wife goes to work. K has become a "house father" who spends much of his time with his children and works on his toy inventions. He attends a pensioner's club regularly. The couple therapy has been discontinued. K visits the Mental Health Office at two month's intervals, receiving low-dose neuroleptic treatment. He says the past year has been the "best since the beginning of his illness", because he has been on better terms with his wife than before.

The first two in-patient periods of N, also a married 38-year-old trained worker, in the Kupittaa Hospital only lasted for 1 and 2 days. He had had paranoid symptoms for at least 3 years previously, which had made him get another job. The symptoms were, however, mostly manifestly expressed only after alcohol intake, being intense and aggressive paranoid outbursts. The first hospitalization took place at his wife's initiative after one of these outbursts. N spoke of eavesdropping at home and at work, shadowing in the streets, and SS men and Nazis breaking up his marriage, etc. He was, however, discharged the following day, because he tried to pull himself together and deny his symptoms, expressing his intense reluctance towards compulsory treatment. The brief re-admission a couple of months later followed the same pattern.

The specialized nurse of the team met N's wife, who told her of her difficulties, crying. The marital relationship had greatly deteriorated along with N's illness. After this, Mrs. N. occasionally contacted the specialized nurse, either visiting her or talking to her on the phone. N refused the help offered to him.

Prior to the last follow-up year, the hospitalizations of N were restricted to these two instances 3 days in total duration. During the 5th year he was re-admitted for treatment that now lasted for nearly 7 months, again in the Kupittaa Hospital. His marriage had ended up in a divorce situation, while N's condition had been aggravated so much that he was no longer able to work. He also had suicidal thoughts. During the re-hospitalization, the patient was given support to help him towards independent life. Nevertheless, the delusional system persisted, being even more massive than before.

At the time of the 5-year follow-up study, N is on a provisional disability pension. He has high-dose neuroleptic medication, which causes slight trembling and mimic poverty. He consults regularly, though at relatively long intervals, the psychiatrist last in charge of him in hospital. He lives alone; the closest "supporter" is still his divorced wife, who comes to see her husband a couple of times a week.

These cases illustrate our notion of the significance of planning that takes into account the case-specific needs of the in-patient therapy of schizophrenic patients in a flexible and versatile manner. Quite obviously, the first hospital and day hospital period of the patient K could have been shorter, if the family-oriented therapy had been undertaken right from the beginning more actively than was the case. Still, we classified K as a patient whose therapy had been well accordant with the case-specific needs (cf. Chapter 7.1.). In the case of N, on the other hand, we can say that the too short hospital therapy, in fact, signified a neglect of treatment at a time when it would have been necessary.

Our hope in the Clinic of Psychiatry was that somewhat longer periods of hospital treatment at the beginning of the patient's treatment would result in a lesser need for hospital treatment in the later years. Is it possible to make conclusions on the basis of the different therapeutic practices of these two hospitals by analyzing the quantities of the patient's later hospital treatments? Any such comparison is somewhat affected by the other factors pertaining to the selection of the first therapeutic unit. Despite the attempts of the hospitals to take care of their "own" patients even at the later stages, the series also includes several patients treated in both hospitals during the follow-up period. We will examine the possible effects of these factors.

The comparison of the correlations of the clinical and psychosocial background variables with the group of patients first treated as in-patients of the Clinic of Psychiatry and, respectively, with those first treated as in-patients of the Kupittaa Hospital indicated that the Clinic of Psychiatry was a more usual treatment unit for female patients, the Kupittaa Hospital for male patients ($p = .003$). More borderline schizophrenics were admitted to the Clinic of Psychiatry ($p = .006$), more schizophreniform psychoses ($p = .013$) and generally patients with shorter duration of psychotic symptoms ($p = .001$) to the Kupittaa Hospital. The Kupittaa patients had more often alcohol problems ($p = .037$) and a reluctant attitude to treatment ($p = .076$). Also admission with judicial sanctions was more common in this hospital (which partly depended on the policy adopted by the hospital administration). Among those admitted to the Clinic of Psychiatry were more patients with earlier psychiatric treatments ($p = .057$), and also the initial insight ability was slightly better in this patient group ($p = .097$).

On the other hand, there was practically no difference between the share of typically schizophrenic patients (the Clinic had 30 such patients, the Kupittaa Hospital 15). The relative amount of regressively disintegrated patients, distinguished by their need for longer hospital treatments, was exactly the same in both hospitals. There also were no differences approaching any statistical significance regarding the social classes of the patients or their primary families, and the same applied to the patients' educational level.

The over-representation of schizophreniform psychoses as well as of the patients with psychotic symptoms of short duration may give rise to the expectation that the need for later hospital treatments could be smaller among the patients whose first therapeutic unit was the Kupittaa Hospital. On the other hand, the amount of borderline schizophrenias was greater among the Clinic of Psychiatry patients. The amount of the most severely ill patients was, however, the same in both samples, so that from a clinical point of view a prognostic comparison between them seems appropriate. Some other background variables (a greater amount of men, the alcohol problems) would possibly emphasize a slightly worse prognostic prediction for the Kupittaa series.

Concerning the *changes in the treatment units* during the later hospitalizations, we found that 6 of the patients who were first treated in the Clinic had later treatments in the Kupittaa Hospital. Of the patients first treated in the Kupittaa, 9 had later hospital treatments in the Clinic of Psychiatry. These figures reflect a moderate degree of "mixing" of the different therapeutic orientations over the follow-up period. Because the number of the patients first treated in the Clinic was clearly greater than in the Kupittaa, the numbers indicate that the patients first treated in the customary way had more often later treatments in the psychotherapeutically oriented hospital than the other way around. This fact may for its part decrease the possibly worse prognostic prediction of the patients first treated in a customary way.

We conclude that *the comparison between the two orientations regarding the subsequent need of the patients for hospital treatment seems to bear certain meaningfulness* despite the selective factors dealt with above.

Figure 4 shows the hospital days of the patients during the follow-up period in such a way that the patients have been divided into groups on the basis of their first therapeutic unit, and the average duration of hospital treatment per follow-up year has been calculated for the patients of each group.

The figure shows that the difference between the two hospitals in the duration of the first period of hospital treatment already begins to decrease when we sum up the in-patient periods of the first follow-up year. Still, there is a statistically significant difference ($p = .021$) for the benefit of the Kupittaa Hospital patients' shorter amount of hospital days. *From the second follow-up year onwards, however, the average for the patients initially treated in the Clinic of Psychiatry is smaller than the corresponding figure for the Kupittaa Hospital.* The difference of the third year is statistically

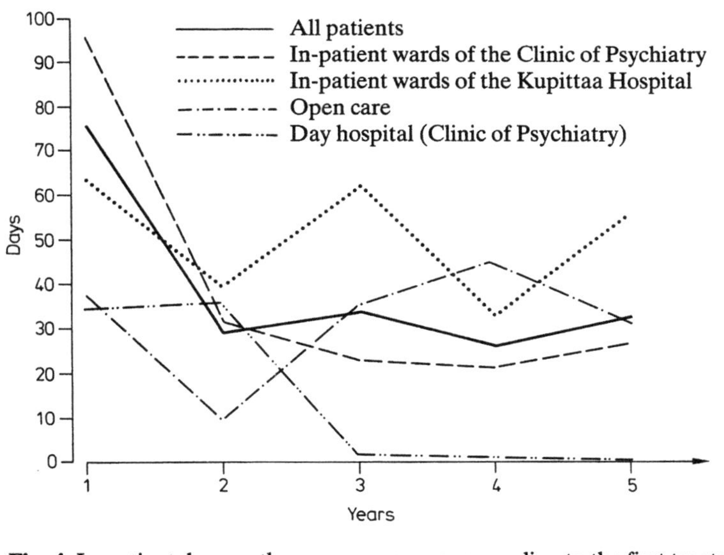

Fig. 4. In-patient days on the average per year according to the first treatment unit

significant (p = .026), and the last follow-up year also confirms the assumption of the lesser subsequent need for hospital treatment among the patients initially treated in the Clinic of Psychiatry at a marginally significant level. The mean annual duration of hospital treatment during the entire follow-up period is 44.46 days for the patients of the Clinic of Psychiatry and 50.08 days for the patients of the Kupittaa Hospital. There is no statistical difference between these figures. There was however, an almost significant difference between the average numbers of hospitalizations required by the patients during the follow-up period, which was 2.83 for the patients initially admitted into the Clinic of Psychiatry and 4.42 (p = .042) for the patients initially admitted into the Kupittaa Hospital.

The assumption that the initial need for longer hospital treatments posed by the psychotherapeutic orientation – compared with the therapeutic orientation relying more heavily on pharmacotherapy and aiming at rapid discharge of the patients – is *compensated for by the lesser need for in-patient treatment over the later years is hence given preliminary support by the present analysis.* Parallel to this is the observation that even the average hospital treatments of the patients initially treated on an outpatient basis increased during the last three follow-up years so as to exceed slightly the corresponding figure for the patients initially admitted as in-patients into the Clinic of Psychiatry. The need for full-time hospital therapy in the initial group of 5 day-hospital patients, on the other hand, disappeared completely during last few follow-up years.

We will return to these questions in Chapter 6.5.

5.1.2 Out-Patient Care

The patients in our series used the out-patient services quite intensively. Although only 21 of our patients were admitted into the study series via an out-patient unit, *merely 7 out*

Table 31. The distribution of the out-patient treatments

Unit	The number of patients	Per cent of the treatments
Turku Mental Health Office	41	28
Out-patient services of the Clinic of Psychiatry	47	35 (47 + 4)
Out-patient services of the Kupittaa Hospital	4	
Psychiatric Out-patient Dept. of the Turku Univ. Central Hospital	16	11
A-clinic of Turku[a]	2	2 (2 + 1)
and its adolescent unit	1	
Mental health offices outside the study area	8	6 (8 + 1)
Out-patient services in other hospitals	1	
Toivola Clinic (sponsored by a private foundation)	7	18 (7 + 19)
Private psychiatrists	19	

[a] An outpatient clinic for alcoholics.

of 100 made no out-patient visits even later on. Six of these 7 had been recommended in the hospital to visit an out-patient unit after discharge. The seventh patient without out-patient therapy was imprisoned upon discharge from hospital and later transferred into criminal-psychiatric hospital. There were 10 other patients whose out-patient periods only comprised of a couple of visits.

Many of the patients in our series were given treatment at more than one out-patient units. *The out-patient treatment of the 93 patients were distributed between the different units as indicated in Table 31.*

The figures do not include the visits made by the relatives separately from the patients for therapeutic purposes.

The numbers of patients indicate that *the Turku Mental Health Office and the Clinic of Psychiatry together were responsible for a majority of the out-patient therapies.* The category of private psychiatrists, together with the Toivola Clinic, constituted the third focal area of out-patient care.

As regards the four most central units, the data on the implementation of psychotherapies (cf. the criteria on p. 93) are shown in the Table 32. The out-patient services of the Clinic of Psychiatry and the Kupittaa Hospital have been combined, as have also been the private psychiatrists and the Toivola Clinic, which represent the private sector.

The mental health office had 2 patients who were given both individual and family therapy, while 4 such patients were treated by the out-patient services of the hospitals. The therapeutic relationships of 8 patients were transferred from the public sector to be continued by the same psychiatrist or psychologist as private consultations or to be carried out in the Toivola Clinic.

The table indicates that the private sector was responsible for a greater number of intensive individual therapies than less intensive ones, while the Mental Health Office and the outpatient services of the hospitals included a slightly higher number of less intensive individual therapies than intensive ones. Even so, the number of intensive individual therapies in each of these two units was of the same order as in the private sector. Most of the family therapies were carried out as outpatient therapies of the Clinic of Psychiatry, but some of them were also implemented by the Mental Health Office and the private sector.

Therapeutic visits which did not include regular psychotherapy were most frequent in the out-patient department of the Turku University Central Hospital. The Mental Health Office also had a relatively great number of patients of this kind, but slightly more than half of our patients who were clients of the Mental Health Office were given regular psychotherapy.

Table 32. Implementation of psychotherapies in the most central therapeutic units

Mode of psychotherapy	Turku MHO	Out-patient services of hospitals	TUCH psych. out-pat. dept.	Private sector
Intensive individual therapy	8	10	—	10
Less intensive individual therapy	11	15	2	5
Family therapies	5	13	—	5
Group therapies	1	1	—	—
No actual psychotherapy	18	15	14	4

The features characterizing the patients of these different units differed from each other with regard to some important background variables. Thus the *Mental Health Office* accumulated more male patients compared with women ($p = .021$ as compared with the total series). A lower-than-average social group of the parents also emerged as remarkable ($p < .01$), while the patient's own social group, their education and the factors associated with their social role lack statistical significance.

Two thirds of *the out-patient activities of hospitals* consisted of continuation of the therapeutic relationships established on the in-patient wards, one third of the therapeutic relationships established by the specialized nurse of our team. There was a tendency to select patients with whom it was easy to set up a therapeutic relationship: patients with a favourable attitude towards therapy, patients who had a better than average insight into their problems and those with interpersonal relationships outside their primary families. In this group female patients were overrepresented compared with men (all these variables, $p < .05$). This group also included a clearly higher-than-average number of patients in the youngest age-group and lack of occupational identity also comes close to statistical significance. However, the selection was not much influenced by the diagnostic background variables. The only exception to this was the group of schizophreniform psychoses, which only included one patient who had been given out-patient therapy in the hospitals.

The *private sector* included clearly more patients from the higher social groups, with regard to the social status of both the patients and their parents (both, $p < .01$). Education, on the other hand, was of lesser significance. It also seems quite understandable that these patients include a higher-than-average proportion of ones who have been given treatment even previously; a certain proportion of the earlier treatments were also given by private psychiatrists. Another selective factor arises from the relatively mild disturbance of the patients: the group of borderline schizophrenias is slightly overrepresented ($p < .10$), and only a few patients had been admitted on the basis of judicial sanctions. The favourable attitude towards therapy and the lack of overtly violent behaviour were also prominent features, associated with a general avoidance of aggressions in this group ($p < .05$). A somewhat astonishing feature was the overrepresentation of unmarried patients.

The group of typical schizophrenias did not reach the level of statistical significance as a selective factor in any of the aforesaid areas of out-patient activities. The patients of this group were slightly more numerous than the average in both the Mental Health Office (26) and the out-patient activities of the hospitals (29), while in the private sector their number was slightly below the average, though still quite notable (11). The representation of the group of regressively disintegrated patients was more or less equal in the three units, being similar to the percentage of these patients out of the total series.

This analysis was unable to illustrate the out-patient activities of the Clinic of Psychiatry in the way that was expected by the team. It seems that, although the therapy of the most seriously disturbed patients was not actually avoided, the therapeutic relationships established in the hospital clearly focussed on the group of patients selected for their favourable characteristics with regard to therapy. This is probably associated with the tendency to favour spontaneity in the creation of therapeutic relationships that was mentioned above. As the out-patient activities are carried out along with the hard work on the in-patient wards at least partly voluntarily

Table 33. Occupational groups of the therapist responsible for psychotherapeutic activities in the most central therapeutic units

Occupational group of therapist	Turku MHO	Hospital out-patient units	TUCH psych. out-pat. unit	Private sector	Other
Specialized psychiatrist	7	5	1	7	
Other physician	–	9	1	8	
Psychologist	4	2	–	5	1
Specialized nurse	13	18	–	–	1
Other nurse	–	1	–	–	
Mental nurse	–	2	–	–	1
Social worker	5	–	1	–	1

(particularly as regards the nurses and mental nurses on the wards), this selection is quite understandable. Nevertheless, it would be more recommendable that the therapeutic relationships to be continued after the in-patient period should focus on the patients who are more difficult to reach therapeutically and less well able to make contacts, and whose capacity and willingness to establish a long-term therapeutic relationship on an out-patient basis is inadequate.

Table 33 shows the *occupational groups* of the therapists who carried out the regular psychotherapies in the most central out-patient units.

"Other physician" always refers to residents specializing in psychiatry, many of whom – similarly to the specialized psychiatrists and psychologists – also had private consultation hours. The mental health office carried out 2 family therapies on home visits, with a specialized psychiatrist and a specialized nurse together acting as therapists.

The greatest difference between the different units was the lack of nursing staff and social workers in the private sector – they had no opportunity for private practice. The role of specialized nurses is particularly conspicuous in both the mental office and the out-patient units of the hospitals.

5.2 Implementation of Psychotherapeutic Treatments

We will next consider the *number of different psychotherapies given in the series during the follow-up period, the therapeutic principles represented by these treatments, and the kind of patients treated in this way.* A logistic regression analysis (cf. 3.3.) was applied to clarify the explaining clinical or psychosocial variables influencing the selection of the patients to the most important modes of therapy. The variables are the same as described in Appendix 1. The statistical connections between these background variables and the most important treatment modes (the treatment variables, Appendix 3) are presented in Appendix 5 (the whole patient series) and in Appendix 6 (the group of typical schizophrenia).

The data on the duration of the therapies and the number of visits made were mostly obtained from the questionnaires which – on the basis of information collected from the epicrises, the patients themselves and their family members – were mailed to the

Table 34. Compatibility between the therapeutic plans made at the basic examination and the therapies given during the first two follow-up years as regards the most central modes of psychotherapy

Mode of therapy	Number of patients planned implemented	planned not implemented	not planned implemented	K
Treatment in psychotherapeutic community	49	14	4	0.63
Couple therapy	12	12	0	0.56
Joint therapy of primary family	6	10	2	0.44
Initial intervention in crisis	15	11	13	0.39
"Intensive individual therapy"[a]	15	11	18	0.31

[a] continued with sessions once a week or more frequently for at least 6 months

therapists in charge of the treatment of the patients at the time of the two-year and five-year follow-up.

In the case of both individual therapies, family therapies and group therapies, it was required that they were not restricted exclusively to the period of hospital therapy, but were carried out on an out-patient basis. The therapeutic relationships *restricted* to the in-patient period were classified as part of the treatment in a psychotherapeutic community. This applies to the "personal nurse relationships", the groups working on the ward, and the family meetings taking place during the patient's in-patient period.

Some findings concerning the psychotherapeutic activities and their effects on the basis of our 2-year follow-up have been published previously (Alanen et al. 1982, 1983) and they are not repeated here. It is, however, interesting to try to find out the *patient-specific agreement between the psychotherapeutic treatments given during the two-year follow-up period and the therapies indicated in the original therapeutic plans.*

The data on this are presented in Table 34. The compatibility between treatments planned and given has been measured with the Kappa (K) coefficient, and the therapeutic modes have been set in order according to the degree of compatibility.

The implementation of therapy is best accordant with the plans in the cases of community treatment. The family therapies carried out were mostly also compatible with the plans, but most of the therapies planned for failed to be carried out. As regards the initial intervention in crisis and the intensive individual therapies, the number of therapies given was accordant with the plans. The number of intensive individual therapies even clearly exceeded the plans – but only about half of the therapies given were compatible with the original indications. The finding clearly reflects the independence of the therapeutic units in carrying out the therapies as well as the fact that the selective processes were also influenced by factors other than those taken into account in determining the plans.

For this monograph, the *data on the psychotherapeutic modes of treatment* applied during the course of the project were compiled into *summaries covering the entire 5-year follow-up period.* The findings presented in Table 35 were obtained.

Table 35. Quantitative implementation of the psychotherapeutic modes of treatment during the five follow-up years

Mode of therapy	Number of patients	
Initial intervention in crisis	26	26
Intensive individual therapy	26	57
Less intensive individual therapy	31	
Intensive family therapy	15	25
Less intensive family therapy	10	
Supportive contact with family member(s)		40
Intensive group therapy	1	2
Less intensive group therapy	1	
Intensive treatment in psychotherapeutic community	25	56
Less intensive treatment in psychotherapeutic community	18	
Intervention in crisis in psychotherapeutic community	21	

The *criteria for the different therapies* were defined as follows:

Initial intervention in crisis = help provided in a psychotic crisis by means of rapidly initiated and frequent, individual or family- and environment-oriented therapeutic visits on an out-patient basis or through brief hospitalization.

Intensive individual therapy = dyadic therapeutic relationship, duration of treatment at least 2 years, at least 80 sessions.

Less intensive individual therapy = dyadic therapeutic relationship, duration of treatment at least 6 months, at least 12 sessions.

Intensive family therapy = therapy given in joint family sessions, duration of treatment at least 6 months, at least 12 sessions.

Less intensive family therapy = therapy given in joint family sessions, at least 3 sessions.

Supportive contact with family member(s) = contact with the patient's family or one family member beyond the bounds of research, whose purpose is to support the family during the therapy of the patients. These contacts included both personal meetings and telephone contacts.

Intensive group therapy = a closed therapeutic group, duration of treatment at least 1 year, at least 24 sessions.

Less intensive group therapy = a closed therapeutic group, at least 6 sessions.

Intensive treatment in psychotherapeutic community = duration of treatment at least 3 months; the following points provided: a) personal nurse relationship, b) situational exploration of the family and the living milieu, and c) involvement of the patient in the group and community processes of the ward.

Less intensive community therapy = the treatment in the therapeutic community was not in all respects equally active as above, but did involve an empathic approach to the patient and his participation in the group and community functions.

Intervention in crisis in psychotherapeutic community = a shorter, more active community therapy in a situation of crisis, including exploration of and intervention in the patient's family and/or social environment.

The intensive and less intensive applications of one and the same mode of the therapy are mutually exclusive. This also applies to the community therapies, excluding the intervention in crisis in therapeutic community. In some cases such intervention was carried out during a hospitalization of a patient who was classified into the category of other community therapies on the basis of his other in-patient period.

Of the intensive *family therapies,* only 5 were joint therapies of the primary family. The other 10 intensive family therapies were carried out with secondary families in such a way that 7 remained purely couple therapies, while 3 therapies (including 2 given on home visits) were also attended by the patient's children. Of the less intensive family therapies, 6 were joint therapies of the primary family and 4 couple therapies.

Some of the patients given individual therapy were treated successively by 2 or more different therapists. These therapies have been combined for the determination of the individual therapy group of the patient. In the family and group therapies the therapist always remained the same.

Of the intensive individual therapies all but one were begun during the first two follow-up years. Likewise all but one of the therapies were continued during the last three follow-up years. Of the less intensive individual therapies 21 were restricted to the first two follow-up years, five had therapeutic sessions during both of the follow-up periods while five were only carried out during the last three years. Of the family therapies, 5 were extended over the two followup periods, while 15 were restricted to the former and 5 to the latter period.

As a conclusion, it can be stated that 51 of the 57 patients given individual therapy started their therapy during the first two follow-up years, while 6 did so after the first two years. The corresponding figures for family therapy were 20 and 5. *Although a majority of the therapies were thus commenced at an early stage, there are 11 regular psychotherapies that were only started more than 2 years after the first admission for treatment.*

5.2.1 Initial Intervention in Crisis

Of the *initial interventions in crisis,* 11 were carried out completely on an out-patient basis and 17 patients were hospitalized for a short period. The therapeutic plans had included 15 out-patient and 11 in-patient interventions. Some attempts to intervene in the crisis of an out-patient failed, and the patient soon ended up in hospital. The figures in table 35 indicate, however, that the patients were not always the same as those intended by the team.

The initial interventions in crisis carried out had a statistical connection with two background variables only: they were more often directed to married than unmarried or widowed and divorced patients ($p = .032$) and to patients who had an empathic relative at home ($p = .084$). Neither of these background variables emerged in the therapeutic plans. Of the background variables noted at that time, overtly violent behaviour, notable impulsive aggressiveness, a tendency to alcohol abuse or other addiction, and classification of the patient into the higher social groups had approached the level of marginal significance.

The therapeutic plans had also assumed that the interventions in crisis would be applied more often to men than to women. The tendency, however, turned out the opposite: the crises of 17 female patients and 11 male patients were intervened in. Intervention in crisis had no correlations with the diagnostic or the psychodynamic subgroups in either the plans or the practical therapies.

The findings can be interpreted in such a way that intervention in crisis at the early stages of the psychosis is clearly aided by the presence of empathic relatives, and that female patients, particularly married women, are easier to reach with this type of intervention at the early stages of the psychosis than males.

It might further be pointed out that the patient's general favourable attitude towards therapy – his willingness to accept all modes of therapy – correlated with crisis intervention at a nearly marginal level.

Intervention in crisis at the early stages of the psychosis remained the only phase of therapy for 5 of our patients. And even of these 5, two or three would have been recommended by our team to continue their treatment on a slightly more long-term basis.

Hence, for example, it turned out at the time of the five-year follow-up that Mr. B, a man who seemed to have managed well in his life and had not had any subsequent psychiatric treatments, still clearly seemed to cling to the delusional notions he had had of his wife during his brief schizophreniform psychosis. He had divorced and re-married, apparently a more satisfactory partner. He had obviously not had new delusions at any stage. Although such "encapsulated" remnant of psychosis probably also was significant for the patient's defences, it would have been a better alternative to work through the problems of the first marriage and the emotional conflicts caused by them, thereby getting rid of them.

Of the crisis intervention patients, 8 later received intensive individual therapy and 19 were classified as "psychotherapy cases". The figures provide good illustration for the team's experience showing that, apart from a few rare exceptions, psychosis must be treated on a more long-term basis than by merely giving the first aid. This does not mean that prompt intervention in crisis in a more intensive and a more family- and milieu-oriented manner than in our series could not significantly diminish the treatment required by several patients, and, first and foremost, the psychologic and social injuries incurred by them.

5.2.2 Individual Therapies

5.2.2.1 The Therapeutic Orientation

Our intensive individual therapies were mostly empathic and supportive long-term therapeutic relationships which, apart from giving support, also included a conscious attempt to increase the patient's insight into his own problems. Two of these therapies (and two of the less intensive individual therapies) were given by therapists who had received or were receiving a psychoanalytic training. Five intensive therapies and one less intensive one were carried out by a therapist who had received a shorter psychotherapeutic training, based on both psychodynamic and learning-theoretical frames of reference. In practice, most of these therapies were accordant with the psychodynamic frame of reference. A majority of the therapies were carried out by staff members who did not have a formal psychotherapeutic training, but were working in accordance with psychodynamically oriented on-the-job training and long-term therapy supervision.

The orientation of our individual therapies can hence be described as psychodynamic.

The epithets given by the therapists themselves confirmed this account. In their replies to the questionnaire, a large majority of the therapists described their individual therapies as being "psychodynamically oriented, supportive therapies". Seven intensive and one less intensive individual therapy were called by the therapists "analytically oriented, intensive therapies", while one intensive individual therapy was described as being based on a "behaviour-therapeutic frame of reference" (and consisting of "conventional out-patient therapy" at the later stages) and four less intensive individual therapies as "conventional out-patient therapies".

An idea of the therapeutic approach propounded in the on-the-job training and supervision in the Turku Clinic of Psychiatry can be obtained from the following description by Alanen:

1. The first task of the therapist is to create a favourable therapeutic relationship with the patient through an empathic, reliable and constant approach.
2. The therapeutic relationship is intensified by interest in the patient as a human being, i.e. his work, hobbies, etc., not merely his symptoms.
3. The healthy aspects of the patient are supported by acting as a "bridge to reality", which includes cautious interpretation of the patient's psychotic thinking towards more sense of reality.
4. The most central focus of the therapeutic communication must always be the analysis of the topical problems and causes of anxiety.
5. This is supplemented – as far as it is possible – by clarification of the connections between the patient's reactions and his human relations in childhood, yet keeping the focus on the contemporary problems.
6. It is good if the patient comes to realize during the course of the therapy that the criticism or feeling of hatred he may show towards the therapist does not risk the maintenance of the therapeutic relationship.
7. It is good if the therapist has been able, at the beginning of the therapy, to get acquainted and create a confidential relationship with the patient's family or other environment and is able, when necessary, to maintain a contact with it, the patient being aware.
8. The therapy is often supported by low-dose neuroleptic medication. If possible, the dosage should be determined in cooperation with the patient, taking into account his suggestions and experiences.
9. The frequency of visits can be increased at stages of crisis.
10. The therapy must be supervised by another therapist.

We illuminate our intensive individual therapies with the following case report. The therapist of the patient was the specialized nurse of our team, who was supervised by a psychiatrist undergoing psychoanalytic training. She describes the therapy thus:

Miss L. is a 25-year old, unmarried office-worker. She was admitted for her first psychiatric in-patient therapy directly from her working place. While in work, she had become absent-minded over the past few weeks, laughing to herself and unable to manage her work, which included service of clients. Particularly when serving male clients Miss L. lost her self-command, feeling that the men were trying to violate her sexually.

It turned out that a few months earlier a male trainee had been employed, with whom Miss L., sudden and regressively, "fell in love". She gradually began to feel that she was "married to this man before the eyes of God", and she began to hear him speaking almost everywhere. The man was merely embarrassed by the situation. The dynamics of the patient's symptoms included marked ambivalence, the counter poles consisting of religious imagery and sexuality.

Miss L. is the youngest of the 7 children of a farming family. Five of the children are living, all but one, the patient, being boys. The parents were relatively old when the patient was born as the "princess of the family". Miss L. has always felt herself to be in a special position as the only daughter of the family. At the beginning of her therapy she told of having always been worried over her old and sickly parents, also thinking that it is her responsibility to care for them when she grows up, as all but one of her brothers had their own families. According to her own statements, it suffices Miss L. that she "was of a family"; she had no male friends and did not dare to think of a marriage of her own even in the future.

Her relationship with her parents was symbiotic and, at the same time, highly contradictory. There was a particularly marked intensive dependence on the father. When the patient was a baby, her mother was very unhealthy, and (according to the mother herself) the baby was not cared for sufficiently. At the age of 2–3 years, the patient "discovered" her father, and the father still tries to take into account all her daughter's needs. Miss L. was also admired by her brothers, but her childhood was lonely, as she was 7 years junior to her youngest brother.

During the first three follow-up years, Miss L. was admitted into the Clinic of Psychiatry altogether 5 times. With the exception of the first in-patient period (167 days), the therapeutic periods were short, no more than 2–4 weeks in duration.[1] After the first in-patient period, the patient was arranged further therapy by a private psychiatrist, but her resistance towards the idea of acknowledging herself as ill was strong, and she discontinued her therapy during the first month. At the time of her second hospitalization about a year later, she consulted herself the specialized nurse she had met previously, wanting to arrange further sessions with her. What was probably significant in the matter, too, was that the specialized nurse had also met the patient's parents and some of her brothers (who had adopted an overprotective attitude similar to that of their parents).

The process of therapy lasted for about 4 years and consisted of 184 sessions. The therapist's opinion was that the therapy remained incomplete. The real male friend the patient met towards the end of the therapy became a new object of dependence for her, and she was reluctant to work through her therapeutic relationship in a satisfactory manner to the end. There remains an agreement that Miss L. can contact her therapist when necessary.

At first the therapeutic visits were relatively intensive (twice a week), while for about half of the time weekly sessions were held, and the frequency of the visits during the last year was even lower.

It was of great significance throughout the therapeutic relationship that the therapist met the patient's parents and brothers when necessary, maintained a contact with the employer and the hospital ward, and also arranged some conversations with the patient and her male friend at the time of crises in their dating relationship. All these contacts were discussed and agreed upon together with Miss L. The patient's sphere of life was hence involved in the therapeutic relationship in a concrete and versatile manner. It can also be said that the patient's important human relations partly served as a bridge and a support between the therapist and the patient.

The patient received no pharmacotherapy except during the inpatient periods. While in hospital, she was given chlorpromazine ad 300 mg/day or perphenazine ad 24 mg/day. After her discharge the patient did not want any medication.

The central goal of the therapeutic relationship was to explore together with the patient the connections and conflicts between her internal fantasy world and the external reality surrounding her. Gradually Miss L. learnt how to delineate her own internal reality and also learnt to identify sensitively the instances when the people close to here were unable to get through to the realities only existing in her own world at that time.

[1] Most of them corresponded to "intervention in crisis in therapeutic community" of the kind described above.

The relatives were advised to be straightforward and to support the patient by making it always clear to her when they were unable to comprehend her.

Since Miss L. had insight into her problems and was motivated to analyze herself, plenty of comprehensible features were found in her fantasy world, when it was examined together, actively following her life course. In several respects, the therapeutic relationship consisted of making a map with the patient – whenever a new point was mutually understood, a new identified area was marked on the "map".

The patient continued her work almost throughout her therapeutic relationship, gradually getting rid of her problems. She also acquired a dwelling of her own and bought a car.

Miss L. has recovered from a serious psychosis in a fairly typical manner: what persists is a weakness of the limits between the ego and the surrounding world and a consequent scantness of the contents of life and a vague feeling of lacking goals. The liability to regression is great, and the patient would probably not be able to tolerate very great upheavals in her life even in the future. The development of the dating relationship is also of notable significance.

As far as I can see, however, the following central goals of the therapeutic relationship were reached: the patient learnt to identify her own sensitive and vulnerable areas, perceived connections between the present and the past, and is now able in her interpersonal relationships to examine the conflicts between her own internal world and the external reality without becoming disintegrated.

5.2.2.2 Number and Frequency of the Sessions

The 26 patients given intensive individual therapy received altogether 4235 hours of individual therapy, the range of variation being 80 to 424 and the *mean per patient* in these therapies 2–5 years in duration being 162.9 sessions. The mean frequency of visits was approximately 1 session per week, but in most cases the frequency of visits was higher at the initial stages of therapy, being 2 or occasionally even 3 sessions per week, and decreased towards the later stages, when the interval between the sessions was usually 2 or even 3 weeks. According to our experience, psychotherapy given once weekly to a psychotic patient suffices to maintain a progressive therapeutic process, if the therapeutic relationship has become intensive enough during the initial high-frequency stage. If, however, the sessions are less frequent than this, the therapy can be said to be – at least practically speaking – a mere supportive contact relationship.

The total number of sessions in less intensive individual therapy was 1735, which makes for an average of 54.2 therapy sessions per each of the 31 patients, the range of variation being 13 to 108. The therapies in this group included some that had session frequencies equal to those used in the more intensive therapies, but were shorter in duration than the latter. These were exceptional, however: a majority of the less intensive individual therapies had a low frequency of sessions – an average of two monthly visits – and hence remained, for this very reason alone, at a purely supportive level.

The figures for the number of visits are based on the duration of therapy and the frequencies of sessions at the different stages reported by the therapists. The average vacations of the therapists have been subtracted from these figures. It has not, however, been possible to take into account the cancelled sessions. This means that the real sessions frequencies are slightly lower than those reported here. Since the cancelled visits are also part of the working time of the therapists, the errors of estimation in e.g. calculating the resources required by the therapies are relatively small.

At the time of the five-year follow-up, 10 of the 26 intensive individual therapies had either been *terminated* or were about to be terminated, The therapies of 16 patients were being continued, though several of them were also approaching their termination. Of the less frequent individual therapies 6 were being continued, some of these having only been started during the later follow-up years.

5.2.2.3 Connections with the Background Variables

As it was already indicated by table 34, the selection of patients for intensive individual therapy was only partly accordant with the therapeutic plans.

In the plans made at the basic study stage, the most significant psychosocial background variables connected with the indication of intensive individual therapy were a higher basic education and the social role of student (both $p < .001$). Subjects belonging to the higher social groups were also indicated for this mode of therapy clearly significantly more often than the average of the series. Among the clinical background variables, a clearly significant connection was found with the subject's insight into his problems and a non-reluctant attitude towards suggested therapy (both $p < .01$).

Of the *patients given intensive individual therapy,* 14 belonged to the group of typical schizophrenias, which corresponds more or less exactly to their percentage of the total series. Borderline schizophrenias numbered 7, schizo-affective psychoses 5, while no schizophreniform psychoses were included in these cases. There were 11 patients with regressive disintegration and only 2 with paranoid disintegration. 12 of the patients belonged to the youngest age group of 16–25 years, 10 to the age-group of 26–35 years, and 4 to the age-group of over 35 years. 16 of these patients were women and 10 men.

The connections of this patient group with the background variables can be seen in Appendices 5 and 6. Of the clinical background variables, *the insight originally shown by the patients turned out to have the highest correlation with the selection for intensive individual therapy* in the whole series ($p = .001$). The other statistically clearly significant correlations were noted for the *lack of acting out behaviour* ($p = .007$) and for a *willing attitude towards admission to treatment* ($p = .010$). An almost significant correlation emerged for *symbiotic contact formation* and the *presence of neurotic symptoms.*

Of the psychosocial background variables, only the marital status – more unmarried subjects, fewer widowed and divorced ones – *correlated significantly with the intensive individual therapy during the five years.*

The initial overestimation of the patient's education and social group as a prerequisite for individual therapy was probably due to a projective identification caused by the team members' own educational level: as it was easier to identify with the life situation of these patients on the basis of one's own experience, they were also expected to be better able to analyze their problems than the others. When the therapies were carried out, the significance of the patients' educational level was reduced by the very fact that the therapies were being given by a more numerous staff with more heterogeneous education than that represented by the team.

Logistic regression analysis of the selection for intensive individual therapy in the entire patient series brought up 5 explaining background variables, and that in the group of typical schizophrenic patients 2 explaining background variables (Table 36).

It should be pointed out here that the explaining background variables both in this logistic regression analysis and those that follow always refer to the findings made at the basic study stage. In addition to the clinical and psychosocial background variables, the first unit of treatment was also taken into account in the analyses (Appendix 1).

Table 36. Implementation of intensive individual therapy: variables influencing the selective processes (Logistic regression analysis)

Explaining variables	R	p
All patients		
Insight ability yes/no	3.42	0.000
Acting out behaviour no/yes	4.86	0.000
Beginning of symptoms acute/slow	2.83	0.008
Neurotic symptoms yes/no	2.06	0.015
Unemployed no/yes	3.38	0.038
Typical schizophrenics		
Duration of symptoms before treatment admission less than 1 month/more than 1 month	3.00	0.009
Mother's severe personality disorder no/yes	2.59	0.061

R = risk; i. e. the relative probability of those differentiated by the explaining variable to be included in the response group.

Even this analysis brings up insight and the lack of acting out behaviour as the most important background variables explaining selection for intensive individual therapy. It can further be seen that an *acute onset of the symptoms* has a significance independent of the other background variables in this selection. The same applies to the presence of neurotic symptoms: they were more frequent in the group of borderline schizophrenias. Of the psychosocial background variables, only the *relative infrequency of unemployment* emerges as having some significance.

The patients selected for intensive long-term individual therapy – or best capable of benefiting from such therapy – were hence characterized by certain clinically favourable background variables, regardless of the fact that the proportion of typical schizophrenics was equally great in this group as in the whole series.

Logistic regression analysis of the selection for intensive individual therapy *in the group of typical schizophrenias* brought up two explaining variables, namely the *short duration of psychotic symptoms prior to admission* for treatment, and, interestingly enough, *lack of any serious personality disorder in the mother.*

The group given *less intensive individual therapy* was clearly more heterogeneous than the group that received intensive individual therapy. It included patients whose therapy was discontinued fairly soon for various reasons – often because of inadequate patient motivation and/or acting-out behaviour – or was otherwise difficult to carry out. The therapies of some other patients, though relatively few in number, were shorter, because there seemed to be no need for further therapy.

The group included 19 patients diagnosed as typical schizophrenics, with 14 patients belonging to the psychodynamic group of regressive disintegration. The conspicuous position of the latter patient group – which was also shown by the significant correlation ($p < .05$) with this mode of therapy – is probably related to their greater-than-average need for therapy, which, in most cases, resulted in an attempt of at least infrequent individual therapy even in the out-patient units.

5.2.3 Family Therapy

5.2.3.1 The Therapeutic Orientation

It has already been pointed out that family therapy as a mode of treatment both in Finland and elsewhere is younger than individual therapy. At the time when our project was launched there was no regular and organized training for family therapy equivalent to that given for psychoanalysis and psychoanalytic individual therapy available in Finland. In the Turku Clinic of Psychiatry, family therapy was taught in seminars, which included case material and through supervision. The direct supervision by means of audiovisual equipment and the associated team work, which have subsequently become common in Finland, had not been started yet.

As regards the orientation of the family therapy given in our series, it can be called psychodynamic and supportive. That was also how most of the therapists described their therapies. The only exceptions in the 2-year follow-up were 3 therapies described by the therapists as "analytic family therapies", while the 5-year follow-up similarly included 3 therapies described by the therapists as "system-oriented family therapies" (including one of the previous analytic family therapies).

The families were seen in joint sessions, and it was considered particularly important for the therapist to create similar empathic contacts with all of the family members.

Because *most of the therapists had relatively little practical experience* of this mode of therapy, their therapeutic attitude was often characterized by mere empathic listening and contact. Particularly *the joint therapies of primary families* involved a notable pressure towards being swallowed up by the family system and becoming part of it.

Both the favourable and the unfavourable aspects of our family-therapeutic approach are illuminated by the therapy which had the highest number of sessions (156) among the therapies of primary families in our series, and which was still being continued at the time of the five-year follow-up. The dynamics of this family were also described in another paper previously published (Räkköläinen and Alanen 1982).

The family background of the patient, the 24-year-old Miss R., was characterized by two early deaths, both matters not discussed at home: the death of the daughter born before the patient at the age of 3, and the death (probably suicide) of the paranoid psychotic father when the patient was 4 years old. Miss R. had a younger sister born some months after the father's death. The life of the mother and her two daughters was characterized by a strong and symbiotic feeling of togetherness, which protected them against the memory of the past losses. The prevailing family myth is described by the words frequently repeated by Miss R.: "We were so happy together".

Miss R. became autistic and disintegrated gradually after her sister married and moved away from home. A dating relationship she had had herself came to an end around the same time. She lost her job because of difficulties of concentration and closed herself up in her home, apathetic and wrapped up in herself, finally almost mutistic.

In hospital, the diagnosis of the symbiotic relationship between the mother and the daughter gave rise to their joint therapy. It turned out that the patient's regressive mental world was notably concerned with the fate of the father and the dead sister; she identified herself with them. Supported by the therapist, the mother also began to disentangle and expose the anxiety-provoking memories and feelings associated with these old tragedies, which she had dammed up inside her, but which now broke out with fresh vividness. Miss R. left her autism and participated intensively in the therapeutic work. She expressed accusations of her mother not revealed before – particularly accusing her mother of never telling her any details of her father's illness and death – and also began to draw a more distinct line between herself and the mystified dead. Her autism and psychotic disintegration disappeared, not returning again.

This stage of progress, however, was followed by a stage of homeostatic resistance to restore the previous situation, which turned out more difficult to work through than the initial stage. The patient had returned home, and her relationship with her mother had acquired a new kind of nearness. The therapist, a young female physician, had, as it were, taken the place of the sister who had left home. This was most clearly reflected by the patient's eager requests to have the therapist visit her home – which she did, too, and whereupon the patient stated that "everything was well again, just as it used to be". The mother also seemed satisfied with the situation, and the attempts to stimulate the patient to separate from her home were met by quiet resistance in both.

At the time of the five-year follow-up, the joint sessions were being continued, though less frequently. Mrs. R. said that they had been talking of terminating the therapy, but that the therapeutic visits had become a kind of "way of life". The patient is not psychotic, but she has remained slightly fearful of the outer world and has not resumed working. She continues to be on a provisional disability pension. The sister lives close to her home, and, after she has acquired independence, she also has a close relationship with her primary family. She keeps contact daily, and one important factor in Miss R's life is to take her sister's children out when the sister is working. Her other contacts outside her home are restricted.

The improvement of Miss R's clinical condition and her subjective satisfaction with her life situation should be appreciated. This may be illuminated by a comparison of Miss R's development with another patient of ours, a man, who also originally had a highly binding and symbiotic relationship with his mother and sisters, but which situation – in an absence of any family-oriented therapy – resulted in mutual "rejection" due to reciprocal frustration and hostility, with the consequence that the patient is exceedingly lonely, paranoid towards his relatives and chronically schizophrenic. But even in the therapy of the family R., new kinds of intervention would now be needed to alter the family system in such a way as to allow Miss R. grow into a more independent life.

The experience of *couple therapies* in our series showed, on the whole, a clearly more favourable course than the joint therapies of the primary family. One reason for this was probably the less serious psychotic condition of the patients – although most of the patients belonged to the group of typical schizophrenics, the clinical conditions were less grave and the ego functions better developed. Marital problems had regularly contributed to the onset of the illness, and it was generally alleviating just to be able to discuss them. Problems pertaining to children were often dealt with in the discussions. We also received confirmation for our suggestion that many of the psychotic patients feel that a joint therapy session together with the spouse increases their security and diminishes their fears of rejection.

The following case description illuminates the effects of successful supportive couple therapy.

The therapist in this couple therapy, which consisted of 29 sessions and went on for about 3 years, was a social worker of the Mental Health Office, who participated in the supervisiongroup for couple therapies conducted in the Clinic of Psychiatry by the head of the project. The patient admitted into our series was a 35-year-old skilled labourer who suffered from serious jealousy paranoia characterized by clearly schizophrenic ideas of reference.[1] Prior to admission for therapy, the family situation had become so difficult that the patient's wife attempted suicide with drugs and two months later the patient did the same, whereupon he was admitted into a psychiatric hospital.

Psychiatric examination revealed quite a typical family-dynamic situation. Mr. P. had disproportionate feelings of inferiority concerning his masculinity, particularly in the sexual region. The wife was a few years senior to him and had, in addition to the two children born of the spouse's wedlock, another child born premaritally. These factors as well as the husband's intense, though ambivalent tendency to dependence suggested that the wife also had the meaning of a mother figure for him. While a child, Mr. P. had always felt himself "rejected". Mrs. P., in turn, was inclined to depression and showed attitudes of provokingly underrating her husband, which had become more exaggerated along with the deterioration of their mutual relationship and the increasing sexual frigidity. She irritated her husband by e.g. going to dances alone although it seems she was never actually unfaithful to her husband. Anyway, this was a source of intense worry for the latter. The problems had resulted in violent encounters, particularly when the husband was under the influence of alcohol.

The initiation of couple therapy immediately demonstrated that the hostility between the spouses served to hide mutual dependence and despair, which began to be alleviated along with the further sessions. The background of both spouses as well as their current problems in e.g. matters pertaining to sexual behaviour were discussed. There were a few difficult sessions, during which the husband insisted on his wife for explanations for his paranoid delusions; as a consequence, however, the lack of confidence gradually subsided and both of the spouses turned out increasingly able to analyze their own attitudes towards the other. Both felt the therapist to be a "parent" whose presence made it possible to have clarifying discussions without uncontrolled quarreling or withdrawal from contact. The dependence on the therapist was shown by e.g. the fact that the increased interval between the sessions suggested by her resulted in a re-aggravation of the spouses' mutual problems and a need to have more frequent sessions again. When the therapy was terminated, the spouses were clearly in better terms with each other, while both seemed to have become more independent.

This impression was unexpectedly obvious when Mr. P. was interviewed at the time of the five-year follow-up. The interviewer reported that "the paranoid ideas have been completely overcome, and the patient is a depressed middle-aged man, who, occasionally showing deep insight, analyzes his life, relating the past to the present". The marriage is by no means unproblematic, but – instead of the previous paranoid adherence – Mr. P. now ponders peacefully whether the spouses will remain together once their children have grown up.

5.2.3.2 Number and Frequency of the Sessions

The figures presented in Table 34 already indicated that the implementation of family therapy was clearly less extensive than was originally planned. Compared with the individual therapies, many of the family therapies were also relatively short. Nevertheless, the total number of sessions in the 15 family therapies defined as intensive was 713, which makes an average of 47.5 sessions per therapy, the range being from 12 to 156. The number of sessions of the 10 less intensive family therapies was 71, which makes an average of 7.1 sessions per therapy. If we combine the intensive and less intensive therapies for joint therapies of the primary family on the one hand and take the therapies of secondary family (the great majority of them being couple therapies) on the other, the average number of sessions in the first group turns out to be 38.5 and that

[1] This patients was one of those originally diagnosed as "severe paranoia" (cf. p. 32).

in the latter 26.5. The frequency of sessions in the different therapies varied greatly. In the therapies with the highest total number of sessions the session frequency, at least initially, was regularly 1 per week, while in the less intensive therapies it was often 1 session per 3 or 4 weeks. At the time of the five-year follow-up study, only two family therapies were being continued, both of them with infrequent sessions.

5.2.3.3 Connections with the Background Variables

Most of the patients whose therapy involved joint therapy of primary family were bound to their homes, unmarried, without an occupational identity, and classifiable to the clinically most serious category of regressive ego disintegration. All these background variables had at least a nearly significant connection ($p < .02$) with this mode of treatment. The number of typical schizophrenics was 8. The background variables were largely the same as in the original therapeutic plans.

It still was interesting that even this group of patients had some clinically favourable baseline characteristics. The personality disorder of the mother or the father were not emphatic among the background variables, nor was the presence of hostile or indifferent family members. A majority of the patients had a tendency to avoid expressing their aggression, and they were also relatively well motivated for the therapy (the background variable indicative of this approached the level of marginal significance).

The patients given *couple therapy* or *conjoint therapy of secondary family* also had largely similar background variables as in the original therapeutic plans. In the selection into this group, the high number of married patients was self-evident: all but one (who was separated) were in marriage. So were also separation from the primary family, a long-term heterosexual relationship and an established heterosexual identity. What was further characteristic of this group was the majority of women in comparison with men, and the social role of having a job or working at home (both $p < .01$). Patients belonging to the older age-groups were clearly more numerous in the couple therapy group than the others ($p < .05$).

This group of 15 patients included 10 patients with typical schizophrenia. There were no statistical connections with the diagnostic subcategories, while exclusion from the psychodynamic group of imminent disintegration had a connection of a marginally significant level.

The background variables of the patients selected for family therapy of the primary or of the secondary family (either intensive or less intensive) compared with the rest of the series can be seen in Appendices 5 and 6 and the results of logistic regression analysis in Table 37.

In the whole series, the most important explaining variables turned out to be *belonging to the group of regressive disintegration* (this was due to the serious disturbances of the patients selected for primary family therapies) and *"normality" of the psychosexual development noted more often than in the rest of the series* (this was due to the cases of couple therapy). Previous psychiatric therapy also emerged as an explaining variable. The group of typical schizophrenic patients selected for family therapy was also characterized by normal psychosexual development as well as the presence of *depressive symptoms*.

Table 37. Implementation of family therapy: variables influencing the selective processes (Logistic regression analysis)

Explaining variables	R	p
All patients		
Ego-dynamic group of regressive disintegration yes/no	2.05	0.042
Psychosexual development "normal"/"abnormal"	1.94	0.012
Earlier psychiatric treatment yes/no	1.90	0.067
Typical schizophrenics		
Depressive symptoms yes/no	3.75	0.006
Psychosexual development "normal"/"abnormal"	2.52	0.050

The latter variable correlated almost significantly with the implementation of the primary family's therapy, but depressive symptoms were also more frequent than the average in the group of couple therapies.

5.2.3.4 Supportive Contacts with Family Members

Beyond actual family therapy, the family-oriented approach in our project also took the form of support given to the family members. The initial interview of the families provided a good opportunity for this, simultaneously creating a contact based on a therapeutic attitude. The specialized nurse of the team, who was responsible for these family interviews, often also acted as a supporter of the families later on, but the same role was, to a lesser extent, also adopted by the other members of the team as well as the staff of the different therapeutic units. Partly these contacts were accordant with the plans made at the basic study stage, while partly they arose spontaneously through an initiative made by the family at some stage of the therapy. An effort was always made to inform the patients of these contacts. It was agreed in several individual therapies that, when necessary, the therapist can be contacted by one of the family members or the family can contact the therapist, but always with the patient being aware of it.

Support to the families or some family members was given in the case of altogether 40 patients. Of the 26 patients given intensive individual therapy, 15 or a majority belonged to this group. There was also a significant correlation ($p = .032$) between intensive individual therapy and the support given to the patient's family. As far as we could see, the contacts made for the purpose of supporting the family were often of great help for both the successful implementation of individual therapy and the alleviation of anxiety in the family members.

We can describe a typical case, where the parents of a young female patient with an acute onset of psychosis of the typical schizophrenia group consulted a psychiatrist member of the team soon after the admission of their daughter. Particularly the father was highly anxious and spoke of a bulge he thought he has noticed on his daughter's forehead and suspected a sign of cerebral disease. The discussion dealt widely with the family's life situation, which was coloured by e.g. the approaching retirement of the father, who was slightly possessively attracted to his daughter. Apart from the daughter's psychosis and the "bulge" on her forehead, the reasons for anxiety appeared to include the religious parents' worry concerning the daughter's possible (actually nonexistent) sexual relationships with men and the feeling of guilt over the daughter's pre-psychotic outburst concerning the excessive possessiveness of the parents.

During the course of the discussion it was pointed out that such problems between two generations are common. The parents' attitude towards the psychiatrist became confident, and they were favourable towards his suggestion that the daughter would begin long-term individual therapy with a psychotherapist to be found during her stay in hospital. The father came to see the psychiatrist once more later on, and the parents phoned him now and then. The patient began her psychotherapy, and although she was once re-admitted into hospital later (during the hospitalization the contact with the parents was re-established), the therapy turned out successful, which was shown by her recovery from the psychosis and the lack of recurrence during the latter follow-up period as well as the fact that she completed her studies, found a job, and got engaged.

Family therapy and support to the family members were also relatively often given in the same cases ($p = .018$). These two activities took place either in succession or simultaneously. The latter procedure was not favoured by the team, who tried to discourage contacts by the family members with their family therapist outside the joint family sessions, but such contacts were taken, nevertheless.

The support given to the family clearly focussed on the family environments of the patients disturbed more seriously than the average. Of the 40 patients whose families were supported, 28 had typical schizophrenia and 17 belonged to the psychodynamic group of regressive disintegration (both $p < .05$). The serious personality disorder in the mother emerged as a marginally significant factor.

The family-oriented therapeutic approach, either in the form of family therapy or in the form of support to the family, or both, was applied in altogether 50 cases, which is exactly half or our series.

Group therapies given to out-patients were so rare in our series that this group cannot be analyzed separately. The lack of group therapy as well as functional group activities taking place on an out-patient basis is one of the shortcomings of the psychiatric therapeutic system in Turku. During the follow-up period, some of our patients had joined pensioners'clubs similar to social clubs.

5.2.4 Treatment in a Psychotherapeutic Community

5.2.4.1 Therapeutic Orientation

The operating principles of our psychotherapeutic ward communities were described fairly widely in Chapter 4.3.5. We will here complete it "from the inside" by quoting the description of the "ego ideals" set by the community for itself as described by the specialized nurse of our team, who has worked on our ward of acute psychoses for a long time (Rasimus in Alanen et al. 1978b):

Therapy does not mean that one does or prescribes something to the patient, but that everything is done in cooperation with the patient. The community can hence be perceived as a system which consciously strives to utilize the potential of the whole staff and the patient body, to reach a goal that has been defined jointly.

The therapeutic quality of the community does not arise from external conditions. If the community is only therapeutic relative to its optimal external conditions, it has merely achieved an ostensibly functional empty shell, which breaks as soon as prerequisites of internal functionality are set for the therapeutic work. Therapeutic and empathic qualities grow from the inside of the human being – through increased self-knowledge, provided that one dares to be open and receptive.

The therapeutic community differs from society in precisely that it provides an opportunity of understanding and analyzing problems that arise when people live together, and that it allows one to live through difficult periods of solving the problems with the help of transference relationships. Thinking of the patient's fragile ego, the general atmosphere should be democratic, hopeful, trustful, willing to solve conflicts, honest and open.

One often hears it said that the hospital is sick – the reason probably being that attention has traditionally been drawn to the abnormality of the patient. The people on the therapeutic side diagnose, report and observe. The therapeutic focus should, however, be elsewhere. Illness has its own life-historical message, and by analyzing and listening to this message, one should find the resources which may allow new growth.

In Turku, we call our psychosis ward a psychotherapeutic community. On this ward, which is particularly suited to the patients with most serious regression, the staff assume the role of a parent relative to the patients. The parent is reliable, firm and safe. In this parental relationship the patient can gradually grow internally and get a contact with his own fragile ego.

What is central particularly at the early stages of the therapy is the holding attitude (Winnicott 1960, Salonen 1976), whereby the therapist holds the patient amidst the overwhelming and exhaustive anxiety. The ward community gives the patient the limits he is lacking – the limits reduce his disintegration and increase security. All the possible means are used to support the patient's fragile self-confidence and to protect the patient against the destructiveness of illness.

Treatment in a psychotherapeutic community in our therapeutic system signifies a maximal use of the resources to help a psychotically disturbed patient out of his regressive and increasingly isolated condition. It was considered indicated particularly for the most seriously ill patients. This was especially the case when the community treatment was continued for a longer period. The originally autistic condition of several patients was thus seen to change soon into openness and confidence towards the environment; withdrawal was seen to hide a symbiotic need for reliance. Miss R., who started family treatment together with her mother, as described above, is a good example of this. In the case of some other patients, social life difficulties were more conspicuous, as was shown by Mr. K. in Chapter 5.1. In such cases the ward therapy often took the form of team work, which was variously extended to the extra-hospital environment.

5.2.4.2 Connections with the Background Variables

The background variables of the patients receiving community therapy in some form corresponded to a notable extent to those specified in the indications. The most significant connections to the treatment in the psychotherapeutic community had belonging to the *ego-dynamic group of regressive disintegration* ($p < .001$), *female sex* ($p < .01$), *and a non-reluctant attitude to treatment* ($p < .020$). Of the diagnostic groups, that of schizophreniform psychoses had a clearly negative connection with community treatment. A marginally significant correlation between borderline schizophrenia and the need for treatment in a psychotherapeutic community noted at the time of making the therapeutic plans was eliminated in the analysis of the actual therapies. The typical schizophrenias numbered 35 ($p = .14$).

Unlike in the case of individual therapy (and also in the couple therapies) the symbiotic or reserved nature of the contact did not emerge in the selection for community therapy: its effects was hence particularly conspicuous in the formation of the therapeutic relationships. Nor did the social group of the patient or his parents contribute to the community therapy that was given any more than the patient's educational level, although there were more students in the group.

The patients who were given a long-term intensive treatment in psychotherapeutic community were among those most seriously ill in our series. The role of regressively disintegrated patients was particularly notable: this group of altogether 25 patients included 16 with regressive ego disintegration ($p = .000$).

It is interesting to note that a willing or passive attitude to the first admission as well as judicial sanctions upon it had no connection with intensive community therapy, although the former factor had some effect on the selection ($p = .12$). *In logistic regression analysis* we *combined intensive treatment in a psychotherapeutic community and intervention in a crisis in a psychotherapeutic community,* examining the background variables that differentiated between this group of patients and the rest of the series (cf. Appendices 5 and 6). We considered these two patient groups to represent best the patient most expediently and actively the target of our psychotherapeutic communities. The modes of therapy were only different with regard to the duration of the community therapy, while the less intensive community therapy differed from these two in being more passive in quality.

In the light of this analysis (Table 38), the explaining variables contributing to the selection for active community therapy turned out to be largely identical with those presented above: *belonging to the group of regressive disintegration* and *female sex* were the most important patient-specific variables affecting the selection. The *primarily favourable attitude towards therapy* also emerged in the analysis of the total series. The logistic regression of merely the group of typical schizophrenias revealed, in addition

Table 38. Implementation of treatment in psychotherapeutic community: variables influencing the selective processes (logistic regression analysis)

Explaining variables	R	p
All patients		
Group of regressive disintegration yes/no	2.58	0.001
Sex female/male	2.09	0.001
Group of imminent disintegration no/yes	3.36	0.031
Refusing treatment in the beginning phase no/yes	1.90	0.049
Typical schizophrenics		
Group of regressive disintegration	2.66	0.002
Quality of interpersonal relationships outside the primary family not stabile/stabile	1.77	0.013
Depressive symptoms yes/no	1.78	0.030

to the group of regressive disintegration, also a *lack of stability in the relationships outside the primary family* and the *presence of depressive symptoms.*

We can probably conclude that community therapy largely focused on patients who were really in need of a comprehensive therapeutic approach which supports their integration and helps them to communicate their feelings. The greater number of women than men in this group was partly due to the different selection of the sexes into the first therapeutic units: more women were admitted via the Clinic of Psychiatry than via the Kupittaa Hospital. But the first unit of therapy was also included among the background variables in the logistic regression analyses, and its exclusion from the group of the ultimate explaining variables seems to suggest that the sex was also significant for the selection in itself.

The significance of the presence of depressive symptoms should probably be interpreted in a corresponding manner: the presence of depressive symptoms was clearly an important indicator of the favourable attitude towards therapy in a schizophrenic patient increasing the possibilities of bringing him into the sphere of therapy.

5.2.5 Group of Psychotherapy Cases

On the basis of the 5-year follow-up findings on the implementation of psychotherapeutic treatments, we discriminated a *group of psychotherapy cases* from the rest of the series. The purpose in this case was

1. *to find out the global coverage of the intensive modes of psychotherapeutic treatments,* and
2. *to get a starting-point for an analysis of the effect of the psychotherapeutic modes of treatment on the patients' prognosis,* also on a global form.

5.2.5.1 Criteria of Inclusions. Combinations of Different Therapeutical Models

We included the patient in the group of psychotherapy cases if he had been given *at least one of the following modes of therapy:*

- *intensive individual therapy*
- *intensive family therapy*
- *intensive group therapy*
- *intensive therapy in a psychotherapeutic community*
- even when none of the criteria for the duration of any intensive modes of therapy were met, *a less intensive psychotherapeutic treatment that was considered sufficient in regard to the patient's disorder and was terminated upon a mutual agreement between the therapist and the patient.*

On the basis of the last of these criteria, the group of psychoterapy cases came to include 7 patients who did not belong to any of the more intensive therapies. They had all been given less intensive individual therapy which had explorative goals and a session frequency comparable with the intensive individual therapies, but was shorter in duration (the number of sessions in these individual therapies ranged from 20 to 76).

Of our 100 patients, 56 were included in the group of psychotherapy cases. Table 39 indicates that a *majority of them had been given more than one mode of psychotherapy.*

Table 39. Combination of psychotherapeutic treatments for the patients of the psychotherapy group

Combination of psycho-therapeutic treatments	Only the intensive treatments considered	Both the intensive and the less intensive treatments considered	Support to the family also considered
The patient only received one mode of therapy	39	10	7
		5 from the group of intensive individual therapy 3 from the group of "sufficient" less intensive ind. therapy 1 from the group of intensive community therapy 1 from the group of intensive group therapy 0 from the group of intensive family therapy	
The patient received several modes of therapy	17	46	49
	3 individual and family therapies 7 individual and community therapies 6 family therapies and community therapies 1 family and individual therapy + community therapy		

17 had received at least two kinds of intensive therapy, and when the less intensive therapies are also taken into account, the number of patients given more than one kind of therapy goes up to 46. And even of the 10 remaining patients, 3 had been given individual therapy supplemented with a supportive contact with family members.

Table 39 indicates that the *most common combination was one of community therapy and the other modes of therapy.* There was only one patient given intensive treatment in a psychotherapeutic community who did not receive additional individual or family therapy even in a less intensive form. This is naturally explained by the fact that the ward communities functioned as therapeutic units where the individual or family therapy was often started or at least arranged as a further treatment for the patient after his discharge. In the case of a few patients the order was the opposite: individual or family therapy had been started in an out-patient unit, but the patient had to be hospitalized later, preferably for intervention in a crisis in a therapeutic community.

A combination of individual and family therapies was also relatively common: 15 patients receiving one of these therapies in the intensive form were also given the other at least in a less intensive form. It would seem logical and recommendable that family therapy should be started first in such cases and individual therapy thereafter, once the bonds of the family situations would have been relieved and the conditions for successful individual therapy improved. It was, however, more common in our series that these therapies were being carried out simultaneously, often by different therapists. In some other cases the intensive individual therapy was supported by less frequent family therapy. But there was also some lack of planning observable in the combination of therapies.

It is interesting to note that of the ten patients given one mode of therapy in this group of psychotherapy cases, only one had been diagnosed as typically schizophrenic, and a supportive contact with the family members had been established even in this case. A majority, 7, of the others suffered from borderline schizophrenias, in addition to which there was one patient with schizo-affective psychosis, and one with schizophreniform psychosis. These figures give a highly illuminating proof for the suggestion that a *combination of several different modes of psychotherapeutic treatment becomes necessary in the treatment of typical schizophrenias in particular* – this was shown by our experience, anyway. Although the long-term individual therapies held a relatively central position in our psychotherapeutic approach, the typical schizophrenic patients further needed either family therapy or treatment in a psychotherapeutic community or both as a supplement for the individual therapy.

5.2.5.2 Connections with the Background Variables

The connections between the group and the psychosocial and clinical background variables are presented in Appendices 5 and 6.

The logistic regression analysis (Table 40) *indicated that the beginning of the treatment either on open care or at the wards of the Clinic of Psychiatry, as opposed to the Kupittaa Hospital, emerged as the first explaining variable both in the whole series and in the group of typical schizophrenia.*

Table 40. Belonging to the group of psychotherapy cases: variables influencing the selective processes (logistic regression analysis)

Explaining variables	R	p
All patients		
First therapeutic unit Clinic of Psychiatry or open care/ Kupittaa Hospital	2.63	0.000
Group of regressive disintegration yes/no	1.97	0.009
Symbiotic contact mode yes/no	1.69	0.015
Unemployed no/yes	1.97	0.014
Typical schizophrenics		
First therapeutic unit Clinic of Psychiatry or open care/ Kupittaa Hospital	2.72	0.024
Beginning of symptoms acute/slow	1.98	0.021
Refusing treatment in the beginning phase no/yes	1.78	0.015

In the whole patient series, four quite different and mutually complementary background variables emerged: besides first therapeutic unit, belonging to the *group of regressive disintegration* (background variable expressive of the clinical features), *symbiotic contact formation* (background variable expressive of the patient's psychologic characteristic), and *exclusion from the group of unemployed* (social background variable). In the group of typical schizophrenic patients, the explaining variables include, apart from the first therapeutic unit, the *sudden onset of symptoms* and the *lack of negative attitude towards therapy* at the basic study stage.

The connections between the first therapeutic unit and inclusion in the group of psychotherapy cases are also shown by Table 41.

Expansion of the psychotherapeutic functions in such a way that the therapeutic responsibility was distributed between all the occupational groups involved in mental

Table 41. Distribution of the patients included in and excluded from the group of psychotherapy cases on the basis of the first therapeutic unit

First therapeutic unit	Therapy cases		Not therapy cases		Total
	number	%	number	%	
Clinic of Psychiatry	35	64.8	19	35.2	54
Kupittaa Hospital	6	25.0	18	75.0	24
Day hospital of Clinic of Psychiatry	3	60.0	2	40.0	5
Out-patient care	12	70.6	5	29.4	17
Total	56	56.0	44	44.0	100

health work clearly diminished the lack of social equality generally associated with psychotherapy. The social groups of patients and parents had no correlation with the group of psychotherapy cases, while basic education showed a marginal correlation. The family-oriented approach, particularly the couple therapies, also contributed to this. Even so, the *widowed and divorced subjects were too often left without therapy.* These groups as well as the patients excluded from working life should be given special attention in the further development of the therapeutic system.

We might further point out that a lack of serious personality disorders in the mother also had a marginally significant connection with the group of psychotherapy cases in the whole series and an almost significant connection among the typical schizophrenic patients.

Of the clinical background variables, the conspicuous position of the *group of regressive disintegration* (23 out of 31 patients; p = .014) is partly explained by the really serious and recurrent need for therapy among the patients of this group. Many of these patients aroused a strong challenge for helping in the therapeutic staff. The *group of paranoid disintegration,* on the other hand, was not in the same way within the reach of therapy, but had negative connection with the group of psychotherapy cases (p = .034).

The high number of regressively disintegrated patients among the psychotherapy cases also shows that the *group of psychotherapy cases consisted of patients who were more ill clinically on the average than the patients not included in this group.* This difference, however, is partly levelled off by *certain psychosocial and also clinical background variables of psychotherapy patients that were more favourable than the average* among the other patients, especially the symbiotic contact formation and an acute beginning of symptoms. Preliminary insight ability and the presence of depressive symptoms had a positive correlation of an almost significant level among the typical schizophrenics and a marginal significance among the whole series with the group of psychotherapy cases.

Of our typical schizophrenic patients, 32 were included in the psychotherapy group while 24 were excluded. The figures indicate that the *typical schizophrenic patients were divided quite evenly between these two groups: 57 % of the psychotherapy cases and 54 % of the others belonged to this diagnostic sub-category.* This gives a good opportunity to compare the prognoses of these patients, although it should be borne in mind that a relatively greater proportion of the typical schizophrenic patients belonging to the psychotherapy cases were regressively disintegrated, while a greater proportion of those excluded from the psychotherapy group were patients with paranoid disintegration. Only 2 (20 %) of the schizophreniform psychoses, 10 (71 %) of the schizo-affective psychoses and 12 (60 %) of the borderline schizophrenias belonged to the psychotherapy cases.

5.2.6 Patients Remaining Excluded from the Psychotherapeutic Treatments

Some psychotherapeutic treatment in a less intensive form had also been given to several patients not belonging to the psychotherapy group. *Of our 100 patients, 20 lacked even any of the less intensive forms of therapy shown in Table 36.* Among these were two patients with whom an effort to therapy – in both cases to intensive individual

Table 42. Lack of any mode of psychotherapeutic treatment: Influence of background variables (logistic regression analysis)

Explaining variables	R	p
All patients		
Depressive symptoms no/yes	3.27	0.005
Basic education elementary school/more	6.00	0.005
Sex male/female	3.875	0.050
Typical schizophrenics		
Ego-dynamic group of paranoid disintegration yes/no	4.92	0.004
Depressive symptoms no/yes	5.29	0.001
Alcohol or other addiction yes/no	2.93	0.108
Unemployed yes/no	3.32	0.124

therapy – was made but discontinued by the patients in the very beginning. Six other patients were included in the cases in which support was given to the family member(s).

We also carried out a *logistic regression analysis* on the background variables of these 20 patients not given any personal psychotherapeutic treatment. The following results were obtained (Table 42):

We can see that the explaining variables emerging in the whole series include a *lack of depressive symptoms, low basic education* and *male sex*. In the group of typical schizophrenic patients, the lack of depressive symptoms remains as an explaining variable, but the *group of paranoid disintegration* and – being somewhat lower in significance – a *tendency to alcohol abuse or other addiction* as well as *unemployment* emerge as new explaining variables. The picture of the patient belonging to the schizophrenia group and not given psychotherapeutic treatment becomes quite distinct in the light of these background variables. It might be pointed out that the first therapeutic unit did not emerge as an explaining factor in this analysis.

5.2.7 Occupational Groups, Psychotherapeutic Training and Supervision of the Therapists

Table 45 shows the numbers of the therapists belonging to the different occupational groups who were responsible for the psychotherapies as well as their psychotherapeutic training.

The calculation only includes the individual therapies, family therapies and group therapies carried out during the five year follow-up period, as shown in Table 35. The

Table 43. The occupational groups and the level of psychotherapeutic trainings of the therapists responsible for the psychotherapeutic treatments

Occupational group	Number of cases	Number of therapists	Level of psychotherapeutic training[a]		
			1	2	3
Specialist in psychiatry	24	13	3	8	2
Other physician	22	10	–	10	–
Psychologist	12	8	5	3	–
Specialized nurse	41	13	–	12	1
Nurse	1	1	–	1	–
Mental nurse	3	3	–	3	–
Social worker	7	4	–	3	1
Total	110	52	8	40	4

[a] 1 = a completed psychotherapeutic special training of 2 – 6 year; 2 = undergoing psychotherapeutic special training, on-the-job training, long-term supervision; 3 = no psychotherapeutic acquaintance.

number of cases, 110, is higher than the number of case-specific therapies, 85, due to the fact that some therapies were successively carried out by several therapists.

One feature that attracts attention in the table is *the high number of therapists:* 52 therapists were responsible for the treatments. *Specialists in psychiatry and specialized nurses were most frequent among the therapists,* both numbering 13. Case-specifically, *the role of specialized psychiatric nurses is clearly the most notable.* The specialized nurse of our team contributed to this by being the therapist in 13 cases. But there were also 12 other specialized nurses attending 28 therapies. *"Other physician"* refers in all cases to a resident of the Clinic of Psychiatry specializing in psychiatry (in two cases in child psychiatry). When they are taken into account, the role of physicians becomes slightly more notable than that of specialized nurses. In addition to these occupational groups, *psychologists* were also responsible for a significant portion of the therapies. Social workers also conducted several therapies, but the participation of nurses lacking special training and – seeing to the large size of the staff category – mental nurses in psychotherapeutic work otherwise except in the psychotherapeutic community remained insignificant.

The psychotherapeutic special training in this table includes completed psychoanalytic training (3 specialized psychiatrists) and two-year training in psychotherapy (5 psychologists). These forms of training prepared the therapists for work in individual therapy. A majority of the therapists classified in column 2 had acquired psychotherapeutic experience through on-the-job training and long-term supervision. Four therapists were considered to lack even this training.

Supervision played an important role in most of the psychotherapies in our series. This is shown by the following figures, which are patient-specific, i.e. pertain to the 85 individual, family and group therapies conducted, not considering the possible change of therapist:

Supervision throughout the whole therapy	25
Supervision for part of the time or upon consultation	31
No supervision	29

Table 44. Occupational group of the therapist patient-specifically in the different modes of therapy

Occupational group of therapist	Intensive individual therapy	Less intensive individual therapy	Family therapy
Specialist in psychiatry	2	7.5	7
Other physician	2.5	6	5.5
Psychologist	8	1	2
Specialized nurse	10.5	12.5	10.5
Nurse	–	1	–
Mental nurse	2	1	–
Social worker	1	2	1
Total	26	31	25

In about 40 % of the cases the supervision was given to individuals, in 30 % to groups and in 30 % upon consultation and/or during the rounds of the senior psychiatrists. The members of the team were responsible for about half of the supervisions. The supervision in the therapies of 5 patients took place outside the communal health care system in the form of additional training financed by the therapist himself.

Table 44 shows the intensive individual therapies, the less intensive individual therapies and the family therapies classified patient-specifically according to the occupational groups of the therapist.

The therapies conducted by specialized nurses were most numerous in all modes of therapy. It is somewhat surprising that the specialists in psychiatry and the other physicians were responsible for a relatively small portion of the intensive individual therapies whereas psychologists conducted mostly this kind of therapies. Two of the intensive individual therapies were conducted by a mental nurse.

If we make a similar patient-specific analysis of the psychotherapeutic training of therapists and the supervision given during the therapies, we get the following findings (Table 45):

Table 45. Psychotherapeutic training of the therapists and supervision of the therapies classified according to the different modes of treatment

Mode of therapy	Psychotherapeutic training of therapist[a]			Supervision given during therapy[b]		
	1	2	3	1	2	3
Intensive individual therapy	8	18	0	2	16	8
Less intensive individual therapy	3	27	2	8	12	12
Family therapy	6	19	0	14	2	9
Group therapy	0	2	0	1	1	0

[a] = see Table 43

[b] 1 = supervision throughout the therapy; 2 = supervision for part of the therapy; 3 = no supervision.

The therapists with actual psychotherapeutic training have conducted relatively more intensive individual therapies and family therapies compared with the less intensive individual therapies. Their psychotherapeutic training did not include training in family therapy, which means that it might be better to ascribe all the family therapies to therapists lacking actual training.

The supervisions of intensive individual therapy were relatively more often given for part of the therapy only, the main reason being the long duration of these therapies. Supervision was usually given at the beginning of the therapy, not towards the later stages. Supervisions covering the whole duration of the therapy were relatively most numerous in the category of family therapies, where they were also needed owing to the inexperience of the therapists. When superivisions covering the whole therapy and part of the therapy are combined, no great differences appear between the different modes of therapy.

It is not unexpected that supervision more often supplements the therapies conducted by therapists lacking psychotherapeutic special training than those carried out by trained therapists. Even so, 5 of the 17 therapies conducted by trained therapists were also given supervision. Supervision was not given to the therapists who were included in group 3 in Table 43.

It turned out too difficult to analyze systemically the connections between the supervision and the outcome of therapies, but regarding the therapists lacking psychotherapy training we could notice that the *successful accomplishment of longer therapies had a clear dependency on the presence of supervision in the therapy of at least some of the therapist's patients.*

5.2.8 Discontinued Therapies

Our data on the discontinued psychotherapeutic treatments have been compiled in Table 46. They are based on the questionnaires mailed to the therapists at the time of the two follow-up studies, and are therefore estimates given by themselves. Not all therapists supplied these data. In the 2-year follow-up, which is more important here, the loss was about 20 %.

The classification of the modes of therapy in the table corresponds to the goals set for the therapy initially. We can see that discontinuation was most common during the first month of therapy, but some of the therapies that had been going on for more than a year were also discontinued.

The heterogeneous quality of the therapies that were discontinued makes it difficult to analyze statistically these findings. A case-specific analysis shows, however, that particularly the patients who discontinued their therapy without starting a new one included several from the *group of paranoid disintegration.* It was even originally difficult to motivate many of these patients to psychotherapy. Some attended the therapy for a longer time, but had a reluctant or ambivalent attitude towards it, dropping out completely later on.

Neither the social background of the patients, nor the occupational group of the therapist seemed to correlate with the discontinuation of the therapy. Nor were there any regularities observable between the occupational group and training of the therapist in charge of the discontinued treatment and the occupational group and training of the therapists who later attended to these same patients.

Table 46. Times of discontinuation of the psychotherapeutic treatments and the therapist's assessments of the therapeutic situation reached.

Type of therapy	Time of discontinuation	Therapist's estimate of treatment					
		2-year follow-up:			5-year follow-up:		
		No therapeutic work	Discontinued early	Began well, discontinued	No therapeutic work	Discontinued early	Began well discontinued
Intense individual therapy	1– 2 mo.	10(6)	–	1	–	–	–
"	3–12 mo.	2(1)	1	3(2)	–	–	–
"	>1 yr.	–	–	–	–	–	1(1)
Less intensive individual therapy	1– 2 mo.	3(2)	1	–	–	–	–
"	3–12 mo.	–	1	1	–	–	–
"	>1 yr.	–	–	2	1	–	2(1)
Family therapy	1– 2 mo.	–	2	–	–	–	–
"	3–12 mo.	–	–	1	–	–	–
"	>1 yr.	1	–	1	–	–	–

The numbers refer to the number of cases. The figures in parentheses indicate the number of patients who later began a therapy with corresponding goals with another therapist.

5.3 Somatic Treatments

5.3.1 Neuroleptic Medication

Of our 100 patients, 98 were given *neuroleptic medication* at some stage of the treatment. Table 49 shows how these patients were distributed *during the first two follow-up years* with regard to the highest daily dose on the one hand and the mean daily dose during the follow-up period and the duration of medication on the other, the

Table 47. Neuroleptic medication of the patients during the first two years of follow-up

Daily dose converted to chlorpromazine[a]	Maximum daily dose	Mean daily dose during the follow-up
>300 mg	46	3
100–300 mg	46	19
<100 mg	6	12
variable doses for more than half of the follow-up period		12
for a few short periods		27
once for a short period		25
no medication	2	2

[a] Besides chlorpromazine, perphenazine, thioridazine, haloperidole, and levomepromazine were the neuroleptics commonly used.

medication being converted to chlorpromazine equivalents (in accordance with Lipton et al. 1978).

Although *the daily dose at its maximum* – generally at the early stages of the therapy – *exceeded 300 mg of chlorpromazine or an equivalent dose of some other neuroleptic for nearly half of the patients,* it appears that *the mean doses of the follow-up period were low,* and that only 34 patients, i.e. 1/3 of the series, received medication throughout the first two years of their therapy. In addition to the two patients without medication, there were 25 patients who only received medication for a short time at one stage.

The medication given *during the last three follow-up years* is shown in Table 48.

Table 48. Medication given to the patients during the last three years of follow-up

Daily dose converted to chlorpromazine[a]	Maximum daily dose	Mean daily dose during the follow-up
> 300 mg	23	11
100 – 300 mg	24	28
< 100 mg	10	18
no medication	38	38

This table does not show specifically the duration of medication, but only gives the mean daily dose of the follow-up period for each patient. It can be seen that during the last three follow-up years, 38 of our patients were without any neuroleptic medication, while 11 continued to receive a mean daily dose equivalent to more than 300 mg of chlorpromazine throughout the period.

During the first two follow-up years the medication given to the patients had strong connections with their clinical background variables. During the last three follow-up years several psychosocial variables in addition to the clinical variables were connected with the medication. The connections of the more-than-average medication during the whole 5-year follow-up period with the background variables are presented in Appendices 5 and 6.

The *logistic regression analysis* produced quite a straight-forward list of the variables explaining the quantity of medication during the whole follow-up period (Table 49).

In the entire series, the quantity of medication was explained by the presence of *regressive disintegration, the first therapeutic unit* (the Kupittaa Hospital versus out-patient care and the Clinic of Psychiatry), and the *presence of hostile or poorly understanding relatives* in the patient's family milieu. In the group of typical schizophrenics, the significance of hostile or poorly understanding relatives was also notable, and the group of regressive disintegration retained its significance. *Male sex* emerged as a third explaining variable.

What was the *mutual connection between medication and psychotherapy?* This question was also approached separately for the first two follow-up years and by analyzing the connections between the therapies conducted during the whole five-year follow-up (Table 35) and the medical treatments of the latter follow-up period.

The most significant observation for the *first two follow-up years* was that *the mean duration of medication during the follow-up and the implementation of psychotherapies*

Table 49. Larger neuroleptic medication during the follow-up years: influence of background variables (logistic regression analysis)

Explaining variables	R	p
All patients		
Group of regressive disintegration yes/no	2.26	0.000
First therapeutic unit		
Kupittaa Hospital/open care	1.66	0.003
Kupittaa Hospital/Clinic of Psychiatry	2.05	
Hostile or poorly understanding relatives yes/no	1.58	0.001
Typical schizophrenics		
Hostile of poorly understanding relatives yes/no	1.88	0.001
Group of regressive disintegration yes/no	1.57	0.003
Sex male/female	1.53	0.008

were positively correlated. Among the different modes of therapy, however, only the less intensive individual psychotherapy (connection of the level $p < .05$) and family therapy (combination of joint therapy of the primary family and couple therapy, $p < .1$) showed this connection, but when we separated the group of 61 psychotherapy cases from the others (as defined in the 2-year follow-up), the statistical connection with the quantity of medication became quite significant ($p = .0012$). The connections with the maximum daily dose were parallel, though less strong, being marginally significant ($p < .1$) for family therapies, community therapy and the group of psychotherapy cases. Of the 33 patients given intensive individual therapy, 17, or one half, had a maximum daily dose of more than 300 mg, and 11 patients included in this group received some medication for the whole of the follow-up period.

The findings give rise to two conclusions: 1) *not even higher doses of medication given at the early stages of the illness prevented the implementation of subsequent intensive psychotherapies,* and 2) *it was common in our series that psychotherapy was supported with neuroleptic medication although the doses remained at a low average level and the medication was discontinued as soon as the patient was no longer considered to need it.*

The connections between the medication received *during the third, fourth and fifth follow-up years* and the psychotherapies were *different* in direction. *The medication of the psychotherapy cases* – as defined on the basis of the mean daily dose of the follow-up period – *was now lesser* in quantity than that of the other patients, though only at a marginally significant level ($p = .097$). *Only one of our psychotherapy patients continued to have high-dose neuroleptic medication corresponding to more than 300 mg of chlorpromazine daily throughout the last follow-up years, whereas 10 other patients in the series had such high doses.*

The negative connections between intensive individual therapy and medication was not of significant level, however, 16 of the patients receiving intensive individual therapy had continued to have low doses and only 10 had been without any medication during the last three follow-up years.

The findings hence *clearly demonstrate that the patients given psychotherapy had less need for heavy psychopharmacotherapy during the latter follow-up period.* However, neuroleptic drugs in lower doses were not uncommon.

When the amount of neuroleptic medication during the whole follow-up period was examined in total (cf. Appendix 3, variable 5), no significant connections between this medication variable and the psychotherapy variables appeared. Nearest to significance was the connection between the group of psychotherapy cases and a lesser-than-average medication in the series of typical schizophrenic patients ($p = .112$). – It should be pointed out once again that – especially in the whole series – many patients excluded from the psychotherapy cases were among the least disturbed and their need for pharmacotherapy was also primarily of short duration.

The therapist's own notions of the significance of medication in the therapy of the patients were analyzed by means of the questionnaires mailed to them. Table 50 shows a summary of their assessments classified according to different modes of psychotherapy.

Even these assessments indicate that therapies were generally supported with medication. Only six therapies lacked any medication, and in 9 cases the medication was considered of no importance, although the patient had been taking his doses. For a majority of the therapies medication was considered useful. The differences between the different modes of therapy were relatively small. Only in three cases was the medication deemed to be of central importance. What attracts attention is that one of these cases belonged to the intensive individual therapies; it was the only therapy of this kind which was reported by the therapist to be based on a behaviour-therapeutic frame of reference.

Table 50. The assessments made by the therapists conducting the psychotherapies concerning the significance of medication in the therapies of the patients.

Therapist's assessment of the significance of medication	Intensive individual therapy	Less intensive individual therapy	Family therapy	Group therapy	Total
Medication of central importance and clearly useful	1	2	–	–	3
Medication important and helpful	7	8	7	–	22
Medication possibly helpful, but not of central importance	12	9	9	2	32
Medication mainly of psychologic significance for the patient, pharmacologic effect possibly not important	1	3	1	–	5
Medication not important	2	3	4	–	9
The patient had no medication during the therapy	3	2	1	–	6
Therapist's assessment not known	–	4	3	–	7

A case-specific analysis shows that the significance of medication was generally greater – even in the group of intensive individual therapies – in the cases where the therapy was slightly less frequent. As to the occupational groups of the therapists, it seems that psychologists had the highest relative number of therapies without medication, while all the three therapies by mental nurses belonged to the group "medication important and helpful".

5.3.2 Other Somatic Treatments

A few of our patients were given *other psychopharmacological medication* besides neuroleptics. Some patients with depressive symptoms were treated with antidepressive drugs. Somewhat greater amount of patients were given benzodiazepines to relieve their anxiety, usually for a shorter period of time. Both of these medications were administered in most cases together with the neuroleptic treatment, as an additional medication indicated by the patient's symptoms. One patient belonging to the group of schizo-affective psychoses was given litium treatment. We did not analyze the use of these medical treatments for different groups of patients more accurately, because we considered neuroleptic treatment essential in the treatment of patients belonging to the schizophrenia group. Moreover the part of patients given other psychopharmaca – especially antidepressants and litium – remained small in our sample and their significance in developing our orientation was peripheral.

Ten patients received *electroshock therapy*, 9 of them at the initial stages of the therapy and one during the latter period. All these therapies were given in the Kupittaa Hospital. Nine of these patients were men and only one a woman. Seven belonged to the group of typical schizophrenias, and one patient from each of the three other diagnostic subcategories received electroshock treatment.

Of the patients given electroschock treatment, 3 belonged to the group of psychotherapy cases. Two of these later received psychotherapeutic treatment (one intensive individual therapy, the other family therapy), in addition to which one patient given intensive treatment in a psychotherapeutic community at the early stages of this therapy was given electroshock treatment during a later hospitalization.

5.4 Social and Rehabilitative Measures

The number of rehabilitative measures carried out in the series is shown by the following table. The two follow-up periods have been considered separately.

Table 51. The social and rehabilitative measures applied to the patients during the follow-up

Quality of the rehabilitative or socially helpful measure	first 2 follow-up years	last 3 follow-up years
Occupational guidance or instruction in occupational or re-training	–	9
Help in getting a job, working experiment or other job-related arrangement	5	17
Financial help from the social welfare office	35	6
Residential arrangements	1	6
Support of psychotherapy by rehabilitation funds	5	2

The social and rehabilitative measures overlapped in several cases. During the last 3 years, altogether 22 patients were rehabilitated for work, and 14 were given other rehabilitative measures.

The need for rehabilitative measures was assessed in the followup study to be clearly greater than the amount of rehabilitation actually carried out. The assessments by the team concerning the need for rehabilitation are shown inTable 52.

Table 52. The assessments made by the team at the time of follow-up studies concerning the need for rehabilitation by the patients

Quality of the social and rehabilitative measure	2 year follow-up	5 year follow-up
Occupational guidance or instruction in occupational of re-training	35	29
Help in getting a job	32	18
Other job-related arrangement	1	2
Financial help	10	4
Residential arrangements	12	17
Help in the family situation	1	1
Other rehabilitative or social help	4	1
No need for rehabilitation	51	51
Dead or no assessment	4	5

The assessments concerning the need for rehabilitation also often overlapped: many of the patients needed several types of rehabilitation. About 45–50 % of the patients were estimated to be in need of various social and rehabilitative measures in both of the follow-up studies.

5.5 Selection of the Mode of Therapy in the Light of the Psychologic Basic Examination

The following account deals with *the connections between some of the findings made in the psychologic basic examination of the series and the selection of the patients for the different modes of therapy during the 5 year follow-up period.* The psychologic examination took place *independently* of the psychiatric basic examination, generelly slightly later, at the time of the patient's first period of treatment. The results have also been analyzed independently, and they are therefore of interest both in themselves and as a standard of reference for the findings based on the psychiatric basic examination.

We analyzed the correlations between *20 pre-selected psychologic variables* and *the implementation and intensity of the different modes of therapy.* The list of variables is presented in Appendix 2. The variables describe the basic personality and the cognitive state of the patient (ego capacities, controls, regression ability, discrimination between self and objects, intellectual capacities) on the one hand and the patient's way of experiencing and organizing his interpersonal relationships ("internalized object relationships") on the other. In accordance with the theory of object relations (e.g. Mahler 1968, Kernberg 1976, Urist 1980), we considered it important for the estimation of the therapeutic opportunities to analyze the world of internal object representations, which refers to the internal object images organized into a relatively constant form during the individual's development and which regulate and control his external behaviour (Blatt et al. 1975). Object representation, which is also called "frame of reference" in cognitive psychology, has turned out to be a sufficiently consistent, analyzable dimension of personality, which helps us to understand the orientation of the individual in social situations. These mental images filter, select and organize experiences and the mass of stimuli on the basis of their essential features, fitting them into an internal, generally highly simplified model. Correspondingly, in a psychotherapeutic relationship and the transference relation involved in it, the internal world of representations becomes activated, whereby even the patient's unconscious images, which are often of very early origin, bring forth their ideal and emotional components. Particularly the more serious psychic disorders have been found to involve fixation and regression into developmentally earlier object images, which are generally characterized by rigidity, stereotypy, inadequate correspondence with reality, decrease of human features, lack of differentiation and poor integration together with associated weak ambivalence and guilt tolerance, and a diminished ability to work through depressive feelings (Blatt et al. 1975, Kernberg 1975, 1976).

5.5.1 Internal Object World and Motivation to Therapy

The patient's conscious, favourable or unfavourable, attitudes towards therapy are often of crucial significance for the implementation of therapy, particularly psychotherapies (as is also pointed out by Benedetti, 1983b). We also noted in our own series that the patients' attitudes recorded at the time of admission were of considerable prognostic value for the implementation of all modes of psychotherapy, and that the effect of these attitudes continued to be of statistical significance as long as two years after the admission. When, at the time of the psychologic examination, we divided the patients into *two groups* on the *basis of the attitudes they showed towards the different modes of psychotherapy*: the groups with favourable and unfavourable attitudes (which were roughly equal in size), notable *differences were seen in their ways of perceiving human objects*. This internal object world was examined by analyzing the responses the patients gave in a projective test (Object Relation Technique, Phillipson) at the time of the basic examination. Protocol raters (advanced undergraduates of psychology) whose inter-rater reliability (.60–.90) turned out satisfactory on all variables – were not aware of the patients' motivation to therapy, nor of the subsequent therapeutic outcome.

When these two groups with different motivations to therapy were mutually compared, it appeared that the patients with a negative attitude typically had vague, impersonal, scant and lifeless mental images. Compared with their controls, these patients typically lacked interest in human objects. The patients who were better motivated to therapy, on the other hand, showed more interest in and need for human contacts, mentally investing objects both libidinally and narcissistically (from the viewpoint of their own needs). They also expressed more affects in their mental images, showing mourning, longing and depression, for example, whereas the patients with a negative attitude responded to the different frustrating situations (separation, loss, loneliness) more often with apparently chronic powerlessness, emotional coldness and denial of sorrow. Their way of expressing emotions was even otherwise scant or non-genuine, external or schizoid. The better motivated patients more often dealt with interpersonal and internal conflicts in their mental images, while the individuals who tended to refuse therapy denied the conflicts or externalized or concretized them. The aforesaid properties made up a dimension of their own in our set of variables (i.e. a factor), and we considered the *central characteristic underlying motivation to therapy to be overall involvement in human relationships or lack of such involvement, which signifies poverty of the object world.*

With regard to their mental world, the patients with a negative attitude towards psychotherapy resemble the psychosomatic patients who have been described with the concept "alexithymia" (Sifneos 1972). They have the same difficulty of recognizing, maintaining and working through emotional states in themselves, as their thinking is more fixed in the concrete reality and their fantasy world is scant. McDougall (1982) has postulated this to be a special psychotic defence, which is even more massive than the other primitive defences. The alexithymic situation would protect the patient against internal life and vividness, which, if fully recognized, would mean a threat to the patient's right to existence, an increased risk of fragmentation, or a possibility of uncontrolled outbursts.

We know from experience, however, that the patients who split emotional and human experience from their reality arouse intense emotions in the people around them, including the therapeutic staff. The feelings of counter-transference are characterized by frustration, boredom and flatness, which often discourage the receiver. Quite understandably, the reactions of the therapist easily result in increased distance, and the therapy remains superficial or external, not reaching the psychotherapeutic level of intensity. Our own findings seem to suggest that the conventional medical model is applied more often to these patients than to the others, which agrees well with the patients' own notion of their illness as a concretized somatic disorder.

5.5.2 Inclusion in and Exclusion from the Group of Psychotherapy Cases

The implementation of psychotherapy is affected by not only the patient's motivation and other subjective properties, but also a number of different environmental and random factors which are difficult to pinpoint in the research arrangement. Despite this, we noted several significant correlations between the implementation of therapy and the patient's characteristics in our series. We also separately compared the group of psychotherapy cases with the rest of the series. *It seems to be of essential importance for the successful implementation of psychotherapy to recognize the significance of human objects for the patient's mental world.* Hence the patients who are autistically indifferent in their object relations remained outside psychotherapy more often than the others. This quality of autistic indifference was conspicuous in 19 % of the psychotherapy cases, but nearly half of the patients not given psychotherapy (45 %, $p = .010$). A parallel observation was also made on the initial motivation to therapy.

A favourable prognostic sign for the implementation of therapy was also subjective loneliness and lack of objects, even when it was described as chaotic and desperate ($p = .032$). The developmental level of the object relations also serves as a discriminatory factor: The patients excluded from the psychotherapy cases were only rarely capable of adult mutuality and consideration for others; this correlation was particularly obvious in the group of typical schizophrenic patients ($p = .002$).

The patients outside the psychotherapy group also appeared to have more fragile ego structures ($p = .074$), and they had difficulties in object differentiation (maintenance of the ego boundaries) more often than the others ($p = .046$). These patients tended to accumulate in the group of abundant neuroleptic medication, as will be pointed out below. They also had a more marked tendency to isolate their problems instead of analyzing them at the psychologic level ($p = .09$).

In order to reveal the possible combined effects of several variables, a *logistic regression analysis* was carried out, which produced a two-variable solution: *According to this analysis, exclusion from the psychotherapy group correlates with two factors, 1) dominance of autistic object relations in the patient's mental world ($p = .017$), and 2) no tendency to symbiotic reliance in his object relations ($p = .003$).* The symbiotic and autistic tendencies in interpersonal relationships were shown by the present findings to be polar opposites, which explain the successful implementation of psychosocial therapies to a notable extent. What is crucial is the significance possessed by human objects in the individual's mental world. It is not equally important, however, whether the object investment is positive (e.g. loving) or negative (e.g. aggressive), or whether it is well developed (adult level love) or regressive (child-like dependence).

5.5.3 Implementation of Individual Therapy

Individual therapies – particularly intensive individual therapy – seem to be the most demanding modes of treatment with regard to the patient's individual-psychologic properties. The group of patients given individual therapy turned out, even initially, to be *more homogenous* than the groups selected for other modes of therapy. Of the different variables examined here, those representing the patient's internal object relations appeared to predict most reliably even the progress of individual psychotherapy. Hence, the patients given individual therapies (both intensive and less intensive) included significantly more individuals with developmentally mature object relations with qualities of adult human relationships, such as equality, mutuality, empathy, caring and more developed affects, e.g. guilt, and an ability to deal with emotions arising in triadic situations, such as envy, competition and jealousy. (As it was pointed out, these patients showed more neurotic symptoms at the time of the basic examination already). Despite their psychosis, they hence also had more developed sectors in their personality.

Of the patients given intensive individual therapy, 27 % were estimated to have object relations of more than average maturity, while the corresponding figure for the rest of the patients was 3 % ($p = .005$). The developmental level of the object relations was, quite consistently, the higher, the more intensive the therapy: in less intensive individual therapy the afore-mentioned figure was 14 %, and in the group not given individual therapy 0 % ($p = .004$). The psychologic examination did not show the psychotherapy patients to have significantly more symbiotic tendencies or any search for narcissistic objects satisfying their own needs, but their repertoire of objects was wider and more versatile in differentation, and they were better able than the others to tolerate even mental images with conflicting affects ($p = .012$). A tendency to paranoid or omnipotent control in the object images, however, significantly reduced the probability of individual therapy ($p = .013$), just as a reserved or suspicious contact in the clinical basic examination was found to be a poor predictive sign. The patients who tended to use paranoid or other controls remained outside individual therapies significantly more often than the others, being given various other supportive contacts ($p = .002$).

Patients showing some insight even initially were selected into the group of individual therapy, which often further endeavoured to increase the patients' insight into their own problems ($p = .019$), and this correlation was particularly clear in the group of intensive individual therapies ($p = .0008$). Unlike the patients not given individual therapy, the patients in the intensive individual therapy group less frequently denied or externalized the conflicts in their interpersonal relationships. The patients given individual therapy were also found to have fewer disorders of the cognitive level (thinking, attentiveness) ($p = .019$); the individuals with no cognitive disorders accounted for 50 % of the group given intensive individual therapy, 39 % of those given less intensive individual therapy, and 6 % of the patients excluded from these groups. The difference between the two extreme groups is statistically significant.

The estimated tendency to psychologic insight also discriminated between the two groups of individual therapy. In the group of less intensive individual therapy, a majority, i.e. 64 %, were individuals with no observable effort to understand matters psychologically (psychological-mindedness).

5.5.4 Selection for Family Therapy

The patients selected into the family therapy group had psychologic characteristics that were different from – partly even opposite to – the characteristics of the individual therapy patients described above. The patients who, together with their families, attended family therapy had a more conspicuous tendency to omnipotent object control and associated reserve in their interpersonal relationships (p = .058). This variable also discriminated best between the family therapy patients and those who were given only individual therapy. Particularly the patients whose families were given special support avoided dependence in their object relations and seldom (only 15 %) showed symbiotic reliance, which was noted in 85 % of the other patients. The patients who ended up in regular family therapy had experienced chaotic internal loneliness and lack of objects more often than the others (p = .030). They also included a large number of patients whose object relations were estimated to be developmentally immature, poorly differentiated, and mostly focussed on a dyadic relationship (p = .050).

It was further observed that family intervention was often used in the case of patients considered to have difficulties in controlling their impulses; the impulse control of 72 % had been estimated as inadequate, the corresponding percentage for the others being 28 % (p = .069). These patients were also found to have fewer cognitive, intellectual means available to control situations: both the estimated potential and the actual intelligence were found to be lower in this group than in the group excluded from family therapy (p = .024). All the patients recommended for therapy of the primary family were more talented than the average, while those recommended for therapy of the secondary family were below the average intellectual level.

The *logistic regression analysis* brought out two explaining factors which were not found to have any combined effect: the *family therapy groups most probably included the patients whose world was characterized by chaotic loneliness,* and who simultaneously were found to have the *fewest cognitive means for coping*. This model fitted quite well to our series (p = .0745).

5.5.5 Selection for Community Therapy

As it is quite understandable, the group of community therapy included a larger amount of patients whose ability to maintain the ego boundaries was more seriously disturbed than in e.g. the group of individual therapy patients (p = .061). The patients who end up in a psychotherapeutic community quite often show a typical tendency in their object relations to seek for supportive need objects, which they often feel to be extensions of their own selves (p = .009). This tendency was particularly clear in the patients of the intensive treatment in psychotherapeutic community, of whom 44 % showed this feature at the time of the basic examination already, while the corresponding property was only recorded in 19 % of the other patients.

Another feature illustrative of the object relations in this group was the lesser tendency to control the external object and to maintain paranoid reserve (p = .013). Clinical paranoia was hence less frequent in community therapy, which seemed to select very clearly patients with regressive disintegration, as it was mentioned above. Object relations coloured by paranoid or omnipotent control were noted in only 13 % of the community patients, but in 38 % of the other patients.

The patients selected for intensive and less intensive community therapy differed from each other in several respects: The patients taken into the intensive community admitted more openly their dependence, helplessness and need, and were also better able to tolerate intimacy. The patients receiving less intensive community therapy were characterized, at least superficially, by better coping: they had serious cognitive disorders and lability less frequently (p = .008), and their overall control of impulses was more stable (p = .009. They also included a large number of patients who emphatically kept up a distance in their object relations. As many as 77 % tended to annihilate the human element in the interpersonal relationships, showing schizoid distance (p = .034).

It was also interesting to observe that the patients in our series who were not estimated to have a capacity for mourning or depression associated with working through problems were at the lower level of community therapy. These patients had solved their problems by limiting themselves to e.g. emotionally cold depression, feelings of narcissistic rage, or by resorting to primitive defences, e.g. denial of feelings of sorrow (p = .023). The ability to experience depression was less common among the community patients (27 %) than among those given individual therapy (50 %), but the difference is not statistically significant. In the group given intensive community therapy, those with and without the ability to experience depression were distributed more evenly. The patients given less intensive community therapy were thus estimated to be a more uniform group, ostensibly able to cope and more independent, but yet not able to tolerate any more detailed and profound analysis of their problems.

5.5.6 Selection for Pharmacotherapy

The amount of neuroleptic medication received by the patient was found to have several correlations with the clinical variables. The average dose of neuroleptic medication could also be predicted with considerable accuracy on the basis of several individual-psychologic variables.

The patients who received higher-than-average amount of medication during the 5 years follow-up period had more disturbances of the basic personality at the time of the basic examination already: the psychologic examinations showed their ability to maintain the ego boundaries to be impaired in several cases (p = .002). Even generally speaking, their ego structures were estimated to be more fragile and they frequently showed extensive fragmentation, helplessness and other ego dysfunctions (p = .002). Their cognitive functions were also more often seriously disturbed and they showed a decline of the intellectual level (p = .003).

In their object relations, these patients showed a tendency to isolation which was characterized by withdrawal into autism and a lack of interest in objects. This correlation was particularly marked in the group of typical schizophrenias, in which all (100 %) of the patients given higher-than-average dose of medication were estimated to lack objects, while the corresponding percentage in the group of low-dose medication was 55 % (p = .001). Many of the patients receiving more medication were also poorly able to tolerate intimacy and liable to maintain a schizoid distance (p = .088). Their object relations were estimated to be generally undeveloped and primitive. This correlation, too, was particularly clear in the group of typical schizophrenic patients (p = .002). The patients on heavy medication even initially showed hardly any tendency to psychologic insight; instead, they more often isolated, concretized or denied the conflicts associated with their interpersonal relationships (p = .020), which tendency is opposite to that noted among the patients selected for individual therapies. The patients who continued to have high doses of psychopharmacas throughout the follow-up period typically gave up their fight against decompensation at a very early stage (p = .019).

The *logistic regression analysis* brings up two variables, one of which describes the object relations and the other the patient's cognitive state. The patients who received more medication throughout the 5 year follow-up period were characterized by: 1) *a notable decline of their cognitive capacities at the time of admission already* and simultaneously 2) *a notable lack of development in their object relations, which were typically narrow and rigid.*

5.5.7 Summary

The clinical basic examination showed that the group of psychotherapy cases consisted of patients with slightly more serious disturbances, and that the regressively disintegrated patients were selected especially for family therapies, community therapies and less intensive individual therapies. The patients selected into a given therapeutic group sometimes had – regardless of their clinical symptoms – certain specific characteristics favourable for that particular mode of psychotherapy. The findings of the psychologic basic examination support these findings in several respects. Despite the differences in the research methods, the positive correlation between the patient's insight and the therapeutic opportunities, particularly in the group of patients given individual psychotherapy, was a parallel finding. The psychologic basic examination evaluated particularly the patient's *ability to deal with his intrapsychic or interpersonal conflicts at a psychologic level*(psychological-mindedness). The patients who showed interest in analyzing their difficulties and seeking for constructive solutions also possessed a conscious motivation for therapy more often than the others and seldom remained outside the reach of psychotherapeutic measures. Opposite to them were the patients who tried to deny or project their problems or analyzed them in a concrete, non-psychologic way and, instead of receiving psychotherapy, were often given neuroleptic medication in higher-than-average doses.

Another finding verified by the two different approaches was that *depressive symptoms* turned out a favourable indicator of the therapeutic outcome. The psychologic examination evaluated the patient's typical reactions to separations, losses and frustrations, showing that the patients motivated to therapy were able to tolerate and express their depressive feelings genuinely and at the affective level more often than the patients reluctant to have therapy. The patients who actively tried to deny depression and sorrow or, instead, were engulfed by manic emotions or feelings of internal rage also showed more resistance to the psychotherapeutic efforts. Even therapies that began as intensive were occasionally discontinued at an early stage in this group of patients.

The psychologic basic examination did not determine the patient's clinical status, but tried to define the ego-level capacities of the patient's basic personality, which may have been relatively stable even before the onset of manifest psychosis. We were able to find *three specific factors illustrative of the ego functions which are somewhat compatible with the chances of psychotherapy in this series:* the overall estimate of ego strength, the quantity of cognitive disorders, and the capacity of object discrimination (the degrees of blurring of the ego boundaries). The patients who had had particularly many difficulties in maintaining their boundaries were more often excluded from the psychotherapy group and received neuroleptic medication in higher-than-average doses. 61 % of the patients in intensive community therapy had been found to have especially marked problems in maintaining their ego boundaries; the patients in the group of less intensive community therapy were distributed more uniformly on this dimension. The patients given individual therapy, in turn, typically had fewer problems pertaining to the ego boundaries. The significance of this variable for the opportunities of therapy is understandable, because the patients, when they feel their identity to be threatened, resort to the typical defences, such as schizoid unemotionality, stereotypic negativism, paranoid distance, or absolute refusal, which constitutes a significant threat to the psychosocial therapeutic effort, although they may fundamentally long for human help. In the cases of these patients, the lack of motivation to therapy often conceals a particular fear of closeness and a threat to existence, and the pathologic defences pose a special challenge for the endurance of the staff.

The situation with regard to the other ego capacities seems to be parallel: the patients with the weakest original ego functions, the most fragmented and helpless in the psychologic examination, seem to be overrepresented among those excluded from the psychotherapy group or receiving higher-than-average medication at the time of the 5-year follow-up examination. In the same way, definite cognitive dysfunctions were seen less frequently in the test results of the patients selected for intensive individual therapy or less intensive community therapy, but particularly often in the group of patients with higher neuroleptic medication. The patients on pharmacotherapy also show the interesting point that a notable proportion of them gave up their attempts at compensation at a very early stage of the therapy. The patient's first unit of therapy and its therapeutic orientation may naturally contribute to this.

Of the different ego capacities, a lack of impulse control was typical of the future family therapy patients. It was particularly conspicuous among the ones whose therapy largely consisted of mere support to the family members. The family therapy patients were found to have a marked tendency to acting out behaviour, lack of persistence and poor control of drive impulses (especially aggressions). The family therapies have thus been carried out on a therapeutically more difficult part of our series. Patients with impulse problems have also been admitted into intensive treatment in therapeutic communities, while the patients who had had less intensive community treatment had better-than-average self-control and adaptation capacity.

According to the psychologic examination, a successful accomplishment of psychotherapy in this series was predicted particularly by the quality of the patient's internal object relations. This is understandable, as we are dealing with modes of therapy based on human contact and interaction. The significance of internalized objects, especially the "positive introjections", has been emphasized particularly for the setting up of the therapeutic relationship and the control of the anxiety associated with this (Giovacchini 1979; Kernberg 1976) The most significant factor in our own series turned out to be the *object investment* and its disturbances. The patients who were predominantly indifferent or only concentrated on themselves were seldom psychotherapy cases and were extremely seldom admitted into the group of intensive individual therapy. They very often belonged, even originally, to the group of patients who had a negative attitude towards psychotherapy and who typically also lacked internal life. The autistic tendency also notably increased the probability of heavy medication. The polar opposite of autism in the present series was the tendency to symbiotic reliance, which generally promoted the opportunities of psychotherapy.

Another phenomenon that posed difficulties to therapy was the tendency to control the object relations, which may take the form of projective identification, reserve and withdrawal into omnipotent attitudes, or an effort to change the object more than one's self. This kind of patients were often left out of intensive individual therapy – sometimes even of the intensive therapeutic community. The method of choice in their case was often support to the other family members. Schizoid distance in the interpersonal relationships was the third, but not equally difficult, hindrance to psychotherapy. Patients with a sterile interval in their human relationships were also given intensive individual therapy, but in community therapy the outcome in their case was quite modest. According to our findings, an effort to utilize the object – even if quite limited – is a more favourable sign of psychotherapeutic success. Particularly the community patients typically strive too seek for need objects to complement themselves.

The developmental level of the internal object relations, which were here measured with projective tests, also clearly correlates with the intensity of therapy, particularly as regards dyadic therapies. Generalizing, we might say that the patient's ability to appreciate the adult features of his interpersonal relationships, such as independence, mutuality and responsibility, has a favourable effect on the progress of the psychotherapeutic relationship.

5.6 Summary and Discussion

This chapter has been dealing with the implementation of psychotherapeutic activities and the factors which contributed to the selection of patients for the different modes of treatment. The latter aspect was explored by means of logistic regression analyses, where the variables under study included 45 variables pertaining to the patients' clinical status and psychosocial background as well as the first therapeutic unit (see Appendix 1).

Same kind of analyses were made regarding the findings of an independent psychological examination (psychologic variables, see Appendix 2). Because this examination was executed somewhat later than the psychiatric basic examination, it is possible that some of its findings were already, in minor amount, influenced by the quality of the patients' first therapeutic encounter in different treatment units.

We are moderately content with the number of psychotherapeutic activities undertaken in our project, although the optimal extent and intensity seeing to the needs of the patients and their families was not yet reached. As we already pointed out in Chapter 1.2. (see Table1), the quantitative staff resources of both our clinic and the entire Turku Mental Health District were relatively modest. This was particularly true of out-patient care: the number of staff in the Turku Mental Health Office per the number of population it was responsible for was notably below the average for the whole country. We can hence conclude that the *qualitative resources are clearly more crucial than the quantitative resources in the development of psychotherapeutic treatment for the patients of the schizophrenia group*. In this respect, the Turku Mental Health District with its university hospital is in a better-than-average position. This does not mean, however, that a corresponding and even more advanced development of therapeutic activities would not be possible in ordinary community psychiatric circumstances both in Finland and elsewhere.

Our *psychotherapeutic orientation is psychodynamic*, being essentially based on psychoanalytic theory formation. This does not mean that our therapeutic activities would be psychoanalytic or that the psychotherapies that were carried out, even as regards the intensive individual therapies, would be predominantly "exploratory and insight-oriented" (Stanton et al. 1984). Our therapies can most pertinently be called *supportive therapeutic relationships based on empathic and reliable contact,* which have variably also included goals of promoting the patient's insight into his own problems and the developmental process taking place in him.

In accordance with the integrated model of illness, we undertook both individual-, family- and community-oriented therapies. At the time when our project was started, the psychiatry in Turku was undergoing an active developmental process in the field of individual therapies, the reason for it being that the psychoanalytic training had become possible in Turku a few years before, psychoanalytically oriented seminars and supervision had been developed energetically in the Clinic of Psychiatry, and interest in the development of the individual therapies of even schizophrenic patients was great. Our psychotherapeutic communities were also being developed actively. The progress of family therapies was slower: although an effort was made also to promote family therapy, the actual boom of development and training in this field occurred in Turku only at the time of the present follow-up examinations.

According to the criteria that we set, we were able to classify 56 of our original 100 patients as "psychotherapy cases". It should be borne in mind that while listing both the individual and family therapies and the group therapies (which were infrequent in our series) we only included the cases where the therapy – though often initiated on a hospital ward – was also continued on an out-patient basis. We supplemented the inadequate community psychiatric resources by cooperating with the private sector, with which we were in close contact for the very reason that many of the psychiatrists and psychologists working in the clinic or another unit of the public sector also had some private office hours. Even so, the private sector only accounted for about 20 % of the therapeutic relationships established with out-patients. The figure was highest in the group of intensive individual therapies, where it covered about one third of the therapies. In the hospitals no beds for private patients existed.

The most central prerequisite for the extent of therapeutic activities now reached was, however, the *extensive participation of the different occupational categories of the staff in the therapeutic activities* in two central units of the community sector, the Clinic of Psychiatry and the Mental Health Office responsible for the out-patient activities. The individual, family and group therapies listed in the follow-up examinations were carried out by altogether 52 therapists. Only 15 % of them had had actual psychotherapeutic training. A majority of the others based their work on intensive on-the-job training and supervision of their therapeutic relationships. Our system of supervision was also inadequate, only covering about 2/3 of the therapies, and half of these partly (including most of the long-term therapies). Within the scope of the present project, it was not possible to analyze systematically the connections between supervision and the therapeutic outcome. Nevertheless, our experience indicated conclusively that a *necessary condition for the adequacy of the therapeutic resources for long-term psychotherapies of psychotic patients is that the therapist is given continuous supervision in the therapy of at least one of his patients*, and that he has an opportunity to discuss, when necessary, even the problems of his other therapeutic relationships with the supervisor.

The largest occupational group among the therapists consisted of psychiatrists and physicians specializing in psychiatry on the one hand and specialized nurses on the other, in addition to which psychologists contributed notably to the therapeutic work, particularly in intensive individual therapies. The standard of specialized nurses is high in Finland. After 2½ years of undergraduate training in nursing they also attend a one-year course of specialized studies, which is markedly psychodynamic in orientation at least in Turku.

The role of social workers and mental nurses with short training was lesser. In addition to the specialized psychiatric nurses, however, the latter group contributed crucially to the work of the psychotherapeutic communities, both in the group activities and as "personal nurses".

A good indication of the significance of personality as well as knowledge of the problems of schizophrenic patients acquired by the nursing staff in their practical work was given by the fact that *no great or systematic differences emerged between the outcomes of therapy in the most central occupational groups*.

To what extent was the need for different modes of therapy met, and what kind of patients were selected for the different therapies?

The results were numerically the best and also (quantitatively) closest to the original therapeutic plans of our team in individual therapies on the one hand and in psychotherapeutic community therapy on the other. As regards family-oriented therapy, the highest figures were reached in separate support given to the family members, while the role of actual family therapy remained less significant. Only two out-patients attended structured group therapy (and even one of these continued participation in the group established on the hospital ward). This shortcoming was, however, partly compensated for by the central role of the different group activities in the psychotherapeutic communities (cf. Alanen 1975) of the hospital and day hospital wards. The facilities for rehabilitation were markedly defective, being quite poorly developed in the Turku Mental Health District in the late 1970's.

These overall conclusions were confirmed by *the estimates of the team and the independent examiner made in the two-year follow-up examination* as to what would have been the actual optimal need for psychotherapeutic treatments in the series. These retrograde estimations are included in the following discussion.

Initial intervention in crisis, the purpose of which was, by means of frequent contacts and often family- or environment-oriented therapy, to prevent the patient from being away from his normal social life sphere for a longer period, was given to 28 patients, which was accordant with our plans. Of these treatments, 11 were given completely on an out-patient basis, while 17 included a short in-patient period. It turned out that treatments of this kind were generally more successful among female patients than among male, in addition to which the therapeutic opportunities, particularly among out-patients, were clearly enhanced if the patient had empathic relatives. In our opinion, the number of interventions in crisis should have been markedly higher, if there had been more resources available for out-patient therapy.

Individual therapy lasting for at least two years and consisting of a minimum of 80 sessions was given to 26 patients of the 100 in our series. Slightly more than half of these therapeutic relationships were being continued at the time of the five-year follow-up examination, though generally with less frequent sessions. 31 other patients were given less intensive individual therapy, which lasted for at least 6 months and consisted of a minimum of 12 sessions.

According to the estimates made by the team in the two-year follow-up examination, 79 of our one hundred patients should have been offered the opportunity of an individual-therapeutic contact to explore the problems that contributed to the onset of their illness and to initiate a possible personal process of development at some stage of the therapy – either at the very beginning or later on. The estimate by the independent examiner was more or less the same: 62 of the 80 patients she interviewed would have been in need of individual therapy or a supportive individual contact. In the light of these figures, the *need for individual therapy in our series was met, quantitatively speaking, in about 70 % of the cases*. Of the patients who were estimated not to benefit from individual therapy even in a less intensive form, part were patients who were most pertinently and adequately treated with family therapy (this was particularly the case with many of the married patients), while another part were individuals whose labile personality or social condition seemed to prevent the creation of any long-term individual contact.

The group selected particularly for long-term individual therapy, here called intensive individual therapy, consisted of patients whose personality features were better suited to this than the personalities of most other patients. According to the *logistic regression analysis*, the two background factors explaining most crucially the selection for intensive individual therapy in the whole series were the *patient's preliminary insight into the connections between his illness and his problems* at the time of the basic examination on the one hand, and the *lack of acting out behaviour* (which often resulted in a break-down of the therapeutic relationship) on the other. The next explaining variables were acute onset of the symptoms and (particularly among the patients with borderline schizophrenia) presence of neurotic symptoms. The independent *psychologic examination* confirmed the significance of insightfulness for the selection for intensive individual therapy and also revealed a connection between the developmental level of the patient's object relationships and the implementation of individual therapy in the series.

The individual therapies often also involved – and their long-term implementation was clearly aided by – support given to the relatives upon the patient's consent.

More intensive *conjoint family therapy* – which corresponded to infrequent individual therapy as to the criteria set for duration and the number of sessions: at least six months, a minimum of 12 sessions – was given to 15 patients in our series, in addition to which at least 3 conjoint family sessions were held in 10 cases. Of these 25 family therapies 10 were given to the patient's primary family and 14 to the procreated "secondary family", mostly as couple therapies of the patient and his or her spouse. One family therapy belonged to both groups: it included the patient, her mother and her separated husband. In 40 cases the *patient's family members* were supported through separate contacts beyond the interviews carried out at the different stages of the project. As many of these belonged to the cases where family therapy was carried out, it can be concluded that *family-oriented therapy in some form was given to altogether 50 patients in our series*.

In the two-year follow-up examination the team estimated that conjoint family therapy or couple therapy would have been needed in 59 cases, and separate support to a family member in yet another 25 cases. The estimates by the independent examiner were clearly lower: for the 80 patients she interviewed, she considered actual family therapy to be indicated in 23 cases and support to relatives in yet other 15 cases. This difference in the estimates is partly due to the fact that, unlike the team, the independent examiner did not meet family member in her interviews.

According to the estimates by the team, the *need for actual family therapy was hence satisfied in more than 40 % cases*, and, even in these, often quite inadequately. *If, however, all the family-oriented activities are considered, the percentage of implementation becomes higher, approaching 60 %*.

The very difference between the estimates of the needs by the team and the independent examiner shows the subjective nature of the estimates of this kind. Our own notion is that psychiatrists still tend to underestimate the need for family-oriented therapy compared with the opinions of the patients and their families concerning the need for such therapy and motivation to it. Aaltonen (1982), who carried out an investigation in the Turku Mental Health Office, found out that of all the first admission patients (not only patients of the schizophrenia group), 61 % of those with a family wished to have family therapy either alone or in combination with individual therapy, when offered this opportunity. The experiences obtained in the Turku schizophrenia project in the 1980's similarly agree to a considerable extent with the estimates presented above by the team concerning both the need for family therapy and the motivation of the patients and their families to it, when the family was already met conjointly and its situation explored at the time of the first diagnostic intervention for planning the therapy.

Of the 28 patients married at the time of the basic examination, exactly half, i.e. 14, were given couple therapy. While making the therapeutic plans, we considered couple therapy indicated for 80 % of these patients. *Implementation of couple therapies in our series corresponded clearly better to the need than did the therapies of primary families. They also turned out to be clearly easier for the therapists lacking family therapy training and resulted in a better outcome*.

In a *logistic regression analysis* where all the patients given actual family therapy were compared as a group with the rest of the series, selection for family therapy in the whole series turned out to be explained most centrally by the background variables of *inclusion in the ego-dynamic group of regressive disintegration* and *stabilized heterosexual identity*. The former of these was influenced by the patients given conjoint therapy of the primary family, the latter by the patients given couple therapy. *The group given conjoint therapy of the primary family included quite seriously ill patients*, who were characterized by both clinical severity of their condition (8 typical schizophrenics, of whom 7 belonged to the group of regressive disintegration) and enmeshment with their families as well as a lack of occupational identity. The patients given couple therapy also included more patients diagnosed as typically schizophrenic than did the group of married patients not given this mode of therapy.

The *psychologic examination* confirmed that the patients selected for family therapy were more seriously ill than those given individual therapy. It showed that the group given family therapy included particularly patients whose internal representational world was characterized by chaotic loneliness and who were simultaneously found to have the fewest cognitive means for coping.

The low percentage of *group therapies* among the therapeutic activities can be partly explained by the amount of other group processes on the wards. The estimates of the team and the independent psychiatric examiner concerning the need for group therapy in the two-year follow-up examination bring out the notion predominantly held within our therapeutic orientation, which suggests that the *significance of group therapy for new schizophrenic patients is more secondary than that of individual and family therapy*: according to the team's retrograde estimate, group therapy would have been useful for 8 patients (the corresponding figure being 10 at the time of making the therapeutic plans), while the independent examiner considered 4 patients to have benefited from group therapy. Our notion of the lesser significance of group therapy compared with individual and family therapy is based on the primary role of individual and family dynamics as a background of the developmental disorder of schizophrenic patients.

3/4 of our patients were admitted via a hospital ward, in addition to which 5 were admitted via a day hospital ward. During the first year already the patients in need of hospital treatment numbered 85, which number further increased up to 88 by the end of the five-year follow-up. Day hospital treatment was given to 24 patients, 3 of them lacking any hospital admissions. *Nearly 2/3 of the patients, i.e. 56, were classified as having received psychotherapeutic community therapy at some stage of their treatment.* The psychotherapeutic communities included the wards of the Clinic of Psychiatry and its small day hospital. For a patient to be classified in this group, however, it was required that – apart from having experienced the empathic approach by the staff, often by a "personal nurse" – he had really actively participated in the group and community processes on the ward. In the other mental hospital of the district, where about 1/3 of the hospital treatments were given, no community therapy exceeding the conventional routine was implemented. The team suggests that, *in principle, the hospital treatment needed by all patients of the schizophrenia group should include treatment in psychotherapeutic community*, if the patients remain on the ward long enough to be able to participate in the community processes.

We have defined the central goals of the therapeutic processes of psychotherapeutic communities for psychotic patients (Alanen 1975) as follows:

1. an empathic orientation shared by the members of the community,
2. an emphasis placed on open communication, and
3. importance of individual therapeutic relationships.

As the development continued, the fourth goal appeared to consist of extending the therapeutic approach to the interactional network of the families and the patient's other subjectively important people, and, generally, extending the work outside the ward boundaries, to support the patients in their life outside the hospital.

The question of the duration of the hospital treatment needed by psychotic patients has been disputed over the past few years. Glick et al. (1976, 1979) in the USA reported findings showing that first admission schizophrenic patients who were in hospital for a relatively long period (90–120 days) were in a better condition after one-year follow-up than patients who were otherwise similar, but had been in hospital for a short time (21. 28 days). No corresponding difference was noted for non-schizophrenic patients. On the other hand, Herz et al. (1977) have been strongly arguing for short-term hospitalization. Caton et al. (1982) saw no difference in the effects of either short or long hospital treatment on subsequent treatment compliance or the patient's subsequent clinical and social status.

According to Glick et al., longer hospital treatment made both the schizophrenic patient himself and the people important to him better accept the need for therapy and permitted better arrangements for long-term out-patient treatment. This agrees with our own experiences, which show that many of the most seriously disturbed patients are only able after a relatively long in-patient period to establish a therapeutic contact which makes it possible to arrange more permanent therapy. The same is also true of the contacts with relatives: it often takes a long time to win their confidence. Even so, we also saw "the other side of the coin" at the initial stages of our therapeutic communities: the excessively long in-patient periods had their drawbacks which were further accentuated by the lack of adequate out-patient facilities. These drawbacks were brought out clearly by the 8-year follow-up study of first admission schizophrenics treated in the Clinic of Psychiatry in 1969 made by Salokangas(1985). He emphasizes that long in-patient periods should be avoided in the treatment of schizophrenic patients, particularly when the functional and rehabilitative activities of the hospital are scant. The findings revealed that the patients who were initially hospitalized for a long period also tended to have long in-patient periods later on.

In our own series, the patients treated on the wards of the Clinic of Psychiatry spent an average of 73.44 days in hospital after the first admission. This period was clearly longer than the 27.0 days of the patients of the Kupittaa Hospital. The difference was levelled off soon, however, and the patients first admitted into the Clinic of Psychiatry spent less time in hospital on an average during the second to fifth follow-up years than did the patients first admitted into the Kupittaa Hospital. The difference was not due to the patients first admitted into the Clinic being clinically more seriously ill, rather the opposite. Among the patients of the Kupittaa Hospital, however, some negative background variables were conspicuous, including the relatively greater proportion of men, who clearly needed more hospital treatment during the follow-up period than women. Nevertheless, we considered it to be demonstrated on the basis of the continuity and consistency of the findings on the need for hospital treatment during the follow-up periods that a *first hospitalization in a psychotherapeutic milieu, whose duration is determined by the therapeutic needs of the patient and his environment, reduces the subsequent need for hospital treatment by the schizophrenic patients*, provided that the period is really used actively for therapy. It should also be recognized that one goal of hospital treatment is always to plan the necessary out-patient therapy in accordance with the patient's needs.

Our psychotherapeutic communities were in charge of seriously disturbed patients. In a logistic regression analysis carried out particularly on the differences between the patients given intensive community therapy or intervention in crisis in a psychotherapeutic community (who mainly differed with regard to the duration of the in-patient period) and the rest of the series, the first explaining variable in both the whole series and the group of typical schizophrenics was inclusion in the *ego-dynamic group of regressive disintegration*. The next explaining variables were the *patient's sex* (female) and *exclusion from the group of imminent disintegration* in the whole series, and *scantness of interpersonal relationships outside the primary family* and *presence of depressive symptoms* in the group of typical schizophrenics. The *psychologic examination* of the same group emphasized the tendency of particularly these patients (despite the serious disturbance of their ego boundaries) in the whole series to seek for supportive need objects, while the patients with a tendency to control external objects and to maintain paranoid reserve received community therapy less frequently. The *selection for psychotherapeutic community treatment was thus also influenced by both a regressive need for help and some of the favourable psychologic qualities of even seriously disturbed patients with regard to the therapeutic opportunities*.

Our group of 56 psychotherapy cases consisted of patients who had been given individual therapy, family therapy or group therapy meeting the criteria set for intensive therapy or intensive treatment in a psychotherapeutic community. Moreover, there were 7 patients who had been given less intensive psychotherapeutic treatment, which was, however, considered adequate seeing to the lesser severity of the patients's disturbance and had been terminated upon agreement between the therapist and the patient. All of the patients who had been included in the series on the basis of the last-mentioned criterion had been given individual therapy.

Of this group of 56 patients, 17 had received at least two kinds of intensive therapy, and when the less intensive therapies were also taken into account, *the number of patients given more than one kind of therapy went up to 46*. The most common combination was between community therapy and some other mode of treatment, but the patients given both individual and family therapy were also relatively numerous. Although the planning of the therapies was partly unorganized, the finding agrees with our notion of a *majority of the patients of the schizophrenia group being really in need of versatile psychotherapeutic treatment capable of flexible mutual integration*. This is particularly conspicuous among the *patients of the nuclear group*, which was also clearly demonstrated by our findings: the 10 patients given only one mode of therapy included merely one typically schizophrenic patient, and even in this case a supportive contact had been taken to a family member.

As it was already pointed out above, different patients were selected for the different modes of therapy. This was also expedient for the patients' needs for therapy as estimated by us.

This gives rise to two conclusions:

1. *Investigations of merely one mode of psychoterapy are really unable to demonstrate fully the opportunities of the psychotherapeutic approach in the treatment of schizophrenic patients, when case-specific needs serve as a basis for the indication for therapy*. It can hence be postulated that many of the American studies of the individual therapy of schizophrenics, for example, include a number of patients with poor motivation and inadequate prerequisites for individual therapy, who would rather benefit from other mode of therapy.

2. *A global and versatile therapeutic approach increases the number of patients of the schizophrenia group given appropriate psychotherapeutic treatment*.

When we applied the *logistic regression analysis* to find out which patients were selected into the group of psychotherapy cases compared with the 44 patients left outside this group, the *first treatment unit* emerged as the most important explaining variable: the patients who started their treatment in the Clinic of Psychiatry or in out-patient care became psychotherapy cases nearly three times more frequently than the patients first admitted into the Kupittaa Hospital, the finding being the same for both the whole series and the group of typical schizophrenics. The next explaining variables in the whole series were *inclusion in the group of regressive disintegration*, *symbiotic contact formation*, and *lack of unemployment* at the time of the basic examination. In the group of typical schizophrenics, the second and third variables explaining selection into the group of psychotherapy cases were *acute onset of symptoms* and *no refusal of any mode of treatment at the initial stage*.

When, in Chapter 6, we compare the patients included in the group of psychotherapy cases and those excluded from it for their outcome, it is useful to underline that the selection into the group of psychotherapy cases was primarily influenced by the therapeutic approach of the patients' first unit of treatment. Apart from this, there were also other contributory factors. *The number of patients included in the group of psychotherapy cases from the group of regressive disintegration*, whose ego functions were most seriously disturbed, *was about twofold compared with the average number of patients included in the other ego-dynamic groups*. Although inclusion in the group of regressive disintegration did not emerge as an explaining variable in the group of typical schizophrenics, it had a remarkable statistical connection with the psychotherapy cases even there ($p = .014$). As we can remember, inclusion in this group influenced particularly the selection for family therapy and community therapy, which is precisely associated with the severity of the patients' disturbances. It might be pointed out at the same time that the prognostically benign schizophreniform psychoses were clearly ($p < .02$) underrepresented in the group of psychotherapy cases in the whole series, while the patients belonging to the ego-dynamic group of paranoid disintegration were marginally significantly underrepresented among the typical schizophrenics classified as psychotherapy cases. *It was clearly more difficult on an average to draw the patients with paranoid disintegration within the sphere of psychotherapeutic activities than to do the same to the patients with regressive disintegration*.

The other aforesaid background variables explaining selection into the group of psychotherapy cases, particularly symbiotic contact formation and the absence of a negative attitude towards treatment, as well as the acute onset of symptoms in the nuclear group, are doubtless associated with a good therapeutic outcome. Selection into the psychotherapy group was hence influenced by both favourable and unfavourable prognostic factors. *The findings of the psychologic examination in the group of psychotherapy cases emphasized the significance of human objects for the patient's mental world:* the dominance of autistic object relations within it correlated with exclusion from the group of psychotherapy cases, while the tendency to symbiotic reliance in object relations correlated with inclusion in it.

But not all of the patients excluded from the group of psychotherapy cases lacked psychotherapeutic treatment. *The number of patients lacking even less intensive personal therapeutic relationship* was 20. Logistic regression analysis of the whole series showed *these patients to be characterized by a lack of depressive symptoms or features* and *lower-than-average basic education;* there was a nearly fourfold number of *men* compared with women. The corresponding explaining variables in the group of typical schizophrenics were inclusion in the *ego-dynamic group of paranoid disintegration*, a lack of depressive symptoms or features, as above, and a *tendency to alcohol or other addiction problems*. The proportion of *unemployed* patients given psychotherapeutic treatment was also lower than average. The first treatment unit was not of equal significance for this selection as it was in the group of psychotherapy cases.

We hence get a very clear idea of the patients for whom it was most difficult to arrange psychotherapeutic treatment: they were male patients with a poor social background who used paranoid defences and denied their depression (and frequently also their illness).

What about the *role of pharmacotherapy* in the treatment of our patients? We do not consider pharmacotherapy an opposite to psychotherapy, but rather a part of the implementation of global treatment on the basis of an integrated model of illness.

Of our 100 patients, 98 received neuroleptic medication at some stage of their therapy, mostly in low or moderate doses. Even so, the maximum daily dose of nearly half of the patients, i.e. 46, exceeded 300 mg chlorpromazine or an equivalent dose of some other neuroleptic. The maximum dose was generally given during the period immediately following admission into hospital, and it also depended somewhat on the hospital: in the Kupittaa Hospital the aforesaid daily dose was nearly the rule at this stage of the treatment, while in the Clinic of Psychiatry it was rather an exception. It should be underlined that the highest daily doses in our series rarely exceeded 450 mg chlorpromazine or its equivalent, and no truly high-dose medication was administered in our series. *When we divided the patients into two groups for examining the medication after the five-year follow-up period: a group with higher-than-average dosage during the follow-up period and a group with lower-than-average dosage, the first group could be said to represent moderate dosage at the most, while the latter group represented low dosage*.

The favourable effect of medication administered in moderate or low doses, particularly at the initial stages of the therapy, was undisputable in most of the patient series. We also found out that not even slightly higher doses of neuroleptics given for short periods at the early stages of the illness eliminated the prerequisites for subsequent intensive psychotherapy. *During the first two years of follow-up there was a positive statistical connection between the continuity of medication and psychotherapy*, which was, however, most conspicuous in the modes of therapy given to the most seriously ill patients (community therapy, infrequent individual therapy, family therapy). The psychotherapy cases were supported with neuroleptic medication at low doses, and the medication was often discontinued when the patient was no longer considered to need it. It has been strongly emphasized in psychopharmacological investigations (e.g. Davis et al. 1983) that there is an increased risk of re-admission upon discontinuation of medication, but this risk was not similarly relevant in the cases where the patient had a regular psychotherapeutic relationship.

During the last three follow-up years the connection between inclusion in the group of psychotherapy cases and the amount of medication given to the patient was negative, though only at a marginally significant level. The *diminishing effect of psychotherapeutic treatment on the need for medication* in the group of schizophrenic patients is shown quite illustratively by the fact that *only one of the 11 patients whose average dose of neuroleptic medication during the last three follow-up years corresponded to more than 300 mg of chlorpromazine daily belonged to the group of psychotherapy cases* (54 patients in the five-year follow-up examination), *while the remaining 10 patients were outside this group* (41 patients in the five-year follow-up examination).

Logistic regression analysis was applied to study the *background variables* which correlated in our series with *more-than-average neuroleptic medication* during the whole follow-up period. In the whole series, this selection was most clearly explained by *inclusion in the ego-dynamic group of regressive disintegration*, the second explaining variable being the *first treatment unit*, (the Kupittaa Hospital versus the Clinic of Psychiatry or outpatient care), and the third the *presence of hostile or poorly understanding individuals among the patients' parents and/or spouses*. In the group of typical schizophrenics the latter variable even emerged as the primary explaining variable; next came inclusion in the group of regressive disintegration and the *male sex*. The finding on the connection between the presence of hostile or poorly understanding relatives and the more-than-average medication given to the patient is parallel to the conclusion of Leff et al. (1981) suggesting that higher EE values of the relatives' critical attitudes towards the patient indicate higher-than-average dosage of medication for the patient, in order that he would not be re-admitted into hospital.

The *psychologic examination* showed that the group of patients with more-than-average medication differed from the rest of the series equally clearly as did the patients selected for psychotherapy. According to a logistic regression analysis based on the findings of the psychologic basic examination, the *patients with more-than-average medication during the follow-up period* were characterized by a *notable decline of cognitive capacities* on the one hand and a *notable lack of development in the object relations*, which were typically narrow and rigid, on the other. Opposite to the psychologic-mindedness of the patients given intensive individual therapy, the patients with more-than-average medication were characterized by a denial or projection of their problems or by a concrete, non-psychologic perception of the problems. This finding clearly suggests that – although the first treatment unit was of notable significance – the *selection for predominantly psychotherapeutic or predominaritly pharmacotherapeutic treatment was also influenced by patient-specific psychodynamic characteristics*.

Our experiences of the implementation of the therapeutic approach also give rise to certain *conclusions concerning the development of the therapeutic organization*, which – similarly to the final conclusions on the indications for the different modes of therapy – will be resumed in Chapter 7. However, it should be pointed out at this stage already that the need for developing psychiatric out-patient care, which has now been recognized globally and justifiably, should not make us deny the *great importance that a ward community functioning in accordance with psychotherapeutic principles still has for the therapy of new – as well as old - schizophrenic patients*. These communities constitute a kind of safe fortress serving as a stronghold needed by the community psychiatric activities intruding more and more into out-patient care and the patient's normal living environment. Particularly in the case of the most seriously disturbed new schizophrenic patients, it still seems that the sheltered hospital or day hospital ward, where a psychotherapeutic atmosphere prevails, is in most cases the best – and in many cases the necessary milieu for commencing long-term treatment.

But *it is of equally great significance that there exists a possibility to continue the patients' psychotherapy on an out-patient basis*. This requires a *system of out-patient care with good qualitative and quantitative resources* on the one hand and *smooth and flexible cooperation between the out-patient system and the hospital wards* on the other. In our own project we achieved this by continuing part of the psychotherapeutic relationships with the ward staff even after the patient's discharge from hospital and by transferring part of them into the mental health office, which was responsible for the out-patient care, as well as to private psychiatrists. If the therapeutic relationships had been started in an out-patient unit or had been transferred there, they were occasionally continued throughout the patient's subsequent in-patient periods, whenever it was considered necessary.

In principle, this model of arrangement turned out successful. The differences between the groups of patients treated by the three central out-patient units – the after-care of the Clinic of Psychiatry, the Turku Mental Health Office and the private sector – do, however, require a few comments.

The patients given aftercare on the hospital wards included clearly more "good and pleasant" patients, ones who may have been regressively psychotic, but had a favourable attitude towards therapy and had better-than-average insight into their problems. It might have been more desirable that the therapeutic relationships commenced on a hospital ward and continued by the ward staff even after the patient's discharge could have been directed, more than was the case now, on the patients with whom it was primarily difficult to make a contact.

The patients of the mental health office, on the other hand, were characterized by a lower-than-average social group of the parents. They also included more patients with no empathic relatives and with refusal from at least one mode of therapy. On the private sector, the patients and their parents had social groups higher than the average, the patients did not show overtly violent behaviour, and patients classified into the group of borderline schizophrenia numbered more than average.

The most central goal of development doubtless seems to be to support the community psychiatric system, particularly as regards the therapeutic resources of the mental health office.

6 Prognosis and the Effect of Therapies on It

We will now examine the prognosis of our patients and the question of what were the outcomes of the different modes of therapy. In this connection it should be pointed out once more that the focus of our investigations lies on the development of the therapeutic activities. We were *not* carrying out a "controlled" prognostic investigation. Compared with their methods, our study of prognoses has its limitations. But, as we demonstrated above, the studies aiming at methodologic correctness also have their restrictions as regards the practical conclusions to be made from their results.

Within our own series, we will mutually *compare the prognoses of the patients included in the group of psychotherapy cases and the patients outside of this group* and *analyze the connections between the implementation of the different modes of treatment and the prognoses*. We will also apply a *multivariate analysis based on logistic regression*, where the prognoses are explained by both the clinical and psychosocial background variables and the central variables of therapeutic activities (treatment variables).

The background variables have been defined in Appendix 1. Since they are based on the findings of the basic examination, they have a predictive character as regards the prognosis. The *treatment variables included the following: inclusion in the group of psychotherapy cases, intensive individual therapy,* either *intensive* or *less intensive family therapy, intensive treatment* or *intervention in crisis in a psychotherapeutic community,* and the *amount of neuroleptic medication received during the follow-up-period*. Of the different psychotherapy variables, it should be pointed out that the family therapy variable is not well comparable with the variables of individual and community therapies, because it includes both the intensive and less intensive therapies, unlike the aforesaid two variables (intervention in crisis in a psychotherapeutic community was also intensive, only differing from intensive community therapy as regards its duration). Inclusion of less intensive family therapy was due to the fact that the number of patients given intensive family therapy was so small as to make statistical analysis difficult, and we wished to obtain some idea of the effects of family therapy, too.

These treatment variables have been defined in Appendix 3.

As it was explained in Chapter 5, the patients given different modes of therapy differed from the whole patient series with respect to some of their baseline characteristics. We will therefore make an effort to *analyze separately the effects of the implementation of comprehensive psychotherapy, i.e. inclusion in the group of psychotherapy cases, and the amount of pharmacotherapy on the prognosis when the background variables explaining the prognosis are kept constant (Chapter 6.7.)*. A corresponding analysis is also made regarding the effects of intensive individual therapy and treatment in the psychotherapeutic community.

6.1 How Was the Prognosis Measured?

6.1.1 Implementation of the Prognostic Study

The clinical status and stage of personality development of our patients as well as their interpersonal relations and social life situation were analyzed both in the basic examination and in the two-year and five-year follow-up examinations. The criteria for the patient's status and situation were the same in all these phases of the study. *The two-year follow-up* was done separately by our own team and an independent psychiatric examiner, Dr. Järvi, who met the patients previously unknown to her in one interview situation. Her knowledge of the patients was less comprehensive than in the examination carried out by the team. In analyzing the results on the prognosis, *this independent psychiatric interview is used particularly for estimating the credibility of the findings made by the team* (6.1.3.) *and partly also for analyzing questions pertaining to the need for treatment and the significance of the therapies* (5.6.).

The five-year follow-up examination was carried out by the team. In both of the follow-up examinations most of the assessments were made and recorded by at least two members of the team, one of whom had met the patient and the other a family member. As to a smaller amount of patients (cf. Ch. 3.2.) we had to be contented with information required from other sources. None of the team members assessed the condition of any patient with whom he had or had had a therapeutic relationship. The criteria for assessing the findings were being continually discussed in the team meetings.

The different hospitals provided data on the time and duration of the hospital treatment of each patient, while the National Pensions Institute provided data on the patient's sickness benefits and pensions.

The most central part of the assessments and analyses of the prognosis and the factors affecting the prognosis presented in this chapter are based on the findings of the five-year follow-up examination. The changes that have taken place in the patient's condition are assessed by comparing the findings made in the basic examination and the five-year follow-up examination which were both graded with the same criteria. Some findings of the two-year follow-up examination will be presented in the same connections mainly descriptively. Some analyses of the two-year findings have been presented in a few earlier papers (Alanen et al. 1982 b, 1983).

6.1.2 Sub-Areas of the Prognostic Study

We analyzed the prognosis of our patients in a multi-dimensional manner. The sub-areas selected for further analysis were the following:

Clinical prognosis (6.2.)

Occurrence of psychotic symptoms
Number of nuclear symptoms of schizophrenia
Suicidal tendencies
Violent behaviour

Psychodynamic prognosis (6.3.)

Psychologic development of personality:
Level of psychosexual development
Way of dealing with aggressions
Development of interpersonal relationships:
Degree of separation from primary family
Number of interpersonal relations outside primary family
Quality of interpersonal relations outside primary family
Insight into one's own problems

Psychosocial prognosis (6.4.)

Working capacity
Disability pension granted on account of psychosis
Development of occupational identity
Loss of grip on life

Need for hospital care (6.5.)

In-patient days during the follow-up period
Treated in hospital during the two last follow-up years

The central prognostic variables and their grading in the statistical analyses are presented in Appendix 4. The criteria for a central part of findings composing the variables have been explained in Chapter 4, where the findings of the basic examination have been presented.

In addition to these central prognostic findings, the condition and development of the patients even in some other respects were analyzed in the follow-up examinations. For example, the patient's symptoms other than psychotic were examined. These and the other additional findings are presented, mainly descriptively, along with the analyses of the different prognostic sub-areas.

We will explore separately the connections between the *development of the patients' family situations* and the connections this had with the therapies (6.6.).

The statistical significances of the connections between the background variables and the major prognostic variables are presented in Appendices 7 and 8, and those between the treatment variables and these prognostic variables in Appendix 9.

6.1.3 Credibility of the Prognostic Findings: Comparison of the Two-Year Follow-up Findings Made By the Team and the Independent Examiner

The team and the independet examiner made parallel assessments using the same scales on the following prognostic variables:

occurrence of psychotic symptoms
number of nuclear symptoms of schizophrenia
suicidal tendencies
violent behaviour
degree of separation from primary family
insight into one's problems
working capacity

The comparison was hence made on four variables for the clinical prognosis, two variables for the psychodynamic prognosis and one variable for the psychosocial prognosis.

At the time of planning the follow-up examination, it was postulated that the assessment of the other psychodynamic prognostic variables would be clearly more difficult for the independent examiner than the team, because she would have to work on a single interview with the patient.

The compatibility between the assessments of the team and the independent examiner was measured with a correlation coefficient, because, in practice, it approaches quite closely the weighted kappa coefficient recommended by Cohen (1968) to be used in measuring the compatibility of the assessments made by two interviewers.

According to Cohen (1968, p. 214), the weighted kappa is suited to measuring compatibility when the differences between two raters need to be weighted according to how marked the difference of discrepancy is. In a psychiatric examination, for example, the examiner probably considers the discrepancy (neurosis <-> psychosis) a more serious difference of diagnostic classification than the discrepancy (neurosis <-> personality disorder). The conventional kappa coefficient considers all discrepancies of equal weight, and is therefore not equally well suited to comparisons of this kind.

If the following assumptions hold, the weighted kappa = correlation coefficient.

1. The marginal distributions are identical, i.e. the distributions produced by two examiners are identical.
2. The discrepancy weights for the table are in agreement with the following model:

	1	2	3	4	5...
1	0	1	4	9	16...
2	1	0	1	4	9
3	4	1	0	1	4
4	9	4	1	0	1
5	16	9	4	1	0
.	.	.	.	.	.
.	.	.	.	.	.
.	.	.	.	.	.

Of these two assumptions, the latter is the more important. The weighted kappa comes very close to the correlation coefficent (r), in practice, although the marginal distributions are not identical.

The comparison between the assessments of the independent examiner and the team naturally only pertained to the 80 patients who were also met by the independent examiner. The following correlations between the assessments were obtained:

occurrence of psychotic symptoms	r=0.659
number of nuclear symptoms of schizophrenia	r=0.679
suicidal tendencies	r=0.647
violent behaviour	r=0.627
degree of separation from primary family	r=0.596
insight into one's own problems	r=0.503
working capacity	r=0.702

The compatibility of the assessments can be considered satisfactory: the correlations for the clinical prognostic variables is of the order of 0.6–0.7, and even in the other prognostic sub-areas it comes up to 0.5 or more. It is particularly interesting to observe that the *assessments of the independent examiner were consistently more optimistic prognostically than the assessments made by the team*. The only exception of this was the assessment of working capacity where no consistent differences were found.

As an example of this, we might give the values on the occurrence of psychotic symptoms. They were defined with the following scale in the follow-up examinations:

1. the patient has marked psychotic symptoms
2. the patient has mild psychotic symptoms
3. no psychotic symptoms are seen, but the patient is suspected to have such symptoms or the patient's personality otherwise appears residually psychotically disturbed
4. definitely no psychotic symptoms
5. data inadequate

Altogether 80 patients were assessed both by the team and by the independent examiner. The following table was obtained:

Assessment by the team	Assessment by the independent examiner 1.	2.	3.	4.	Total
1.	8	3	4	1	16
2.	1	3	3	8	15
3.	0	1	1	2	4
4.	1	0	6	38	45
Total	10	7	14	49	80

The team hence estimated that marked psychotic symptoms were seen in 16 patients, while the independent examiner saw symptoms of this kind in 10 patients, the corresponding figures for mild psychotic symptoms being 15 and 7. This means that the team diagnosed definitely psychotic symptoms in altogether 31 patients and the independent examiner in 17 of the interviewed. However, the independent examiner suspected 14 patients to have symptoms, while the corresponding figure for the team was clearly lower, i.e. 4. As a consequence, the assessments of the patients definitely lacking psychotic symptoms were very close to each other: the team reported 45 patients of this kind and the independent examiner 49.

There are at least 3 possible reasons for the differences between the assessments made by the team and the independent examiner: firstly, the limits of assessment may have been different, secondly, the two interviews were carried out with some interval in time, and thirdly, the team had been dealing with the patients for a longer period and also had data from sources other than the patient interviews. It seems quite probable that the last of these factors, i.e. the teams's more comprehensive knowledge of the patients, was of crucial significance for the differences made in assessing the occurrence of psychotic symptoms. It was probably also of crucial significance for the differences in the assessments of the other prognostic variables. An exception to this were the assessments of insight ability, which were otherwise quite parallel, but differed notably at the end of the scale favourable for insight: the team regarded only 6 patients to have the best possible insight into their problems ("sees his problems and symptoms as part of himself and endeavours to solve them"), while the independent examiner classified 33 patients into this category, whereas the corresponding figures for the next best category ("has some insight into his own role in the development of his problems or symptoms") were opposite: 44 for the team and 20 for the independent examiner. No numerical findings suggesting a distinct difference of the scale of assessment were made in estimations other than that pertaining to insightfulness.

We considered these experiences to suggest that the assessments by the team provide a sufficiently reliable and, at the same time more profound view of the patient's condition than can be given by the separate interview conducted by an independent examiner. The independent examination was therefore not repeated at the time of the 5-year follow-up examination. – It should be pointed out, however, that a follow-up examination will be conducted by investigators outside the team 8 years after the admission of our patients, with the purpose of comparing the prognosis with previous patient series from Turku (Salokangas 1977, 1985; see the overall plan for the schizophrenia project in Turku presented in Chapter 1.2.).

As a conclusion, it can be said that the *comparison shows the mutual inter-rater correlation to be satisfactory.* We can also conclude that the team seems to have avoided the risk of making unduly optimistic assessments of our patients. We might rather ask whether the awareness of this possible source of error may have even made the team excessively critical in setting the line for the most optimistic assessments in the prognostic scales of some sub-areas. This was probably also reflected in the fact that the assessments made by the team and the independent examiner concerning the significances of the therapies (not published here) differed from each other in the same direction as the prognostic assessments: the independent examiner estimated the significance regularly more often as "highly favourable" than the team.

6.2 Clinical Prognosis

6.2.1 Patients Who Died Or Were Not Reached for the Follow-up Examination

At the time of the two-year follow-up, it turned out that *three of our patients had died, all through suicide.* Two of them belonged to the group of typical schizophrenias, one to the group of schizo-affective psychoses. One of these patients belonged to the group of psychotherapy cases: he had been treated with intensive therapy in a psychotherapeutic community. Attention was attracted to the fact that all of these patients had had exceptionally intense sensations of being rejected.

In the case of two patients the sensations of rejection were associated with the breakdown of marriage, in one case before the onset of the psychosis, in the other during the psychotic period. The third patient was unmarried and very lonely, a student from very poor conditions in northern Finland, whose contacts with both the relatives and the fellow students were practically non-existent. He committed suicide soon after discharge from hospital, while the other two were still registered in-patients at the time of the suicide.

At the time of the 5-year follow-up, no new death cases were found. There was one patient in the case of whom we were not even able to contact the relatives, who – similarly to the patient – had moved to another locality in Finland. The possibility of suicide is hence not excluded in the case of this patient, either, even if it seems very unlikely.

6.2.2 Occurrence of Psychotic Symptoms

The occurrence of psychotic symptoms is one of the most essential points to be assessed in the prognosis of schizophrenic patients. Since all of our patients had been diagnosed for psychotic symptoms at the time of the admission, the lack of psychotic symptoms at the time of the follow-up examinations could also be taken as an indicator of recovery, whose correlations with the therapies given to the patient served to illustrate the effect of the therapies.

Adequate information on the occurrence of psychotic symptoms was obtained from 97 patients in the two-year follow-up examination (all except those who had died) and 92 patients in the five-year follow-up (in addition to the patients who were dead or "lost", there were three for whom the assessment could not be made).

In the two-year follow-up the team saw psychotic symptoms in altogether 35 patients, of whom 28 belonged to the group of typical schizophrenias. 62 patients (including 26 typical schizophrenics) were not found to show any psychotic symptoms. The corresponding figures at the time of the five-year follow-up examination were 28 (including 26 typical schizophrenics) and 64 (25).

We divided the psychotic symptoms seen in these follow-up examinations into severe symptoms – which were obviously detrimental for the patient's coping – and mild ones. The hospital record data and the assumably reliable information provided by the relatives on the occurrence of symptoms were also taken into account. Moreover, in the group of patients without psychotic symptoms, we discriminated between a sub-group where we considered the appearance of psychotic symptoms at least transiently possible and a sub-group with definitely no psychotic symptoms. Both of these groups should, in practice, be considered asymptomatic.

In Table 53, the findings made by the team are presented as percentages separately for each diagnostic sub-category.

As it can be seen, *psychotic symptoms were noted in 36 % in the two-year follow-up examination and in 31 % in the five-year follow-up examination. The corresponding figure for the typical schizophrenic patients was about 50 % in both of the follow-up*

Table 53. Occurrence of psychotic symptoms in the different diagnostic categories in the two-year and five-year follow-up examinations. The figures are percentages

Diagnostic category	2-year follow-up (N = 97) I	II	III	IV	5-year follow-up (N = 92) I	II	III	IV
Typical schizophrenia	37	15	11	37	18	33	16	33
	52		48		51		49	
Schizophreniform psychosis	–	–	20	80	–	–	11	89
Schizo-affective psychosis	–	15	8	77	–	–	17	83
Borderline schizophrenia	–	25	5	70	–	10	10	80
Total	21	15	10	54	10	21	14	55
	36		64		31		69	

I = marked psychotic symptoms; II = mild psychotic symptoms; III = no psychotic symptoms observable, but transient symptoms formation is suspected or the patient's personality appears otherwise possibly psychotically disturbed; IV = definitely no psychotic symptoms.

Table 54. Occurrence of psychotic symptoms in the different ego-psychologic groups in the five-year follow-up examination. The figures are percentages

Ego-dynamic group	I		II	III		IV
Imminent disintegration (N = 21)	0		10	5		86
		10			90	
Acute disintegration (N = 24)	0		12	21		67
		12			87	
Regressive disintegration (N = 29)	21		24	14		41
		45			55	
Paranoid disintegration (N = 18)	17		39	17		28
		55			45	

examinations. Marked symptoms were, however, clearly fewer in the latter follow-up examination. The figures are somewhat higher if we include the patients who were not found to have any psychotic symptoms, but were postulated possibly to have some from time to time.

The presence of psychotic symptoms was *notably more common in the group of typical schizophrenias than in the other diagnostic subcategories*. The difference between the typical schizophrenias and the other sub-categories had further increased during the period between the two-year and five-year follow-up examinations. The latter revealed mild psychotic symptoms in only two patients with borderline schizophrenia out of all the other sub-categories.

It is interesting also to analyze the occurrence of psychotic symptoms separately in our *ego-dynamic groups*. Table 54 presents the results of a comparison of this kind in the light of the five-year follow-up findings.

The groups that were the most seriously ill were the groups of regressive disintegration and paranoid disintegration, of which the group of regressive disintegration showed a somewhat higher frequency of conspicuous symptoms, whereas the overall frequency of psychotic symptoms was higher in the group of paranoid disintegration. The other two groups also included a couple of patients with mild psychotic symptoms.

Table 55. Occurrence of psychotic symptoms at the time of the five-year follow-up: influence of background and/or treatment variables (logistic regression)[a]

Explaining variables	risk	p
All patients		
Diagnostic category typical schizophrenia	1.94	.000
Onset of symptoms slow	1.58	.001
Medication: more than average	1.78	.020
Typical schizophrenics		
Medication: more than average	2.17	.008
Onset of symptoms slow	2.63	.035

[a] The grading of the explaining variables: see Appendix 1.

The correlations between the *background variables* and the disappearance of psychotic symptoms were analyzed on the basis of the five-year follow-up examination. In order to make logistic regression analysis possible, the patients were divided into two groups: the ones with psychotic symptoms and the ones without symptoms.

The logistic regression analysis, which took into account both the clinical and psychosocial background variables defined in the basic examination and the treatment variables, showed that the variables explaining the *persistence of psychotic symptoms in the whole series consisted of inclusion* in the *diagnostic category of typical schizophrenias, slow onset* of the symptoms, and *higher-than-average dosage of medication* during the follow-up period (Table 55). In a separate analysis of the group of typical schizophrenic patients, the latter two variables retained their position, though in a reversed order. The prognostic significance of the clinical variables hence turned out more pronounced here than the significance of the psychosocial variables.

We thus found a clear connection between the clinical background variables and disappearance of psychotic symptoms. The female patients had psychotic symptoms less frequently (22.7 %) than males (37.5 %), but the difference between the sexes was marginally statistically significant only in the group of typical schizophrenia.

Two of the *treatment variables* were connected with the disappearance of psychotic symptoms in the whole series: *intensive individual therapy* had a positive connection ($p = .049$) and *higher-than-average dosage of medication* a negative ($p = .000$). The positive connection of intensive individual therapy remained completely the same when only the typical schizophrenics were included in the analysis. *Inclusion in the group of psychotherapy* cases also now emerged as an almost significant positive factor ($p = 029$, 19 asymptomatic and 12 symptomatic patients with typical schizophrenia). The dosage of medication continued to have a negative connection ($p = .006$), while family therapy and community therapy had no connection with the persistence or disappearance of psychotic symptoms.

6.2.3 Occurrence of Nuclear Symptoms of Schizophrenia

The development that took place in the occurrence of the nuclear symptoms of schizophrenia is shown in Table 56.

Table 56. Occurrence of the nuclear symptoms of schizophrenia in the patient series at the times of the basic examination and the follow-up examinations. The figures are percentages

Nuclear symptoms	basic examination	2-year follow-up	5-year follow-up
Autism	40	11	3
Schizophrenic thought disorder	99	33	28
Hebephrenic affective disorder	11	6	5
Schizophrenic auditory hallucinosis	25	11	12
Somatic sensations of being influenced	20	6	5
Psychic sensations of being influenced	19	11	15
Catatonic symptoms	8	2	1
Sensations of depersonalization and derealization	28	19	15

Compared with the basic examination, the number of nuclear symptoms is notably smaller in the follow-up examinations. The two-year and five-year follow-up examinations do not differ much, though most of the nuclear symptoms have continued to decrease. A particularly favourable trend can be seen in the gradual disappearance of autism.

Altogether 29 patients appeared to have one or more nuclear symptoms at the time of the five-year follow-up examination.

Six patients had 4 or more different nuclear symptoms, and 17 had 2–3 nuclear symptoms.

Of the different nuclear symptoms noted in the basic examination, only autism had a definite predictive connection with the occurrence of psychotic symptoms in the five-year follow-up examination: they were seen in 43.2 % of the autistic patients, and 21.8 % of the others ($p = .029$). Of the 11 patients with an initial hebephrenic affective disorder, surprisingly only 5 had psychotic symptoms at the time of the five-year follow-up.

We also analyzed the connections between single nuclear symptoms and some other central prognostic variables. Autism noted in the basic examination turned out to have a highly significant connection with disability to work and reception of disability pension and an almost significant connection with loss of the grip on life (see Ch. 6.4.3.) at the time of the five-year follow-up examination. The patients classified as autistic in the basic examination also had an almost significantly higher number of days spent in hospital (262.4 days) during the follow-up period than the rest of the series, but the group did not differ from the others even marginally as regards the number of patients treated in hospital during the last two years. Of the other nuclear symptoms noted at the time of the basic examination, hebephrenic affective disorder had a connection almost significant with the number of days spent in hospital during the follow-up period and a significant connection with having an in-patient period during the last two years, but none with the other prognostic variables. A parallel, though only marginally significant, finding on the hospitalization during the last two follow-up year was made for the patients with somatic sensations of being influenced. Auditory hallucinosis was not significantly connected with any of the prognostic variables analyzed, nor did catatonic symptoms, psychic sensations of being influenced or depersonalization noted at the time of the basic examination.

The connection between the number of nuclear symptoms and the background and treatment variables at the time of the five-year follow-up was analyzed with a three-step scale (0–1 nuclear symptom, 2–3 nuclear symptoms, 4 or more nuclear symptoms). The close connection between the persistence of nuclear symptoms and the group of typical schizophrenias emerged at a highly significant level in this analysis ($p < .001$). The psychosocial variables also now had somewhat greater prognostic significance than they had with the persistence of psychotic symptoms as such.

It is particularly interesting to analyze the *connections between the decrease of nuclear symptoms during the follow-up period and our background and treatment variables*. We compared the patients who had moved downwards on our three-step scale during the five follow-up years (58 patients) with the patients who showed no corresponding decrease of nuclear symptoms (16 patients). The patients who only had one nuclear symptom at the time of the basic examination were excluded from the comparison.

Logistic regression analysis yielded the following results on the factors contributing to the *decrease of nuclear symptoms* (Table 57).

The factor that most notably *explains the decrease of nuclear symptoms* in the whole series is *exclusion of the patient from the group of typical schizophrenics*. The explaining

Table 57. Decrease of the nuclear symptoms of schizophrenia during the five-year follow-up period: influence of background and/or treatment variables (logistic regression analysis)

Explaining variables	risk	p
All patients		
Not included in the diagnostic category of typical schizophrenia	1.41	.002
Separated from the primary family	1.39	.006
Intensive individual therapy	1.33	.004
Typical schizophrenics		
Separated from the primary family	1.61	.001
"Psychotherapy case"	1.63	.004

variable second in importance is *separation from the primary family prior to the basic examination*, which retains its position even when the analysis is restricted to the typical schizophrenic patients. In addition to this, one treatment variable emerges as an explaining factor in both cases: *intensive individual therapy in the whole series* and *inclusion in the group of psychotherapy cases in the sub-series of typical schizophrenic patients*. The analysis thus brings out the favourable effect of psychotherapy on the clinical prognosis of schizophrenic patients.

Of the other treatment variables, it should be pointed out that *intensive therapy or intervention in crisis in a psychotherapeutic community* also had a marginally significant positive connection with the decrease of nuclear symptoms in the group of typical schizophrenic patients. The connection between higher-than-average dosage of medication and favourable development, in turn, was marginally negative in the whole series, but not in the group of typical schizophrenias.

Family therapy also turned out to have a marginal positive connection with the decrease of nuclear symptoms at the time of the two-year follow-up examination, but no longer at the time of the five-year follow-up examination.

6.2.4 Suicidal Tendencies and Violence

Table 58 indicates the development of *suicidal tendencies* in our series.

Table 58. Development of suicidal tendencies in the patient series. The figures are percentages

Quantity of suicidal tendencies	Basic examination N = 100	2-year follow-up N = 98	5-year follow-up N = 92
Committed suicide		3	–
Attempted suicide or self-mutilation	17	13	5
Serious thoughts of self-destruction	10	13	11
Less serious suicidal tendencies or delusional fears of destruction	40	12	24
No suicidal tendencies	33	58	59

Table 59. Development of violence. The figures are percentages

Degree of violence	Basic examination N = 100	2-year follow-up N = 98	5-year follow-up N = 92
Violent behaviour	15	9	11
Threats of violent behaviour	7	12	10
Less serious aggressive features or delusions	15	5	10
No aggressive tendencies	63	74	65

The more serious suicidal tendencies decreased especially between the two-year and five-year follow-up examinations. Nevertheless, 5 patients had attempted suicide even during the latter three follow-up years.

The five-year follow-up findings showed the suicidal tendencies (including the 3 uppermost lines of the table) to be clearly most frequent in the diagnostic category of typical schizophrenics and the ego-psychologic group of regressive disintegration ($p < .05$ for both groups compared with the rest of the series). Of the other background variables, acting out symptoms correlated almost significantly with the persistence of suicidal tendencies, as did also the youngest age group, male sex, and separation struggle from the primary family at the time of the basic examination. The same level of significance was also reached by unemployment.

The logistic regression analysis showed that the *decrease of suicidal tendencies* in the whole series was explained by the patient's *sex (female)*, *lack of acting out symptoms*, and *exclusion of the youngest age group*, in this order, while the explaining factors in the group of typical schizophrenic patients were *admission with judicial sanctions* and *family therapy*.

The *development of violence* is shown in Table 59.

The change in aggressiveness is smaller than the change that took place in the suicidal tendencies. The five-year follow-up findings on *violent tendencies* showed them to be particularly conspicuous in the group of typical schizophrenics, among male patients and among the patients whose life course prior to the basic examination was found to have been characterized by difficulties of social adjustment (all $p < .01$).

The most serious act of violence in our series was represented by a patient who was – having been considered non-responsible because of his psychotic symptoms – referred to a criminal mental hospital for homicide. He had killed a drinking mate while under the influence of alcohol himself. The patient suffered from typical schizophrenia and had not had any kind of psychotherapy. Even before inclusion in our series, he had been punished for assault.

6.2.5 Other Observations on the Patient's Clinical Status. Phenomenon of Defencelessness

The follow-up findings on the development of *symptoms other than the psychotic ones* are presented in Table 60.

All but the neurotic symptoms showed a declining tendency, while the neurotic symptoms were slightly more numerous in the follow-up examinations than in the basic examination. Our other findings indicated that neurotic symptoms in psychotic

Table 60. Development of the symptoms other than psychotic in the series. The figures are percentages

Quality of symptoms relationships	Basic examination N = 100	2-year follow-up N = 97	5-year follow-up N = 95
Conspicuous neurotic symptoms	25	35	35
Depressive symptoms	63	54	52
Acting out symptoms	27	18	18
Tendency to alcohol or other addiction	35	13	18

patients are clearly favourable prognostic predictors. At the basic study stage they were most numerous in the group of borderline schizophrenias, while the typical schizophrenic patients lacked any such symptoms.

In the follow-up examination we also gave attention to the occurrence of *some symptoms or personality features not included in our basic examination questionnaire*.

Our team considered particularly interesting the finding of an *unusual psychic openness, the lack of psychologic defence mechanisms of some patients* in the two-year follow-up examination. These patients rarely had any overtly psychotic thoughts any longer – though some had –, but they did not have any neurotic defences, either. They, as it were, lacked the normal distance to the interviewer, which gave an impression of a kind of child-like character and simultaneous openness towards the developmental process, possibly even vulnerability. There were 16 patients of this kind. Diagnostically speaking, 11 of them were typical schizophrenics, while 5 had schizo-affective psychosis; the groups of schizophreniform psychoses and borderline schizophrenias included no such patients. Many of these patients belonged to our group of psychotherapy cases ($p = .038$) and had been given particularly intensive individual therapy ($p = .016$).

In the five-year follow-up examination, 22 patients, or one fourth of our series, showed a lack of defence mechanisms. These patients, however, appeared somewhat different from what the corresponding group had been at the time of the two-year follow-up. The lack of defences now was connected with the treatment variables of intensive therapy or intervention in crisis in a psychotherapeutic community ($p = .011$) and higher-than-average dosage of medication ($p = .015$). Inclusion in the group of psychotherapy cases also retained its marginal connection with this group. But the most conspicuous connections emerged between defencelessness and two clinical background variables based on our ego-dynamic grouping: of the altogether 22 defenceless patients, as many as 15 ($p = .000$) belonged to the group of regressive disintegration, while none belonged to the group of paranoid disintegration ($p = .007$).

Psychosomatic symptoms were seen in 10 patients in the two-year follow-up and in 14 patients in the five-year follow-up. Similarly to neurotic symptoms they were most frequent in borderline patients and least frequent in typical schizophrenic patients.

6.2.6 Summary and Discussion

The *percentage of suicides* in our series, 3 % during the five-year follow-up period, corresponds to the findings of several investigations carried out during the past few decades, which range from 1 % to 11 %, partly depending on the length of the follow-up period (Rennie 1939, Alström 1942, Johanson 1958, Jakobson 1967, Bleuler 1972; cf. Miles 1977). In the Finnish investigations with follow-up periods roughly similar to ours, the suicide frequencies of schizophrenic patients have varied within 2–4 % (Achté et al. 1980, Niskanen and Pihkanen 1971, Salokangas 1977, 1985). What attracts attention, however, is that the suicide frequencies in some Nordic studies (Hermansen 1968, Marinow 1972, von Sivers 1973, 1983) have been markedly higher, 8–18 % (the five-year follow-up figures being 50–80 % of these). In the American series analyzed by Harrow et al. (1978), 8 % of the patients committed suicide during a follow-up period of 2.7 years.

Juel-Nielsen (1985) recently stated that the increasing rate of suicides in the psychiatric services is a price to be paid for the liberalization of the atmosphere in psychiatric hospitals and the shift of the focus of therapy on out-patient care. If this is true, the apparently increased risk of suicide among schizophrenic patients can be taken as one justification for increasing the efficacy of family- and milieu-oriented therapy. It is difficult to say whether our own therapeutic approach was of favourable significance for the prevention of suicides in our series. We might postulate this to be indicated by the finding of the logistic regression analysis showing family therapy to be an explaining variable for the decrease of suicidal tendencies among our typically schizophrenic patients.

The percentage of patients who had recovered from their manifest psychotic symptoms by the end of the five-year follow-up period was about 70 % in our whole series and 50 % in the group of typical schizophrenics. The figures were nearly the same in the two-year follow-up examination already, although the focus of psychotic symptoms had shifted from more severe to milder symptoms during the latter follow-up period.

Among the asymptomatic patients, we discriminated a group suspected to have mild symptoms transiently or observed to have a personality that appeared possibly psychotically or residually psychotically disturbed despite the lack of overt symptoms. When these patients are taken into account, the percentage of definitely asymptomatic patients comes down to 55 % in the whole series and 33 % in the group of typical schizophrenics. It should be pointed out, however, that the group of patients with manifest symptoms also included the individuals who were reliably known to have symptoms on the basis of hospital documents or relatives' reports, although the symptoms were not observable at the time of the patient's interview. Our criteria can hence be considered quite strict, and the patients with suspected symptoms or psychotic personality features were, in practice, asymptomatic. This is also suggested by the comparison of the findings made by the team and the independent examiner on the psychotic symptoms in the parallel two-year follow-up examinations, which was presented in Chapter 6.1.3.

The comparison of our findings with other results concerning clinical recovery is rendered difficult by differences in the definition of recovery, the diagnostic criteria for inclusion in the series and the age limit (many of the series have no upper age limit). Moreover, nearly all of the other series that would otherwise be comparable only include patients admitted into hospital, whereas our own series also included patients admitted via the out-patient system. It is true, however, that the number of patients given mere out-patient treatment was no more than 12 % during the first follow-up year, being even somewhat lower thereafter (9 %, in the group of typical schizophrenics 7.4 %).

With these reservations, however, the comparison supports the notion that the clinical prognosis of our patients was relatively good. This seems obvious if, for example, we compare the recovery of our patients with the 3 series collected by Achté and his co-workers in Helsinki, where the criteria of the clinical prognosis and the follow-up period were more or less the same as in our work. After a five-year follow-up period, the patients classified as "recovered" or "apparently recovered" accounted for 37 % of the group admitted in 1950, 40 % of those admitted in 1960, and 42 % of those admitted in 1965. Achté only discriminated the patients affected with typical schizophrenia in the first two of these samples (they accounted for 45 % of the 1950 series and 51 % of the 1960 series). After the five-year follow-up period, 7 % of these patients in the 1950 series and 20 % in the 1960 series were "recovered" or "apparently recovered". Only first admitted hospital patients were included in these series, and the second difference compared with our series was the absence of age limits: 8–15 % of these patients from Helsinki were 50 years or older upon admission (Achté 1967, 1980; Niskanen & Achté 1972).

In the 7½-year follow-up of patients first admitted into hospital during 1965–67, which was carried out by Salokangas (1977, 1978) as part of the schizophrenia project in Turku, 48 % of the whole series and 38 % of the typical schizophrenics lacked psychotic symptoms, whereas "extensive" psychotic symptoms were seen in 24 % and 34 % of the patients, respectively.

In the review presented by Stephens (1978), the percentages of "recovered" patients after a minimum follow-up of five years in populations delimited with a diagnostically narrow concept of schizophrenia, often defined as populations of process schizophrenia, were clearly below 30 %. In an extensive Norwegian series described by Astrup, Fossum and Holmboe (1966), 15 % of the "narrow concept" schizophrenic patients were asymptomatic after 5–22 years. In Stephens' own series only 7 % of the patients were completely asymptomatic, and in the series of first admission schizophrenics with a good social prognosis described by Brown et al. (1966) (56 % of the patients had recovered socially) only 9 % were considered as "fully recovered" after five years. The figures are notably lower than ours.

We can, however, also ask whether such low recovery rates may have been indirectly influenced by the "incurability" considered characteristic of process schizophrenias on the basis of the etiological hypotheses. Some of the recent prognostic findings, which are more optimistic than has been the case previously, may speak in favour of this assumption. The diagnosis of schizophrenia in these works has generally been set on the basis of symptomatologic descriptions. In a series collected by Bland (Bland et al. 1976, 1978) in Canada for the purpose of analyzing the 10-year prognosis of first admission schizophrenics admitted in 1963, 58 % of the 88 patients were classified as "recovered, no social or intellectual deficit". In the British series of Watt et al. (1983), which met diagnostically the PSE criteria, a similar 58 % portion of the 48 first admission schizophrenics had "a good outcome" after five years, by which the investigators mean one or several episodes of illness "with no or minimal impairment". In the American series of Harrow et al. (1978) 36 % were asymptomatic after 2.7 years. In a follow-up study conducted by von Sivers (1983) in Sweden on 111 schizophrenic patients first admitted into a clinic of psychiatry in Stockholm during 1961–65 after a follow-up of 6–11 years, 44 % the patients were found to be asymptomatic. The patient series was not representative of the whole catchment area, and seriously ill patients were probably overrepresented among those excluded from the series compared with less seriously ill ones.

We conclude that *the prognosis for recovery from psychotic symptoms in our series can be considered good compared with most other corresponding works with similar follow-up periods.*

Although the finding on recovery can probably be considered good particularly in our diagnostic nuclear group, nearly all of the patients who had symptoms after five years belonged to this nuclear category. In this respect, our findings confirm the notion that *patients with typical schizophrenia have a clearly poorer prognosis than other patients of the schizophrenia group.*

As to the ego-dynamic groups, it was interesting to observe that the patients with psychotic symptoms after five years were more numerous in the group of paranoid disintegration than in the group of regressive disintegration, where the primary degree of disintegration was deeper. Marked symptoms were, however, slightly more frequent in the latter group. Of the 12 regressively disintegrated patiens who were asymptomatic after five years, 11 belonged to the group of psychotherapy cases.

Our logistic regression analysis of the variables explaining the persistence of psychotic symptoms did not yield any unexpected findings. In addition to inclusion in the group of typical schizophrenics, two variables emerged in the analysis of the whole series which also retained their significance in a separate analysis of the nuclear group: *slow onset of the psychotic symptoms* and *more-than-average neuroleptic medication during the follow-up period.*

The logistic regression analysis also showed that the variables explaining the *decrease of nuclear symptoms* in the whole series were exclusion from the nuclear group of schizophrenia, separation from the primary family by the time of the admission, and intensive individual therapy. The explaining variables in the group of typical schizophrenics were similarly separation from the primary family and inclusion in the group of psychotherapy cases. *Separation from the primary family as a baseline characteristic hence turned out an important predictor for an optimistic clinical prognosis of schizophrenia.* At the same time these analyses *confirmed the notion of the favourable effect of psychotherapy on the clinical prognosis of schizophrenic patients.* More-than-average medication did not emerge as an explaining variable here, nor did it correlate significantly with a poor clinical prognosis in the group of typical schizophrenics.

Of the other findings we made, we might mention the *clearly better prognosis of women compared with men,* which, however, was marginally significant in the group of typical schizophrenics, not in the whole series. A parallel finding was also made in the series described by Bland et al., Watt and von Sivers. The differences between the different age groups, on the other hand, were small. Of the social background variables recorded in the basic examination, unemployment was most significant, while the factors of social group and educational level lacked any significance, unlike in the American study by Astrachan et al. (1974), for example.

The connections between single schizophrenic symptoms and the subsequent prognosis in our series were relatively insignificant.

Autism noted at the time of the basic examination was of most predictive significance for the persistence of the other nuclear symptoms as well as for the other prognostic findings, despite the fact that this symptom in itself turned out unexpectedly liable to disappear in our series. Of the other symptoms, hebephrenic affective disorder and somatic sensations of being influenced had some connections with the prognostic findings, mainly the subsequent need for hospital treatment.

The presence of *neurotic symptoms* in patients admitted because of a psychosis of the schizophrenia group was clearly significantly connected to recovery from psychotic symptoms during the follow-up period in our series. A finding parallel to this was the minor increase of patients with neurotic symptoms during the follow-up period. In other words, there were patients who, after recovery from psychotic symptoms, developed symptoms indicative of the emergence of neurotic defence mechanisms.

A different development had been taking place in the patients whose unusual psychic openness, *psychologic defencelessness*, attracted our attention at the time of the two-year follow-up. It took the form of nearly child-like confidence and a lack of the normal distance in the interview situation. Many of these patiens belonged to our psychotherapy cases, especially the group given intensive individual psychotherapy, and they had been characterized by a lack and/or lability of significant interpersonal relationships at the time of the admission. We therefore concluded that the phenomenon reflected the intermediary stage which some psychotic patients – particularly ones withdrawn from interpersonal relationships – undergo during the development initiated by psychotherapy. This was partly supported by the observation that many of the defenceless psychotherapy patients had a clearly more integrated personality at the time of the five-year follow-up examination and could no longer be included in this group. The new follow-up examination did reveal defenceless patients, even more, in fact, than did the two-year follow-up examination, but these patients now had the strongest connections with inclusion in the group of regressive disintegration. Of the treatment variables, the lack of defences was now connected with more-than-average medication and intensive therapy or intervention in crisis in a psychotherapeutic community. At this stage of the follow-up, defencelessness thus appeared to be connected, most of all, with increasing regressive chronicity of serious schizophrenic illness. However, the experience of an empathic ward community may also have been making the patients liable to this development, as an opposite to autistic withdrawal. It was interesting that while an overwhelming majority of the patients classified as defenceless in the five-year follow-up examination belonged to the group of regressive disintegration, none of the patients with a typical paranoid defensive system as a baseline characteristic (the group of paranoid disintegration) were defenceless.

6.3 Psychodynamic Prognosis

The psychodynamic development and prognosis of psychotic patients has been investigated much less than their clinical and social prognosis. Even so, aspects of psychodynamic development, e.g. the ability to establish satisfactory relationships with other people, are of essential importance in the lives of all people and even more important in the lives of psychotic patients, because they have experienced particularly severe frustrations and problems in this respect even before the onset of their illness. The illness makes their position even more exposed to threats, which easily increases both their own tendency to withdraw from society and the tendency of other people to withdraw from their company. In any analysis of the outcome of psychotherapy the evaluation of psychodynamic development is of notable significance, because the main focus of the therapy lies on the field of it.

Significant work on the psychologic effects of the psychotherapy of psychotic patients has been carried out by e.g. Schulz (1975, 1976) who developed a scale for self and object differentiation for this purpose. Pao (1979) considers precisely the internal developmental process that results in an improvement of the schizophrenic patient's self- and object-representational world the most central aim in the psychoanalytically oriented individual therapy of psychotic patients.

Gunderson and his co-workers (Gunderson and Gomes-Schwartz 1980, Gunderson 1982) developed a four-dimensional system of measurement mainly intended for the assessment of the results of intensive exploratory individual therapy, where the dimensions are: longitudinal awareness (insight into the origin, consequences and continuity of one's problems throughout one's life), insightfulness (mainly into the actual field of problems), object relatedness, and subjective experience.

Mc Glashan and Miller (1982) divided the fields of influence of psychoanalysis and psychoanalytic psychotherapy as follows: developmental level (e.g. separation – individuation and sexuality), aspects of the self, object relatedness, reality acceptance, fullness of experience, coping mechanisms, integrative capacity, self-analytic function and symptomatology.

While planning the psychodynamic methdods of assessment in our own project, we were, for several reasons, content with more modest and less specific goals. We investigated the outcome of psychotherapy in a more global way, not limiting ourselves to the more specific nature of the individual therapeutic process. We made an effort to base our prognostic investigation on *relatively unsophisticated and unambiguous assessments to be derived from our questionnaires*, which, as far as we could see, could be made quite reliably on the basis of the experience of our team. The development of our patients as well as the effects of the clinical and psychosocial background variables and therapies were examined by *analyzing the changes that took place in the patient's developmental status between the basic examination and the five-year follow-up examination,* taking into account only the unambiguous and easily defined findings of progress or regression. *The changes were verified as shifts on the scale of questionnaire for each field from one point to another, reducing the shifts at some points in such a way as to ignore the relatively small and laboriously definable shifts.* In this way, adequate information could be gathered through interviews with the therapists or family members even of many patients who were not met personally.

6.3.1 Psychosexual Development

While examining the psychologic personality development of our patients we attached special attention to psychosexual identity on the one hand and balanced control of aggressions on the other at the time of the basic study already. Measurement of prognostic development turned out easier on the former field than on the latter.

The data on the *development of concrete heterosexual relationships* of our patients are shown in Table 61.

Table 61. Development of the heterosexual relationships of our patients during the follow-up period. The figures are percentages

Presence of heterosexual relationships	Basic examination (N = 100)	Two-year follow-up (N = 97)	Five-year follow-up (N = 94)
No relationships	23	39	31
Only transient relationships	11	15	22
Long-term relationships	64	45	45

We can clearly see the *negative influence of illness on long-term relationships*: the patients had clearly fewer long-term relationships during the follow-up periods than prior to the basic examination. The *number of patients without sexual relationships, in turn, had increased particularly during the period between the basic examination and the first follow-up examination, after which the difference levelled off somewhat* along with the increase of transient relationships.

We selected, however, the patient's *level of psychosexual development* (see Ch. 4.1.3.1), not the presence of actual heterosexual relationships, as a sub-factor of the prognostic study. We considered it to reflect better the real progress, status quo or regression that had taken place in the personality development than the concrete relationships. We found no greater difficulties in estimating whether a patient who had lost a long-term relationship had also undergone a distinct regression of the psychosexual development or not. The results are shown in Table 62.

The figures indicate that regression of psychosexual development had taken place in several patients particularly during the period between the basic examination and the two-year follow-up examination, while the situation seemed to have improved somewhat between the two-year and five-year follow-up examinations. The observations are hence parallel to those made for concrete and heterosexual relationships.

An established heterosexual identity had been *reached* between the basic examination and the five-year follow-up examination by *13 patients who lacked it at the time of the basic examination*. Of these patients, 7 had been diagnosed as typical schizophrenics, which means that favourable development was relatively equally frequent in the group of typical schizophrenics as in the rest of the series. The condition of 24 patients was unchanged (including 15 typical schizophrenics).

Table 62. The results on the assessment of the patients' level of psychosexual development at the different stages of the project. The figures are percentages

Level of psychosexual development	Basic examination (N = 98)	Two-year follow-up (N = 97)	Five-year follow-up (N = 94)
Delayed	17	23	16
Chaotic or characterized by identity crisis	20	25	21
Established homosexual identity	–	–	–
Established heterosexual identity	62	51	61

Table 63. Achievement of established psychosexual identity during the follow-up period in the group of patients lacking such identity at the time of the basic examination; effect of background and/or treatment variables (logistic regression analysis)

Explaining variables	R	p
All patients		
Father's personality not seriously disturbed	2.76	0.35
Sex: female	4.66	0.58

According to the *logistic regression analysis*, the tendency to progress (Table 63) was explained by two psychosocial background variables: *lack of serious personality disorder of the father and female sex*. A more detailed analysis indicated that the lack of personality disorder of the father and the change in the psychosexual development were mutually associated in the group of female patients, while no corresponding association was seen in the male group.

Of the treatment variables, only less-than-average medication had a marginal connection with developmental progress. Of the 7 patients who had reached an established heterosexual identity during the follow-up period and had been diagnosed as typical schizophrenics, 4 had been given intensive individual therapy; 6 of them belonged to the group of psychotherapy cases.

The *established level of heterosexual identity* noted at the time of the basic examination had been *lost during the follow-up* period by 11 patients (including 9 typical schizophrenics) and retained by 46 (including 22 typical schizophrenics). In the group of typical schizophrenics adverse development had taken place almost significantly ($p = .05$) more often than in the rest of the series. The explaining variables consisted of 3 background variables: *unmarried civilian status*, *tendency to alcohol or other addiction*, and *slow onset of symptoms*.

Furthermore, regression appeared to be highly significantly connected with the lack of separation from the primary family at the time of the basic examination and almost significantly connected with the male sex and the serious personality disorder of the mother. Of the treatment variables, only the more-than-average medication correlated significantly with regression ($p < .05$).

Overtly violent behaviour by the patient was seen in 20 cases during the first two follow-up years and in 18 cases during the latter three years. Compared with the data

Table 64. Loss of achieved stabilized heterosexual identity during the follow-up years. Influence of background and/or treatment variables (logistic regression analysis)

Explaining variables	risk	p
All patients		
Unmarried	5.33	.003
Alcohol or other addiction	5.71	.013
Onset of symptoms slow	3.36	.001

Table 65. Changes in the patient's characteristic way of dealing with aggressions. The figures are percentages

Way of dealing with aggressions	Basic examination (N = 97)	Two-year follow-up (N = 96)	Five-year follow-up (N = 94)
Avoids aggressive behaviour	65	63	55
Impulsive	33	38	35
"Normal"	2	2	10

collected at the basic examination stage (26 patients), some improvement had taken place.

In the same way, the patients' characteristic way of *dealing with their aggressions* appeared to be classifiable as "normal" slightly more often in the five-year follow-up than in the previous examinations (for the criteria, see 4.1.3.1.).

Table 65 indicates that the tendency to avoid aggressive behaviour did, however, remain characteristic of more than half of the patients even at the time of the latter follow-up examination.

A shift from the avoidance of aggressions to their impulsive expressions was associated with an optimistic prognosis in some cases and with a pessimistic one in some others. Both for this reason and because the number of patients who began to control their aggressions in a "normal" way was small, the development of the control of aggressions could not be taken as a prognostic indicator in our work. It is interesting, however, to note that 8 of the 10 patients whose ability to control aggressions was normal at the end of the follow-up period belonged to our psychotherapy cases.

6.3.2 Development of Interpersonal Relationships

The development taking place in the field of interpersonal relationships was evaluated by means of three prognostic indicators. They were based on the degree of the patient's psychological separation from his primary family, the number of interpersonal relationships they had outside the primary family, and the quality of these relationships.

Separation from the primary family as an indicator of prognostic changes was more restricted than the other two indicators in that it was most relevant for the patients who were enmeshed in their primary families at the time of the basic examination or were

Table 66. Changes in the patient's psychologic separation from their primary families during the follow-up period. The figures are percentages

Relationship to primary family	Basic examination (N = 100)	Two-year follow-up (N = 97)	Five-year follow-up (N = 95)
Strongly enmeshed	16	20	22
Separation struggle	35	35	28
At least ostensibly successful separation	49	45	50

undergoing a separation struggle, while it was less relevant for e.g. married patients. But we already observed in the basic examination that even some of the married patients were continuing their separation struggle from their primary families; and some of the patients who divorced during the follow-up period resumed their dependence on their parents. For these reasons, we also included the married patients in the analyses.

The development that took place in the relations between our patients and their primary families is shown in Table 66.

The changes appear to be very small. The number of patients strongly enmeshed in their primary families had slightly increased, while the number of patients undergoing the separation struggle had correspondingly decreased. Not even the increased age of the patients had had any notable promoting effect on the psychologic separation processes during the follow-up period in the whole series.

A favourable development, e.g. *progress in the separation process,* had taken place in 14 patients (including 8 typical schizophrenics), while the previous situation persisted in the case of 37 patients (including 23 typical schizophrenics). The *logistic regression analysis* of the variables explaining the favourable change turned out the following (Table 67).

The first explaining variable for the progressive development that had taken place in the whole series turns out to be that *no* family therapy had been given to the patient, while the second consists of female sex. In the group of typical schizophrenics the female sex emerges as the first explaining variable, while less-than-average medication comes up as the second.

The better development in the female group than in the male group was also conspicuous in several other analyses of prognosis. The inverse effect of being given family therapy, however, is surprising in particularly this prognostic criterion. We cannot consider it a random phenomenon, but rather an indication of the truly modest outcome of our family-therapeutic efforts in this series.

The family therapies of primary families were partly carried out in very difficult family situations, and, owing to the lack of system-oriented interventions, they were unable to alter these situations. The case of Miss R (see Ch. 5.2.2.) serves as an example of family therapy, where the situation of the patient, who was strongly enmeshed in her primary family, relative to

Table 67. Progressive development of separation from the primary family during the five follow-up years: effect of background and/or treatment variables (logistic regression analysis)

Explaining variables	risk	p
All patients		
No family therapy	uncalculable[a]	.004
Sex: female	3.04	.003
Typical schizophrenics		
Sex: female	4.81	.008
Neuroleptic treatment: less than average	4.09	.017

[a] Progressive development found by 36 % of those who did not receive family therapy but none to whom this mode of therapy was given.

her parents (in this case the mother) was improved – as the situation of living at home became better tolerable – but no progressive development of separation was achieved.

None of the treatment variables other than those presented in Table 67 had any statistical connections with the separation development. There was, moreover, only one other variable in the whole series that had an almost significant connection with favourable development, namely the fact that the patient did not have an established heterosexual identity at the time of the basic examination. A comparison of the prognostic variables indicated that achievement of heterosexual identity during the follow-up period had a significant (p = .008) connection with the progress of the separation development.

Regression of the separation process had taken place in the case of 16 patient (including 13 typical schizophrenics), while 64 patients showed no regressive development (there being 33 typical schizophrenics among them). The *logistic regression analysis* of the variables explaining the regression of the separation process turned out the following (Table 68):

Table 68. Regression of separation from the primary family during the five-year follow-up period: effect of background and/or treatment variables (logistic regression analysis)

Explaining variables	risk	p
All patients		
No occupational identity	3.87	.003
Not admitted to treatment of his own will	2.60	.035
No social deviances in family background	2.20	.058
Typical schizophrenics		
No occupational identity	6.55	.001

The most important factor explaining the regressive development is the *lack of stabilized occupational identity at the time of the basic examination* in both the whole series and the group of typical schizophrenics. In other words, the patients who had better abilities to find themselves a place in the working life, gained support from this for their independent coping even after the onset of their illness.

The regression of the separation process was significantly connected with inclusion in the group of regressive disintegration (p = .007) and inclusion in the two highest

Table 69. Development in the number of significant interpersonal relationships established by the patients outside their primary families during the follow-up period. The figures are percentages

Number of significant relationships	Basic examination (N = 99)	Two-year follow-up (N = 95)	Five-year follow-up (N = 95)
No significant relationships	21	49	38
One significant relationship	36	25	30
Several significant relationships	42	26	31

social groups (p = .004). The latter finding was repeated in the group of typical schizophrenics (p = .021). Regression was especially marked in the group of patients who had graduated from senior secondary school (or at least completed the junior secondary school), but had not reached the goals of occupational training compatible with their basic educational level.

The development in the number of significant interpersonal relationships established by the patients outside their primary families is shown in Table 69.

The figures show quite obviously that the *onset of psychosis often results in a loss of friendship relations*. At the time of the basic examination, about one fifth of the patients lacked any significant relationships outside the primary family, but the corresponding figure at the time of the two-year follow-up accounted for half of the series. *More favourable development had, however, taken place during the latter follow-up period.*

The number of significant interpersonal relationships had increased during the five-year follow-up in the case of 19 patients (including 8 typical schizophrenics). No increase was found in the case of 35 patients (21 typical schizophrenics).

The *logistic regression analysis* of the whole series (Table70) showed the increase of the number of interpersonal relationships to be explained by the following factors: the patient *was not unemployed* at the time of the basic examination, the patient had *schizo-affective psychosis*, and the patients *lacked alcohol problems*.

None of the *treatment variables* were connected with the progressive development that had taken place. Intensive therapy or intervention in crisis in a psychotherapeutic community came closest to statistical significance (in the group of typical schizophrenics p = .12). In the two-year follow-up examination we had noted a distinct positive connection between community therapy in particular and the development of the number of interpersonal relationships (r = .30). The psychotherapeutic community apparently served as a favourable milieu for the increase of interpersonal relationships, but its influence was short-lived in this respect in most cases.

Of the patients who had more than one significant interpersonal relationship at the time of the basic examination, *15 had remained at this level* (including 6 typical schizophrenics), *while 24 patients* (including 17 typical schizophrenics) *showed a regressive trend.*

Table 70. Increase of the number of significant interpersonal relationships outside the primary family during the five-year follow-up period: effect of background and/or treatment variables (logistic regression analysis)

Explaining variables	risk	p
All patients		
Not unemployed	5.17	.016
Schizo-affective psychosis	2.40	.042
No alcohol or addiction problems	2.66	.025
Typical schizophrenics		
Psychosexual development delayed or chaotic	4.24	.022

Table 71. Decrease of the number of significant interpersonal relationships outside the primary family during the five-year follow-up period: effect of background and/or treatment variables (logistic regression analysis)

Explaining variables	risk	p
All patients		
Neuroleptic treatment: more than average	2.57	.001
No individual psychotherapy	1.90	.040

The strongest statistical correlation emerged between regression and *more-than-average neuroleptic treatment* ($p < .001$). It also turned out the most important explaining factor for the decrease of interpersonal relationships in the *logistic regression analysis* (Table 71). The second explaining variable was also a treatment variable, namely the fact that the *patient had not been given intensive individual therapy.*

The *group of typical schizophrenic patients* had a marginal connection with the decrease of interpersonal relationships. A separate analysis of this group further emphasized the *connection between intensive individual therapy and the lack of regressive changes in the number of interpersonal relationships* (Fisher's exact test 0.008). No logistic regression analysis could be carried out in this group because of the small size of the group.

The development of the quality of the interpersonal relationships is shown in Table 72.

The tendency is the same as in the qualitative development of the interpersonal relationships: the *group of labile and short-lived relationships has increased considerably*, while the other two have decreased in size.

We considered it most expedient in the statistical analysis to combine the classes of labile and short-lived relationships and the relationships coloured by repeated conflicts, and to analyze the correlations of the changes between this combined group and the group of stable and long-lived interpersonal relationships to the background variables. After all, achievement of stable and long-lived interpersonal relationships in particular could here be considered an indicator of "normality".

When this method of comparison was applied, it was found out that in the whole series *definite qualitative improvement of the interpersonal relationships,* i.e. achievement of stable and long-lived interpersonal relationships, during the follow-up period had only taken place in the case of 10 patients who lacked such relationships at

Table 72. Qualitative development of the patient's significant interpersonal relationships outside the primary family during the follow-up period. The figures are percentages

Quality of relationships	Basic examination (N = 95)	Two-year follow-up (N = 91)	Five-year follow-up (N = 91)
Labile and short-lived	30	58	58
Coloured by repeated conflicts	37	26	23
Stable and long-lived	33	16	19

Table 73. Qualitative improvement of interpersonal relationships during the five-year follow-up: effect of treatment and/or background variables (logistic regression analysis)

Explaining variables	risk	p
All patients		
Avoidance of aggressions	5.71	.023
Presence of empathic relatives	3.09	.058

the basic examination stage (including 4 typical schizophrenics). A progressive development was not found in the case of 47 patients (26 typical schizophrenics). *Regression* of stable and long-lived interpersonal relationships, in turn, had taken place in the case of 21 patients (including 13 typical schizophrenics), while 7 patients (including 3 typical schizophrenics) had retained the qualitative level of their interpersonal relationships.

The *logistic regression analysis* (Table 73) revealed the tendency *to avoid aggressive behaviour and the presence of empathic relatives* in the patient's family to be the explaining variables of a qualitative improvement of interpersonal relationships. This finding suggests that even inhibited control of aggressions provides a better basis for the development of interpersonal relationships into a more stable form than impulsive expression of aggressions.

In the group of typical schizophrenic patients the qualitative improvement of the interpersonal relationships had an almost significant connection with two background variables: lack of stabilized heterosexual relationships at the time of the basic examination, and inclusion in the youngest age group. Moreover, there were marginal connections with two variables: intensive individual therapy and lack of serious personality disorder of the father. The number of cases being so small, logistic regression analysis could not be carried out.

The loss of the stable and long-term interpersonal relationships noted at the time of the basic examination correlated most strongly with the background variable of *serious personality disorder of the mother* in the whole series (Fisher's exact test $p < .01$). A marginal connection of opposite direction emerged for intensive individual therapy.

6.3.3 Insight and Sense of Illness

The patient's insight at the time of the basic examination was analyzed by estimating *to what extent they were able to perceive their own role in the development of their problems and symptoms and ready to make an effort to solve them.* Within the group of patients lacking any such insight, we divided between two groups: the patients who *completely denied their illness and problems*, and the patients who *admitted having problems, but considered them to have been caused by others.* In the follow-up examination we noted that, apart from the latter group, who explained their problems in a paranoid and projective way, there were also patients who lacked insight into the connection between their illness and life, but yet *considered themselves ill without projectively accusing other people or their social environment.* Some of them considered their illness mostly "congenital", while some others attributed it to somatic causes and yet some other had

Table 74. Development of the patient's insight and sense of illness during the five-year follow-up. The figures are percentages

Insight and sense of illness	Basic examination (N = 100)	Two-year follow-up (N = 97)	Five-year follow-up (N = 95)
Denies completely one's illness and problems	20	8	4
Admits there are problems, but deems them to be caused by others	29	22	17
Has a sense of illness, but lacks insight into the connections between illness and the problems of one's life	(–)	6	25
Has some insight into one's own role in the development of one's problems and/or symptoms	48	54	41
Sees one's problems and symptoms as part of oneself and tries to solve them	3	6	13

assumed, even less specifically, the role of being ill, which often also involved some secondary benefit, e.g. a pension. By the time of the five-year follow-up examination, the number of these patients had continued to increase.

Our table for sense of illness and insight (Table 74) thus came to include a new group in the follow-up examinations; this group was located between the insightful patients and the patients tending to externalize their problems projectively. With regard to the lack of insight, these patients were comparable to those using the defences of denial and projection.

We can see that the projective externalization and the *denial of illness has decreased during the follow-up period*, while the *number of patients who are intensely aware of their problems* on the one hand and *patients who have a "non-specific" sense of illness* without insight into its essence on the other *has increased*.

We can naturally ask whether it would have been possible to find patients with a "non-specific" sense of illness at the time of the basic examination already, if attention had been given to this point at that time. This is possible, although a mutual comparison of the follow-up examinations indicates that the number of these patients has increased particularly during the latter follow-up years.

At least some insight into their problems or symptoms was shown in the five-year follow-up by 51 patients. The number of patients in this group was the same as in the basic examination, but the patients were not quite identical. A majority (69 %) of the patients classified as insightful in the basic examination were still insightful, and a majority of those lacking insight (62 %) continued to be in the same situation. The statistical correlation between the patients classified as insightful in the five-year follow-up examination and those classified correspondingly in the basic examination was clearly significant ($p = .003$).

Insightfulness at the end of the follow-up period had the strongest, highly significant connections, both in the whole series and in the group of typical schizophrenias, with two treatment variables: intensive psychotherapy and inclusion in the psychotherapy cases. The connection of both of these therapeutic variables with insightfulness at the time of

Table 75. Increase of insight during the five-year follow-up period: influence of background and/or treatment variables (logistic regression)

Explaining variables	risk	p
All patients		
Psychotherapy case	3.53	.001
No alcohol or addiction problems	3.22	.008
Socially deviant family background	1.86	.008
Typical schizophrenics		
Intensive individual therapy	4.57	.001
No alcohol or addiction problems	6.47	.004

the five-year follow-up examination were of the level of $p < .0005$ in both the whole series and the group of typical schizophrenias. Of the patients given intensive psychotherapy, 84.6 % showed insight in the whole series and 78.6 % in the group of typical schizophrenias, the corresponding figures for all psychotherapy cases being 70.4 % and 59.4 %. As regards the other psychotherapy variables, the insightfulness of the patients given intensive therapy or intervention in crisis in a psychotherapeutic community was marginally significantly better in the whole series and almost significantly better in the group of typical schizophrenias than the insightfulness of the other patients, while the family therapy cases showed no corresponding development.

Of the typical schizophrenic patients, 33 lacked insight, while 21 were insightful (38.9 %, compared with the rest of the series there was a negative connection of the level of $p < .001$). The other highly significant connection in the whole series emerged between *lack of insight* and *serious personality disorder of the mother* noted in the basic examination.

The significance of the therapeutic variables also emerged strongly in the *analysis of the changes* that had taken place *in the patient's insightfulness during the five follow-up years*. The *logistic regression analysis* was focussed on the *increase of insight* (Table 75). The patients were divided into three groups: the ones without insight (the top three lines in Table 74), the ones with some insight into their problems (the fourth line in Table 74), and the fully insightful ones (the bottom line in Table 74). The insightfulness of 27 patients (including 13 typical schizophrenics) was found to have increased, while no increase was seen in the case of 65 patients (including 41 typical schizophrenics). Only three patients, who were already classified as having the best possible insightfulness at the time of the basic examination, were excluded from the analysis.

The most powerful explaining variable was inclusion in the group of psychotherapy cases in the whole series and intensive individual therapy in the group of typical schizophrenics. These two psychotherapy variables were highly significantly connected ($p < .001$) with the change of insightfulness particularly in the group of typical schizophrenics. Inclusion in the group of psychotherapy cases had a connection of nearly the same level ($p = .0012$) in the whole series, too, while the corresponding connection of intensive individual therapy was slightly lower ($p = .025$). *Intensive therapy or intervention in crisis in a therapeutic community* also had a clearly significant connection with the development of insight both in the whole series and in the group of typical schizophrenic patients. Lesser-than-average medication had an almost significant connection with the increase in the group of typical schizophrenic patients.

The second variable explaining the increase of insight was the *lack of alcohol or other addiction*. The effect of this background variable is easy to understand, if we interpret the alcohol problem as an escape from other problems, while the third explaining variable that emerged in the whole series, *social deviance in the family background*, remained enigmatic for us.

The *decrease of insight* was only analyzed in the whole series, because no more than 16 patients showed a decrease of this kind. The only clearly significant connections with this prognostic assessment were noted for more-than-average medication during the follow-up period and unemployment at the time of the basic examination.

6.3.4 Summary and Discussion

The criteria we used for estimating the psychodynamic development and prognosis of our patients were relatively unsophisticated, but unambiguously definable and, as far as we can see, therefore also reliable. They were based on notions and information obtained from the clinical interviews. Some findings based on psychologic test methods will be published separately later on.

The comparison of our findings with other results is more difficult here than in the case of the prognostic findings on the clinical status, since the other investigations have generally given less attention to the psychodynamic prognosis, and the works for which there are findings available have utilized criteria that have not been identical with ours.

Our general observation is that wherever the follow-up of the psychodynamic prognosis in our series dealt with the patient's interpersonal relationships, obvious regressive development had taken place especially between the basic examination and the two-year follow-up examination. Such a tendency was seen in both the quantity and quality of the patients' interpersonal relationships outside their primary families and their concrete heterosexual relationships, and it was also reflected in the figures associated with the assessment of their level of psychosexual development. This clearly reflects the *negative effect of the illness on the patient's interpersonal relationships in their environment*, which is influenced not only by factors associated with the illness, but also by social isolation (in-patient periods, dropping out of working life, etc.) and the development of the attitudes of both the patients and the other parties in their interpersonal relationships. It was gratifying to find out that there had been a turn towards the better in the developmental tendency in these respects – though more moderate – during the latter follow-up period. This was most apparent in our estimates of the development of psychosexual identity. It should be noted that what happened was not always, and not even mostly, that patients who had been in a better condition earlier would have returned to their old position, but there were also many patients who had progressed relative to the situation that had prevailed at the time of the basic examination.

The findings on the patients' psychologic separation from their primary families also showed the kind of tendency described above, though less markedly: the changes between the different stages of the investigation were small, and no levelling change between the two-year and five-year follow-up examination took place in the number of patients strongly enmeshed in their primary families. Nor did the increased age of the patients bring about any change in this. We may keep in mind that the finding of a lack of separation from the primary family at the time of the basic examination was a factor predictive of a poor clinical prognosis.

The findings on the patients' *insight* into the connection between their illness and their problems constituted another item behaving differently from the other prognostic variables. The number of patients who showed at least some insight into their own role in the development of their problems and/or symptoms slightly increased between the basic examination and the two-year follow-up, whereas the number of patients denying their illness diminished. During the period between the two-year and five-year follow-up examinations the number of patients whose insight into their problems was graded as maximal on our scale, i.e. who saw their problems and symptoms as being in integral psychologic connection with each other, continued to increase. Nevertheless, we still estimated the number of such patients to be relatively low, 13 %. The total number of patients with at least partial insight into their own role, however, remained closely parallel to the baseline findings. The number of patients denying or externalizing their problems had further declined, while the number of patients who admitted being ill, but lacked insight into the connection between their illness and the problems in their life, increased.

The psychodynamic development of the patients diagnosed as typically schizophrenic in the basic examination was slightly less favourable on all these prognostic dimensions than the corresponding development of the other patients. However, the *developmental progress between the basic examination and the five-year follow-up examination was more or less equally frequent in the group of typical schizophrenic patients as in the rest of the series, while developmental regression was more common in the group of typical schizophrenics.*

How much did the changes depend on the treatment given to the patients on the one hand and on their baseline characteristics on the other? Logistic regression analysis was again applied to find this out. Separate analyses were carried out on the patients showing progress and on those showing regression in their development during the period between the basic examination and the five-year follow-up. The number of patients in each analysis was often quite small, especially when the group of typical schizophrenics was analyzed separately. Logistic regression analysis therefore had to be given up on some prognostic dimensions in this group, and the small number of patients makes even other findings subject to provision.

The most obvious, and highly convincing, connection emerged between the psychotherapeutic modes of treatment and increase of insight. Both inclusion in the group of psychotherapy cases and intensive individual therapy were connected highly significantly with the increase of insight in the group of typical schizophrenics, and inclusion in the group of psychotherapy cases also had a connection of nearly the same level in the whole series. Logistic regression analysis showed inclusion in the group of psychotherapy cases in the whole series and intensive individual therapy in the group of typical schizophrenics to be the most crucial variables explaining the change towards improved insight. There was also a third psychotherapy variable, intensive therapy or intervention in crisis in a psychotherapeutic community, that had a clearly significant statistical connection to the favourable development of insightfulness in both the whole series and the group of typical schizophrenics.

The effect of psychotherapy on insight has also been noted in some other investigations of schizophrenic patients. In the works by May (May et al. 1976), the only difference between a psychotherapy plus drug group and a group given merely medication emerged on this variable. Gunderson et al. (1984), who used the same rating scale (Camarillo Insight Scale) saw no difference in this respect between their patients given exploratory insight-oriented (EIO) and reality-adaptive supportive (RAS) therapies. Even so, the development of the EIO patients was better than the development of the RAS patients precisely (and only) as regards the ego functions, which according to the authors' definition ("more able to delay, understand, modulate and express impulses and emotions"), clearly also has connections with the development of insight ability. The favourable effect of psychodynamic psychotherapy – e.g. our therapies – on the patients' insight ability is easy to understand in itself; one central goal of the therapy is to help the patients by increasing their insight into their problems.

Of the other logistic regression analyses, only two psychotherapy variables emerged as explaining variables: in the whole series, separation from the primary family proceeded better if the patient had *not* been given family therapy; and the decrease of interpersonal relationships was prevented by intensive individual therapy given to the patient. The latter finding also pertained to the whole series, but appeared especially conspicuous in the group of typical schizophrenics, though logistic regression analysis could not be carried out separately in this group.

The aforesaid finding on family therapy is somewhat regrettable. It reflects the qualitative underdevelopment of our family-therapeutic activities on the one hand, and the selection into the conjoint therapies of primary families cases with an extremely rigid family homeostasis, which were unable to change with our therapies. The couple therapy patients, whose therapies were relatively more successful, were, in turn, separated from their primary families at the stage of the basic examination already.

Another statistically significant connection was seen between intensive individual therapy and the favourable qualitative development of interpersonal relationships, particularly in the group of typical schizophrenics, where no logistic regression analysis could be carried out on this factor.

On the whole, the effects of psychotherapy on the development of the psychodynamic prognosis were shown by these analyses to be relatively modest, with the exception of the estimates of insight. The effects of intensive individual therapy were still obvious on some other psychodynamic prognostic variables.

More-than-average medication during the follow-up period emerged as the most important explaining variable in the logistic regression analysis carried out on the decrease of interpersonal relationships in the whole series. It also had a clearly significant connection with the patients whose insightfulness decreased during the follow-up period.

Of the background variables defined in the basic examination, psychosocial variables were of clearly greater predictive significance for the development of the patients' psychodynamic prognosis than were the clinical variables. Hence, favourable development of the psychosexual identity was particularly frequent among female patients whose father had no serious personality disorder. Baseline characteristics contributing to loss of an obtained heterosexual identity included unmarried status, presence of alcohol problems, and slow onset of symptoms. Also, regression in this respect was more common among male patients than among female ones, and among the patients who had mothers with seriously disturbed personalities, although these two connections did not emerge as explaining variables in our series. Female sex also appeared as a variable explaining the progress of separation from the primary family in both the whole series and the group of typical schizophrenic patients, whereas lack of occupational identity at the basic examination stage was the most important explaining variable for the regression of the separation process. A typical portion of the group with a regressive separation process and without occupational identity consisted of college students whose illness began halfway through their studies.

The background variables explaining the increase of interpersonal relationships in the whole series included absence of unemployment and alcohol problems at the basic examination stage as well as inclusion in the group of schizo-affective psychoses. In the group of typical schizophrenic patients, the ones lacking heterosexual identity at the basic examination stage showed most increase of interpersonal relationships; the achievement of heterosexual identity during the follow-up period and the creation of significant interpersonal relationships were mutually connected.

The variables explaining the qualitative improvement of the interpersonal relationships outside the primary family consisted of two variables in no way conspicuous in the earlier analyses: avoidance of the expression of aggression and presence of empathic relatives in the family. It should be borne in mind that the interpersonal relationships outside the primary family also included the marital relationships, and that the empathic relatives of several patients were their spouses. The most marked predictor of the qualitative deterioration of the interpersonal relationships outside the primary family was shown by our analysis to be serious personality disorder of the mother.

Besides the psychotherapy variables, the variable most crucially explaining the increase of insight was the absence of alcohol or other addiction problems at the time of the basic examination. The tendency to alcoholism hence turned out to be inversely proportional to motivation and/or ability to internal work and awareness of one's problems.

6.4 Psychosocial Prognosis

The studies of the psychosocial (or social) prognosis of schizophrenic patients have traditionally focussed, first and foremost, on the patients' *working capacity* and *participation in working life*. Our analysis will also concentrate on these aspects. But in addition to the working capacity, *pensions*, and some other questions pertaining to adjustment to working life, we will also consider the development of the *occupational identity* of our patients, which was already referred to in the basic examination. Moreover, we will also describe the development of the *social roles* and *dwelling conditions* among our patients.

While conducting the two-year follow-up examination, our team made up a new concept, which we consider quite appropriate precisely for describing the life course of schizophrenic patients: *maintenance or loss of the grip of life*. As a prognostic variable, this concept belongs to the range of psychosocial prognosis, although it also has points of contact with the patient's psychodynamic situation.

Table 76. Patient's working capacity in the different diagnostic categories in the two-year and five-year follow-up examinations. The figures are percentages

Diagnostic category	Two-year follow-up (N = 96)			Five-year follow-up (N = 95)		
	I	II	III	I	II	III
Typical schizophrenia	34	22	44	33	20	47
Schizophreniform psychosis	60	30	10	78	22	0
Schizo-affective psychosis	54	23	23	50	25	25
Borderline psychosis	50	30	20	50	40	10
Total	42	25	33	43	25	32

I = normal working capacity; II = reduced working capacity; III = unable to work.

Of the psychosocial prognostic variables, only the development of the occupational identity is analyzed as a change taking place between the basic examination and the five-year follow-up examination. The other prognostic variables are based on the patient's condition at the end of the follow-up period.

6.4.1 Working Capacity

The patients' *working capacity* was evaluated at the time of the two-year and five-year follow-up examinations. The evaluation was made with a three-step scale: the patient was considered fully able to work, his working capacity was considered poorer than normal, or he was considered completely unable to work. The classification was not based on the patient's contemporary working situation, i.e. whether he was working or not, though it is naturally quite closely associated with this classification. The intermediary group of poor working capacity included some patients on disability pension who were not, however, considered completely unable to work by us, but also patients who had at least transient jobs or were studying, but had clearly lost their working capacity of the normal level.

A summary of the findings on working capacity is shown in Table 76, where they are presented as percentages for each diagnostic sub-category.

The follow-up findings are quite parallel: No changes in the patients' working capacity seem to have taken place between the two examinations. The findings also give

Table 77. Working capacity in the different ego-psychologic groups in the five-year follow-up examination. The figures are percentages

Ego-dynamic group	I	II	III
Imminent disintegration (N = 21)	57	33	10
Acute disintegration (N = 25)	56	24	20
Regressive disintegration (N = 30)	27	27	47
Paranoid disintegration (N = 19)	37	16	47

I = fully able to work; II = reduced working capacity; III = unable to work.

rise to a conclusion that the *prognosis for the working capacity of our patients is relatively less optimistic than the prognosis for the psychotic symptoms*.

Although the nuclear group includes more patients completely unable to work, it is noteworthy that the *differences between the diagnostic sub-categories are unexpectedly small, being clearly smaller than the differences in the disappearance of psychotic symptoms*.

It is pertinent also to analyze the *ego-dynamic groups* separately here. We will carry out this analysis on the basis of the five-year follow-up situation (Table 77).

The difference between the patients with more serious illness (regressive and paranoid disintegration) and the ones with less serious forms of illness (imminent and acute disintegration) is obvious, but smaller than in the disappearance of psychotic symptoms. These findings suggest that the prognosis of working capacity is clearly also affected by variables other than the clinico-diagnostic ones.

This comes quite clearly in the *logistic regression analysis of the factors contributing to the working capacity*, where the patients fully able to work in the five-year follow-up examination constituted one group and those with a reduced working capacity or unable to work made up another. The variable explaining the maintenance of working capacity are shown in Table 78.

All of the explaining variables except the first in the group of typical schizophrenics, the amount of neuroleptic medication, are psychosocial background variables. Unemployment and the *lack of occupational identity emerge as factors predictive of a poor working capacity* particularly in the whole series. *Basic education* is – contrary to nearly all of our other analyses – of favourable explaining significance for working capacity. In direct cross-tabulation, however, its connection with working capacity was less significant than the connections of the other explaining variables, as it does not quite reach the level of being almost significant either in the whole series or in the group of typical schizophrenics. The significance of basic education as a factor contributing to the maintenance of working capacity was especially notable among the patients who

Table 78. Working capacity at the time of the five-year follow-up. Influence of background and/or treatment variables (logistic regression)

Explaining variable	risk	p
All patients		
Not unemployed	10.66	.000
Stable occupational identity	1.81	.003
More basic education	1.56	.008
Female sex	1.66	.023
No hostile or poorly understanding relatives	2.03	.031
Typical schizophrenics		
Neuroleptic treatment: less than average	4.78	.000
Female sex	4.38	.013
More basic education	2.11	.006
No alcohol or other addiction problems	9.17	.079

were not unemployed at the time of the basic examination. *Working capacity was clearly better among female patients than among males* ($p = .003$ in the whole series, $p < .001$ in the group of typical schizophrenias). *Alcohol problems* also were connected statistically with the loss of working capacity both in the whole series ($p < .05$) and in the group of typical schizophrenias ($p = .001$), in which only about 10 % of those having these problems had maintained their working capacity.

The finding on *poorly understanding or hostile relatives* had a clearly significant connection with the loss of working capacity both in the whole series and in the group of typical schizophrenics. Some other family variables also were connected with working capacity: empathic relatives positively, seriously disturbed personality of the mother and even seriously disturbed personality of the father (in the group of typical schizophrenia) negatively. The social group of the patient or the parents was not of significance, however.

Of the treatment variables, only the lower-than-average amount of medication emerged in the logistic regression analysis. Its connection with the maintenance of working capacity was equally obvious in the whole series as in the group of typical schizophrenics ($p < .001$). But the *psychotherapy variables were also connected with working capacity,* although they did not emerge as explaining variables. Inclusion in the *group of psychotherapy cases* had an almost significant connection with good prognosis in the whole series and a clearly significant one ($p = .002$) in the group of typical schizophrenics. Both *intensive individual therapy* and *intensive therapy or intervention in crisis in a psychotherapeutic community* were also connected with the maintenance of working capacity by typical schizophrenics (former $p = .028$, latter $p = .021$) but their influence in the whole series did not reach the level of statistical significance.

Working capacity was thus one of the prognostic variables where the significance of psychotherapeutic treatments was conspicuous especially in the group of typical schizophrenics. Numerically, 52 % of the psychotherapy patients in the whole series remained able to work, as compared with 32 % in the group of patients not included in the group of psychotherapy cases. The corresponding figures in the group of typical schizophrenics were 50 % and 10 %. *Only two of the patient in the nuclear group not included in the psychotherapy cases had remained completely able to work, the corresponding figure in the psychotherapy group being 16.*

Table 78 indicates that *unemployment* at the time of the basic examination had a notable influence of the prognosis of working capacity. Of the 22 patients who were unemployed at the time of admission, 20 were interviewed in the five-year follow-up examination, and only one was able to work normally.

During the first two follow-up years, 17 patients had been unemployed for at least 3 months. The corresponding figure for the period between the two-year and five-year follow-up examinations was 8. Of these 8, 4 were the same as the ones noted previously, which means that altogether 21 patients had had unemployment problems during the whole follow-up period. Among them, there were 12 male patients and 9 female ones. Men thus had unemployment problems more frequently than women, but the difference was small and not apt to declare their worse psychosocial prognosis.

Table 79. The patient's social roles and disability pensions at the times of the basic examination and the follow-up examinations

Social role	Number of patients					
	Basic examination (N = 100)		Two year follow-up (N = 97)		Five year follow-up (N = 95)	
Student	20		6		5	
Permanent job		45	37	43	35	41
Temporary job			6		6	
Works at home (the spouse responsible for the home or otherwise)	12		7		7	
Unemployed	22		8		1	
On pension for psych. reasons	–	1	31	33	39	41[a]
On pension for somatic reasons	1		2		2	

[a] Of these, 2 were long-term in-patients of a psychiatric hospital and 1 patient of a forensic psychiatric hospital.

6.4.2 Social Role and Disability Pensions

The *social roles* of our patients at the time of the basic examination on the one hand and at the time of the follow-up examinations on the other are presented in Table 79. This table also shows how many of the patients received *disability pension* on the basis of their illness.

The table indicates that the *number of patients working permanently or temporarily had declined only slightly,* whereas *a notable reduction had taken place in the group of unemployed patients* and – during the first follow-up period – *in the group of students.* The number of housewives or patients otherwise working at home also clearly diminished during the first two follow-up years. The group on pension increased correspondingly: *nearly one third of our patients, 31, had been granted a disability pension on the basis of their psychic illness during the first two follow-up years already, and the number had further increased by the time of the five-year follow-up examination, being 39.* Moreover, 2 other patients were receiving a pension for a physical illness.

One of these two, who suffered from rheumatoid arthritis, was on a disability pension at the time of the basic examination already. He was included in our series because of short-term schizo-affective psychosis with good prognosis. The other pension granted for physical illness had been given to a patient with torticollis spastica, who was classified as having borderline schizophrenia.

A more detailed analysis indicated that of the 22 patients unemployed at the basic examination stage, 16 were on pension at the end of the five-year follow-up period. One was working permanently, one was working temporarily, one patient (who had got married in the meantime) was working at home, and one continued to be unemployed, in addition to which one of these patients had died and another was lost to the five-year follow-up examination.

Of the students, 5 continued their school or college at the time of the five-year follow-up examination. Four had found a permanent job and 2 a temporary job, while 8 were on disability pension and 1 had died. Of those who had found a permanent job,

2 had completed their studies successfully prior to that, one in a university, the other in a college. The situation was hence clearly better in this group than in the group of unemployed patients, but the figures do not give a very optimistic picture of the study performance of our patients.

We now analyze the *inclusion in the group on disability pension at the end of the five-year follow-up period* in the same way as we have analyzed our other prognostic variables, elucidating the connections between the disability pension and the background and treatment variables. Before we do that, however, it is useful to explain briefly the system of pensions applied in Finland.

The system of sickness insurance and disability pensions in Finland is subject to the National Pensions Institute and well developed. Sickness insurance daily allowance can be paid to subjects aged 16–64 years who are "unable to do their ordinary work or work comparable to that because of illness" on the basis of disability that has lasted for 7 days. A certificate given by a physician is required. Daily allowance, however, is only paid for a maximum of 300 days. If the disability continues beyond that, the subject must apply for a disability pension on a basis of a physicians' certificate and the same grounds as above. The maximum period of 300 days includes the days for which sickness insurance daily allowance has been paid during the two years preceding the beginning of the disability; the period hence need not be uninterrupted. Previous episodes of illness are not considered, however, if the patient has been able to work for at least a year since the previous episode of disability.

The withdrawal on pension after the 300-day period of disability is of ambiguous value for the schizophrenic patient, whose therapy often requires a long time. The pension is often granted even in cases where the patient's condition is clearly improving. It is usual, however, that the physician recommends the pension to be granted provisionally, but generally for a year.

After that the situation is re-estimated, and the patient can either be considered able to work or be granted a further pension either provisionally or on a more permanent basis.

The good social security also has its negative aspects: the disability pension can become a "secondary benefit" difficult to give up even after recovery. This is particularly true of cases where the patient, even when his condition is good, continues to feel uncertain about the maintenance of his working capacity – as is often the case in psychic illness. The uncertainty is especially notable during periods of unemployment. The patient's family may also support this secondary benefit, which also applies to the family, and thereby help the patient to maintain his role as sick. The practical criteria for granting disability pension on the basis of illness in Finland became clearly less strict over the 1970's.

Table 80. The social roles of our patients and the estimates of their working capacity in the five-year follow-up examination

Social role	Working capacity			
	incapac-itated	affected	normal	total
Student	2	0	3	5
Working temporarily	0	4	2	6
Working permanently	0	3	32	35
Working at home	0	3	4	7
Unemployed	0	1	0	1
On pension	27	12	0	39
On pension for somatic causes	1	1	0	2
Total	30	24	41	95

The pension policy was doubtless greatly influenced by the increase of unemployment that began in the early 1970's and restricts severely the possibilities of rehabilitating patients for work. In borderline cases, continuation of disability pension granted on the basis of illness is a more popular solution than registration in the unemployment files.

Did the group of patients granted disability pension in our series include ones for whom the pension could not be considered justifiable? To elucidate this question, we *compared the social roles of our patients* at the time of the five-year follow-up examination *and our assessments of their working capacity*. The results are shown in Table 80.

The comparison indicates that *none of the patients on disability pension were considered to be able to work normally, although about one third were estimated to have merely partly affected working capacity*. On the other hand, there were 2 patients, both of them students, who were unable to work, but were not on disability pension. Of the patients working temporarily, 4 out of 6 had affected working capacity, as did also nearly half of those working at home. The group with permanent jobs, however, had only a few patients with affected working capacity relative to the total number of patients in this group.

According to these findings the disability pension can be considered justifiable in at least 70 % of the cases in which it was granted. The situations of the other 12 patients on pension estimated to be able to work at an affected capacity appeared variable, and the justification of the disability pension was not easy to evaluate.

The group included some patients in quite a good condition clinically, but with a possibility of a relapse of psychotic symptoms in working life. In the case of one mother of two children, a housewife, the pension had the practical justification of giving the patient a financial independence of her husband, who treated her quite badly.

Nevertheless, the *group of patients with an affected working capacity receiving a pension included several for whom intensive rehabilitative measures would have been clearly indicated*, even regardless of possible resistance by the patient. The same can be stated of some patients estimated as unable to work.

The *disability pension* of one patient had been *discontinued* during the first follow-up period already, and the pensions of 5 other patients were discontinued during the latter follow-up period. According to our estimate, the favourable development was, at least partly, due to psychotherapeutic treatment in 5 cases.

Table 81 contains a summary of the *diagnostic categories of the patients on disability pension* at the time of the five-year follow-up examination, showing both the absolute

Table 81. Distribution of the patients on disability pension into the different diagnostic categories

Diagnostic category	Number of patients on pension	%
Typical schizophrenia	30	55.6
Schizophreniform psychosis	2	20
Schizo-affective psychosis	3	25
Borderline psychosis	4	20
Total	39	40.6

Table 82. Variables explaining disability pension at the end of the five-year follow-up period. Influence of background and/or treatment variables. Logistic regression

Explaining variables	risk	p
All patients		
Neuroleptic medication: more than average	5.78	.000
No empathic relatives	2.36	.006
Alcohol or other addiction problems	1.58	.006
Typical schizophrenics		
Neuroleptic medication: more than a average	4.88	.000
No empathic relatives	2.01	.012
Alcohol or other addiction problems	2.11	.018

numbers and the percentages of the patients in each category. Only the pensions granted on the basis of psychic illness are included.

As expected, disability pensions were most common in the group of typical schizophrenics, where slightly more than half of the patients were receiving disability pension. Nine patients on pension were outside the nuclear group. Statistically speaking, *inclusion in the group of typical schizophrenic patients had a significant connection with pension* (p = .002). Of the different ego-dynamic groups, the regressively disintegrated patients had a significant connection with being on pension, whereas no statistical connection with the group of paranoid disintegration was found.

The logistic regression analysis (Table 82) brought out pension to be explained by variables other than those based on the clinical categorization, however. Both in the whole series and in the group of typical schizophrenic patients, the most important explaining variable was *more-than-average neuroleptic medication*, the next being *lack of empathic relatives*, and the third presence of *alcohol or other addiction problems* at the time of the basic examination already.

No other treatment variables apart from neuroleptic medication had connections with disability pension. What came closest to statistical significance was the negative connection between inclusion in the group of psychotherapy cases and pension in the group of typical schizophrenics (p = .12). The *first unit of treatment*, however, *had a significant connection with pension.* The percentage of patients on pension was 23 % among those first admitted into out-patient care, 34.5 % among those first admitted into the Clinic of Psychiatry, and 71 % among those first admitted into the Kupittaa Hospital (p = .003; p = .008 in the group of typical schizophrenics). Equally important was the patient's sex: only 12 of the female patients were on pension, while 27 of the male patients were on a similar pension (p = .009). The difference was largely due to the group of typical schizophrenics (22 male and 8 female patients were on pension, p = .003). There were no differences between the different age groups.

6.4.3 Dwelling Conditions

The table below shows the data on the dwelling conditions of our patients at the times of the basic examination and the two follow-up examinations.

Table 83. Patient's modes of dwelling at the time of the basic examination and the two year and five-year follow-up examinations

Mode of dwelling	Number of patients		
	Basic examination (N = 100)	Two-year follow-up (N = 97)	Five-year follow-up (N = 95)
Alone	28	27	25
With parents	25	25	21
With own family	35	29	32
With other relatives	7	6	3
With a friend or acquaintance	4	5	7
In a residential home	–	2	4
Chronically in hospital	–	–	3
In prison	–	2	–
In another institution	–	1	1
Other mode of dwelling	–	1	–

The changes are small: the numbers of patients living alone or with their parents remained almost unchanged. The number of patients living with their own families declined during the first two follow-up years, but increased slightly during the latter period. Living with other relatives became less common, while living with a friend or acquaintance (which regularly referred to at least short-term sexual partnership) increased. Four patients lived in a residential home at the end of the follow-up period.

6.4.4 Occupational Identity and Its Development

The occupational identities of our patients were assessed in the basic examination and in the five-year follow-up examination. The development that took place in it is shown in Table 84.

We can see that *regression of the occupational identity was clearly more common among our patients than corresponding progress during the follow-up period*. Many of the patients who had dropped out of working life felt they had also lost their occupational competence and the consequent status in society.

The stable occupational identity was less common among the typical schizophrenic patients: at the end of the follow-up period, 19 patients of this group had a stable

Table 84. Development of the patient's occupational identity between the basic examination and the five-year follow-up examination. The figures are percentages

Degree of occupational identity	Basic examination (N = 100)	Five-year follow-up (N = 95)
No occupational identity	24	35
Developing occupational identity	15	19
Stable occupational identity	61	45

Table 85. Stabilization of occupational identity during the five-year follow-up period: effect of background and/or treatment variables (logistic regression analysis)

Explaining variables	risk	p
All patients		
Intensive individual therapy	3.05	.014
No interpersonal relationships outside primary family	2.86	.009

Table 86. Deterioration of occupational identity during the five-year follow-up period: effect of background and/or treatment variables (logistic regression analysis)

Explaining variables	risk	p
All patients		
Serious personality disorder of the mother	3.22	.006
Neuroleptic medication: more than average	2.18	.027

occupational identity, 10 had a developing identity, and 25 lacked even that, while the corresponding figures for the other patients were 25, 8 and 8 ($p = .017$). The situation was worst in the group of regressive disintegration ($p < .001$), while the group of paranoid disintegration did not differ at all from the average for the whole series in this respect.

Of the patients who lacked a stable occupational identity at the time of the basic examination, 12 had *reached* such identity by the end of the five-year follow-up period (including 10 patients with typical schizophrenia), while 23 patients continued to have an unsatisfactory situation in this respect (including 15 typical schizophrenics). *Regression* from the stable occupational identity reached by the basic examination had taken place in 24 cases (including 16 typical schizophrenics), whereas 36 patients (including 13 typical schizophrenics) had retained their occupational identity. It is interesting that both progress and regression were hence relatively more common in the group of typical schizophrenics than in the rest of the series.

The *logistic regression analysis* of these changes could only be carried out in the whole series. The results are shown in the Tables 85 and 86.

We can see that the most central variable contributing to the *stabilization of the occupational identity* was *intensive individual therapy.* The group included 11 patients who had received intensive individual therapy, and 7 of them showed stabilization of occupational identity. Inclusion in the group of psychotherapy cases also had a parallel, though statistically marginal, connection with the stabilization of the occupational identity. The other explaining variable was the *lack of interpersonal relationships outside the primary family* at the time of the basic examination. The occupational identity particularly in the diagnostic nuclear group had hence developed favourably among the patients whose interpersonal relationships had simultaneously also increased compared with the basic examination.

The most important variable explaining the *loss of an occupational identity once established* was a background variable pertaining to the family milieu: *serious personality disorder of the mother. More-than-average neuroleptic medication* emerged as another explaining variable.

6.4.5 Maintenance or Loss of the Grip on Life

The concept of maintenance or loss of the grip on life was based on some observations made by Räkköläinen et al. (1979) in the follow-up examination of a former series of psychotic patients. By *maintenance of the grip of life* we mean that the *patient continues, at least in his thoughts pertaining to the future, to maintain his effort to achieve the goals and modes of satisfaction associated normally with the interpersonal relationships and social life of an adult human being (or the patient's age mates)*. The loss of the grip is manifested as an abandonment of the objectives associated with the adult role and pertaining to other people – particularly other family members and sexuality – as well as in the attitude towards working life in general, where the loss of the grip on life is indicated by more permanent attitudes towards pensions, sick leaves, hospitalization and other factors providing passive-regressive satisfaction.

It is important that neither the presence of psychotic symptoms, nor the patient's being on disability pension as such are taken into account in this assessment. It is true, of course, that the loss of grip is often clearly due to increasing chronicity of the psychotic illness. Even so, there are some markedly psychotic patients who have retained their effort towards functional activity and have not lost their grip on life in the sense we mean here. For some others, on the other hand, a tendency to a regressive mode of life may serve as an alternative to psychosis. This can guarantee for the patients such supportive structures in their interpersonal environment which are essential for their ego's capacity to prevent repeated or continuous disintegration. This threat may be felt by these patients to be increased through efforts at adult-level interaction. The loss of the grip on life generally involves feelings of apathy and hopelessness, but it may also, through such regressive reliance on other people and/or the help provided by society, become a situation accepted by the patient himself. *In contrast to our other psychosocial variables, the assessment of the maintenance or loss of the grip on life focusses on an attempt to comprehend the patient's subjective notion of his situation and his relationships with the world outside himself.*

As far as we could see, it was not difficult in the follow-up examination to identify the patients who had lost their grip on life by means of both empathic observation and/ or objective examination of their mode of life. *At the time of the two-year follow-up examination* there were 64 patients who had maintained their grip on life and 31 who had lost it. The corresponding figures in the *five-year follow-up examination* were 67 and 28. In the light of these figures, the number of patients who had lost their grip was slightly lower in the latter follow-up examination than in the former.

Case-specifically, the five-year follow-up assessment included 20 patients estimated as having lost their grip who had already been classified thus in the two-year follow-up examination. There were 11 patients with favourable development and 8 patients who had lost their grip during the period between the follow-up examinations.

The *logistic regression analysis* of the background and treatment variables explaining the maintenance of the grip on life gave the following results:

Table 87. Maintenance of the grip on life at the end of the five-year follow-up period. Effect of background and/or treatment variables. Logistic regression analysis

Explaining variables	risk	p
All patients		
Neuroleptic treatment: less than average	1.14	.000
No unemployment	2.71	.001
Occupational identity stabilized	1.37	.003
Not diagnosed as typical schizophrenia	1.62	.009
Typical schizophrenics		
Neuroleptic treatment: less than average	2.41	.000
No unemployment	8.31	.006
Empathic relatives	2.10	.028

The analysis thus indicates that the *factors explaining the maintenance of the grip* in the whole series include one treatment variable: *less-than-average neuroleptic medication*, two psychosocial background variables: the patient's *not being classified as unemployed at the time of the basic examination* and *stabilized occupational identity*, and one clinical variable: *exclusion from the diagnostic nuclear category.* In a separate analysis of the typical schizophrenic patients, the variables based on lesser neuroleptic medication and lack of unemployment retained their significance, and the finding of *empathic relatives* at the time of the basic examination emerged as a third favourable background variable.

Higher-than-average medication hence was very strongly connected with negative development even on this psychosocial prognostic variable. The psychotherapy variables unexpectedly had no significant connections with the maintenance or loss of the grip on life. The variable that came closest to statistical significance was the favourable effect of the psychotherapeutic community in the group of typical schizophrenic patients ($p = .100$). Of the psychotherapy cases, 74 % had maintained their grip while the corresponding figure for those given intensive individual therapy was 81 %.

Of the variables pertaining to the *family background*, both the presence of empathic relatives and the lack of poorly understanding or hostile relatives were clearly significantly ($p < .01$) connected with the maintenance of the grip on life in the whole series as well as in the group of typical schizophrenics. The females in both the whole series and the group of typical schizophrenics had retained their grip almost significantly better than the male patients, while the age group did not matter in this respect.

6.4.6 Summary and Discussion

Of all the patients in our series, *43 % were found to be fully able to work*, 25 % *partly able to work, and 32 % unable to work* at the time of the five-year follow-up examination. The corresponding percentages for the typical schizophrenics were 33, 20 and 47 %. The figures were more or less the same in the two-year follow-up examination.

Although the patients of the nuclear group had a poorer average prognosis for working capacity than the other diagnostic categories, the difference was clearly smaller than those seen in the findings on the disappearance or persistence of psychotic symptoms. This is also shown by the figures for the disability pensions granted on the basis of psychic illness. 39 patients were on pension in the whole series (40.6 % of those interviewed in the five-year follow-up examination), the corresponding figure being 55.6 % in the group of typical schizophrenics and 20–25 % in the other diagnostic categories. When we remember that manifest psychotic symptoms outside the nuclear group at the same stage were only noted in 2 patients with borderline schizophrenia, we can conclude that even some of the patients without psychotic symptoms were on pension.

The number of disability pensions in the five-year follow-up examination had increased by 8 from 31 recorded at the time of the two-year follow-up examination, which is also in contrast to the finding on the slightly improved general clinical status of the patients. All these factors suggest that the *maintenance or loss of working capacity by the patients was also connected to factors other than their clinical condition.*

The findings made in other Finnish investigations seem to suggest that the number of schizophrenic patients on disability pension has tended to increase over the past two decades. The findings by Achté and his co-workers show that the percentage of surviving first admission schizophrenics from Helsinki on pension after five years was 39 % in the group admitted in 1950, 28 % in the 1960 group, 32 % in the 1965 group, and as high as 43 % in the 1970 group. In the Turku series analyzed by Salokangas, 31 of the patients admitted during 1965–67 were on pension after 7½ years, which accounts for 34 % of those interviewed in the follow-up examination, while the corresponding percentage in the group admitted in 1969 was 44 % (Achté 1967, 1980, Niskanen & Achté 1972, Salokangas 1977, 1985).

According to Lehtinen (1975), who carried out an investigation of a sample of 1000 persons in some parts of southwestern and northern Finland during 1969–72, 10 % of those unable to work because of psychic reasons were unjustifiably without a disability pension. The situation seems to have changed thereafter, one reason being the increasing unemployment. Parallel to this, the criteria for granting disability pensions have also been made less strict. Many of the patients are granted, almost automatically, a provisional disability pension after they have been incapacitated by illness for 300 days. As the employment situation is poor and restricts the opportunities of rehabilitating patients for work, continuation of the pension often remains a more popular solution than transfer of the patient into the unemployment files, despite the favourable development of the patient's condition. The pension may also become a factor realistically increasing the patient's financial security and the permanence of his interpersonal relationships.

Of the 39 patients on pension in our series, we classified 12 as not completely incapacitated. Their working capacity was, however, considered to be declined, which means that none with a normal working capacity received disability pension. There were 6 patients in our series who had returned to regular working life (or studies) after having been on a provisional disability pension. Five of these patients belonged to our group of psychotherapy cases.

Any comparison with investigations carried out elsewhere is difficult because of differences on both the diagnostic criteria and the criteria of working capacity. We might, however, present some findings of the studies also described in Chapter 6.2.6. In the series collected by von Sivers (1983) Sweden, 48 % of the male patients and 67 % of the female patients admitted in the early 1960's were in full-time or part-time jobs 6–11 years later; 43 % of the male and 22 % of the female patients were on disability pension. In the Canadian series analyzed by Bland (1976), the patient's economic productivity was good or fair in 59 % of the cases and poor in 35 %. In Harrow's (1978) American sample the working capacity after a 2.7-year follow-up period was good in 36 % of the cases, equivocal in 34 % and poor in 30 %. Of the male patients, 3/4 had at least some difficulty in this respect. In the series studied by Strauss et al. (1972), 40 % of the patients were fully employed after a follow-up period of two years; the second best category (the patients who were able to work for more than half of the latter follow-up year) included 20 % of the patients. In another American series analyzed by Stephens et al. (1978) good functioning after 10 years was seen in 39 % of the cases and poor functioning in 44 %. The diagnostic criteria in these populations were relatively close to ours. When we further point out that the length of the follow-up period did not seem (even in our series) to have any great effect on the development of the working capacity, we can conclude that our findings are roughly parallel to the results of these studies. The comparison also confirms our notion of the clinical prognosis of our own patients being relatively better than their prognosis for working capacity.

Gam (1980) published a 5-year retrospective investigation of all first admitted schizophrenics to Danish psychiatric institutions during one year in 1970–71. In this material, 68 % of the patients had a disability pension at the end of the follow-up period, and only 12 per cent supported themselves by ordinary work. Compared with our material, the diagnostic limits in this study were rather strict.

The psychosocial background factors contributed particularly conspicuously to the maintenance of our patient's working capacity. All the explaining variables except the first in the group of typical schizophrenia, a less-than-average neuroleptic medication, pointed out to their influence. The significance of unemployment was especially remarkable in the whole series: of the patients with unemployment as a baseline finding, only 10 % were able to work after the five-year follow-up period, a majority of the others being on disability pension. Among the patients not initially unemployed, the loss of working capacity was most crucially due to the *lack of occupational identity.* This was also one of the few points in our analyses where *basic education* emerged as significant. The *better working capacity of women in comparison with men* is accordant with the findings made by von Sivers and Harrow as well as by Salokangas. In our series, 54 % of the female patients and 33 % of the male patients were fully able to work, the corresponding figures in the group of typical schizophrenia being 58 % and 13 %.

Lassenius et al. (1973) in Sweden postulated that poor employment conditions would increase the unemployment problems of especially men, thereby impairing their psychosocial prognosis. This postulation did not receive much support from our own findings. The prognosis of male schizophrenic patients seems, in general, to be less good than that of female patients, but this discrepancy is particularly conspicuous in the prognosis of working capacity. It is possible that the greater expectations applied to the psychosocial role of men more generally affect the prognostic development of schizophrenic male patients.

According to our logistic regression analysis, *disability pension* at the time of the five-year follow-up examination was explained in both the whole series and the group of typical schizophrenics by the same variables in the same order: *more-than-average medication during the follow-up period* and the *baseline characteristics of a lack of empathic relatives and the presence of alcohol or addiction problems*.

More-than-average neuroleptic treatment hence emerges as a notable parallel factor for both unability to work and being on disability pension. What attracts attention is that this is especially true of the group of typical schizophrenic patients, for whom neuroleptic medication is generally considered particularly indicated, often as continuous treatment.

The lack of empathic relatives (and also the presence of hostile or poorly understanding relatives, which clearly correlates with disability pension) reflects in this prognostic dimension the significance of family milieus for the prognosis, which has also turned out important in many other ways.

Although inclusion in the group of *psychotherapy cases* did not emerge as an explaining variable in these analyses, it correlated with the maintenance of working capacity almost significantly in the whole series and clearly significantly in the group of typical schizophrenics. In the nuclear group, there was also an almost significant parallel connection with intensive individual therapy and intensive therapy or intervention in crisis in a psychotherapeutic community. With regard to the disability pensions, inclusion in the group of psychotherapy cases did not reach a statistical connection. It turned out, however, that of the patients who started their therapy in out-patient care or in a psychotherapeutically oriented hospital, only one half compared with those given more conventional hospital treatment initially were on disability pension after 5 years.

There is no doubt that a better view would have been obtained of the effect of psychotherapeutic treatments if the working capacity of the patients had also been assessed at the time of their admission. This was not done, because most of the patients were unable to work at the time of the basic examination. A retrospective assessment of their working capacity during the preceding year would have been possible, however, by using e.g. the criteria developed by Strauss and Carpenter (1972, 1977) for this purpose, but the team was not aware of these criteria at that time.

The degree of the *occupational identity* of the patients was determined both in the basic examination and at the time of the five-year follow-up examination. In the former assessment 61 % of the patients had a stabilized occupational identity, while 45 % of the patients had a corresponding identity in the latter assessment.

According to the logistic regression analysis, the *achievement of a stable occupational identity* during the follow-up period was explained by *intensive individual therapy* and a *lack of interpersonal relationships at the time of the basic examination* in the whole series. *Regression* of the occupational identity, in turn, was explained by a *serious personality disorder of the mother* and *more-than-average neuroleptic medication*. No separate analysis could be carried out in the group of typical schizophrenias. Since, however, the group which gained occupational identity during the follow-up period consisted largely of patients of the nuclear group, we can conclude that favourable development was especially typical of patients of the nuclear group with a previous tendency to isolation who had been given intensive individual therapy. Inclusion in the group of psychotherapy cases also had a positive, though only marginally significant, connection with stabilization of the occupational identity.

As a new psychosocial background variable, we analyzed the patient's subjective experience of *maintaining or losing his grip in his efforts towards the ordinary goals and modes of satisfaction* in adult life (or in the life of his age-mates) during the two follow-up sub-periods. The term is based on the observations made by Räkköläinen et al. (1979) in a previous follow-up survey of schizophrenic patients in Turku (cf. also Alanen et al. 1983). The term "optimistic/integrated attitude" used by Gunderson et al. (1984) probably comes close to it in some respects. *The loss or maintenance of the grip is mainly a matter of the extent to which the patient continues, at least in his thoughts of the future, to strive towards the kind of interpersonal relationships and goals of working life he originally used to have, which are accordant with the norms of his cultural milieu.* The premise for this assessment are hence more concrete than those for the more general definitions of attitudes. The common opposites to the maintenance of the grip are withdrawal into an autistic psychotic world on the one hand and assumption of a given-up regressive social role on the other.

In a dichotomous, and therefore relatively unsophisticated, assessment, we found out that 33 % of our patients had lost their grip by the two-year follow-up examination and 30 % had done so by the end of the five-year follow-up. The loss of the grip was clearly more common in the diagnostic nuclear category than among the other patients (44 % in the five-year follow-up examination). Even so, the number of patients maintaining their grip was higher than the number of ones who had lost it in this group, too.

The background variables explaining the maintenance of the grip on life were largely parallel to those found in the analyses of working capacity and disability pensions. Less-than-average neuroleptic medication was particularly influential, baseline findings of a lack of employment problems emerging as next. The presence of empathic relatives was significant especially in the group of typical schizophrenia. Of the psychotherapy variables, however, only intensive therapy or intervention in crisis in a psychotherapeutic community reached the limit of marginal statistical significance in the group of typical schizophrenic patients.

6.5 Prognosis in the Light of Hospital Treatments

The need for hospital treatment is considered one of the most important measures of the prognosis of schizophrenic patients. Its significance is underlined by the economic aspect: hospital treatment constitutes the greatest economic burden on society caused by schizophrenia, as it is more expensive than out-patient care. In addition to the direct cost of hospital treatment, we must also take into account the economic losses incurred by society as a consequence of the loss of the potential contribution to productive life by the individuals who end up as chronic inmates of institutions.

Calculation of the days spent in hospital, however, is an ambiguous prognostic indicator, particularly in the short run. Hospital treatment is not an exclusively negative matter – even from the viewpoint of the costs to society. Its purpose, after all, is to improve the patient's condition and, if possible, rehabilitate him as a functional and working member of the community. This goal is particularly emphatic in the case of first-admission psychotic patients. We already demonstrated above (Chapter 5.1.1.2.) that in our own series the need for later hospital treatments decreased in the group of patients whose first in-patient period was relatively long (at the average) and psychotherapeutically oriented, compared with patients treated shorter at more conventionally oriented hospital wards.

Hospital treatments as a prognostic indicator must therefore be examined over a period of several years. We accomplished this in two ways:

1. *We calculated the number of days spent in hospital annually by our patients and analyzed their connections with our background and therapeutic variables.* The actual prognostic variable consisted of *the total number of in-patient days during the five-year follow-up period* in the groups discriminated on the basis of the background and treatment variables.
2. We compare the groups differentiated on the basis of the background and treatment variables with the rest of the series also on the basis of *how great a portion of the patients* in each group *were in hospital at least once during the last two follow-up years.* The number of such patients in the whole series was 31.

The first of these prognostic variables gives us an idea of the total amount of time spent on the hospital treatment of our patients and the factors affecting it. This prognostic variable is hence also directly related to the costs of the hospital treatment of our patients. The second prognostic variable, in turn, gives an idea of the long-term developmental tendency, indicating the background and treatment variables that determined whether the patient was still in need of hospital treatment during the last two follow-up years or not.

6.5.1 In-Patient Days During the Follow-up Years

The data on the duration and number of in-patient periods during the follow-up years in the whole series and the different diagnostic and ego-dynamic groups were given above in Chapter 5.1.1.1. (cf. Figures 2 and 3 pp. 82 and 83).

The group of typical schizophrenics did not differ from the rest of the series significantly during the first two years, but the differences of the third, fourth, and fifth year as well as the overall difference during the entire follow-up period were highly significant. Of the ego-dynamic groups, the group of regressive disintegration had a highly significant connection with a greater-than-average need for hospital treatment throughout the follow-up period.

Of the treatment variables, only *more-than-average neuroleptic medication* had a definite and continuous connection with the number of in-patient days, which was highly significantly greater than the average in this group. The *group of psychotherapy cases, however, did not differ statistically from the rest of the series* in this respect, with the exception of the first follow-up year, when the psychotherapy cases had marginally significantly more in-patient days in the whole series than the other patients. Only during the last follow-up year was the number of in-patient days smaller in the group of psychotherapy cases than among the other patients, more clearly so in a separate analysis of the typical schizophrenics. The development of the number of in-patient days in the group of psychotherapy cases is shown in Figures 5 and 6.

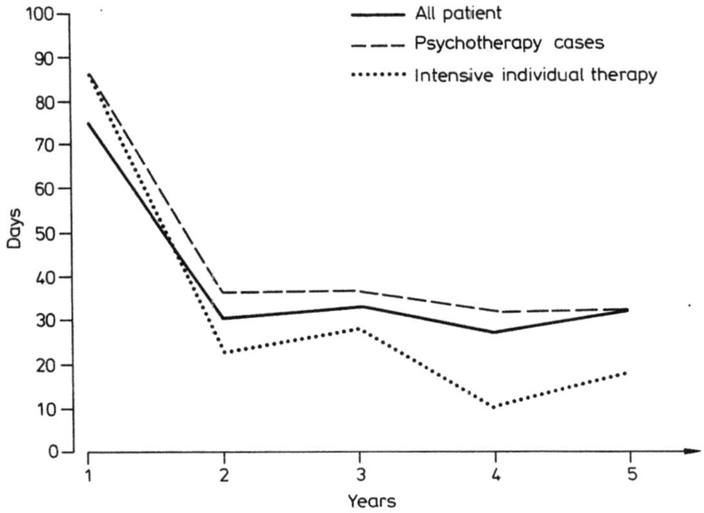

Fig. 5. In-patient days on the average per year in the whole patient series: All patients, the group of psychotherapy cases and the patients given intensive individual therapy

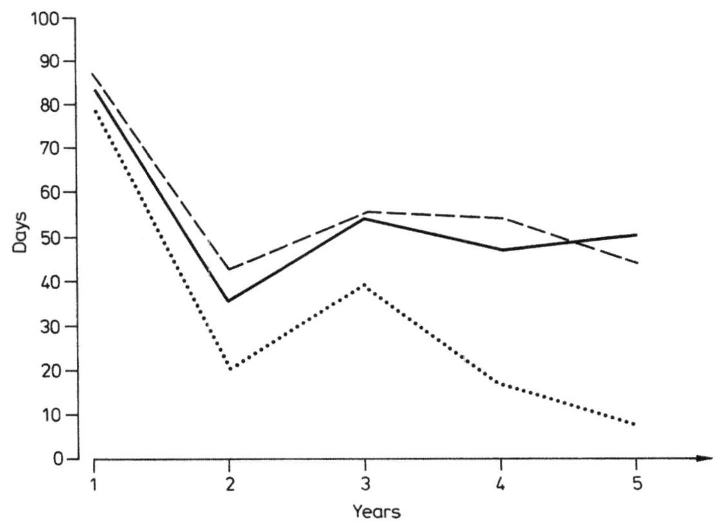

Fig. 6. In-patient days on the average per year in the group of typical schizophrenic patients: all patients, the group of psychotherapy cases and the patients given intensive individual therapy

The Figures also include the average level of the number of in-patient days among the patients given *intensive individual therapy.* We can see that the need for hospital treatment decreases more rapidly in this group than in the group of psychotherapy cases. Nevertheless, the difference between this group and the patients not given intensive individual therapy is only almost significant during the last follow-up year in the group of typical schizophrenic patients and marginally significant in the whole series during the fourth follow-up year. *The total number of in-patient days during the follow-up period, however, remains without statistical significance even in this group* compared with the other patients, although it comes close to marginal significance relative to the typical schizophrenics ($p = .13$).

The patients given family *therapy* had an almost significantly greater-than-average number of in-patient days in the whole series during the first follow-up year, but the figure then came down below the level of statistical significance, yet being marginally significantly greater ($p = .083$) than the corresponding figure for the rest of the series in the overall analysis of the whole follow-up period. In the group of typical schizophrenic patients, no differences were seen between the patients given and not given family therapy.

The patients given intensive therapy or intervention in crisis in a psychotherapeutic community had an almost significantly greater-than-average number of in-patient days during the five follow-up years ($p = .013$). In the group of typical schizophrenic patients, however, even this treatment variable lacked differences of even marginal significance already during the first follow-up year.

The *connections* of these findings *with the level of primary clinical disturbance of these patients appear unambiguous.* The groups with more-than-average medication, intensive community therapy and family therapy included patients with more-than-average severity of the illness as did also the whole group of psychotherapy cases. Inclusion in the group of regressive disintegration was one of the explaining variables for the distribution into all these groups in our whole series. In the group of community therapy, the number of in-patient days was further increased by the fact that this type of therapy was given on hospital wards. The group with intensive individual therapy who needed less hospital treatment, in turn, included somewhat less disturbed patients than the average.

But attention should also be given to another factor that clearly contributes to the total sum of in-patient days: *particularly during the latter follow-up period, a majority of the in-patient days accumulated on a few patients*, and *such patients in need of long-term hospital treatment were included in both the group of psychotherapy cases and the rest of the series.* Hence two of the four patients who were in hospital for more than two years altogether during the follow-up period (cf. Ch. 5.1.1.1.) belonged to the group of psychotherapy cases. Both were suffering from typical schizophrenia and had been classified as regressively disintegrated; one had been given both intensive family therapy and community therapy, the other intensive community therapy and infrequent family therapy, and an effort at an individual therapeutic contact had been made in both cases, yet without success.

The in-patient days of these two patients accounted for 22.5 % of all the in-patient days of the psychotherapy cases during the five follow-up years in the whole series and 30.4 % in the group of typical schizophrenics.

Another significant factor is the *gradual favourable development of the connections between the psychotherapy variables and the number of in-patient days over the follow-up years*. This is clearly observable in the group of the patients given intensive individual therapy.

The connections between the first therapeutic unit and the number of days spent in hospital was already analyzed in Chapter 5.1.1.2. (Fig. 4, p. 87).

Of the background variables, especially the *difference between the number of in-patient days in the female and male patient groups* attracts attention. Over the entire follow-up period the difference in favour of the female patients is no more than marginally significant (p = .097), but in the group of typical schizophrenic patients it is almost significant (p = .028). The importance of this difference is emphasized by its stability: the tendency was relatively slight during the first year of follow-up, but marked and stable during the rest of the follow-up period (in the group of typical schizophrenic patients the significance continued to be of the level of p = .03–.06). *The other background variables that had a similarly stable effect on the number of in-patient days from one year to another* included *acting out tendencies* (the number of in-patient days was higher than the average, total series p = .052, group of typical schizophrenics p = .032), *unemployment* at the time of the basic examination (in the whole series p = .055, group of typical schizophrenics p = .040), and *lack of occupational identity*, whose effect on the increase of in-patient days was only significant in the whole series, though it was all the more considerable there (p = .003).

In the case of *some other variables*, however, it is notable that they *begin by correlating clearly with the number of in-patient days during the early follow-up, but decline in significance, losing it completely by the last follow-up year*. The variables included the *patient's age*. In the whole series, the need for hospital treatment during the second and third years is highly significantly greater in the youngest age group compared with the two oldest age groups, but during the fourth year the difference declines to become almost significant, losing its significance completely during the fifth year. *During the whole follow-up period, however, the number of in-patient days is significantly (p = .004) higher in the youngest age group than in the others*. In the group of typical schizophrenics, on the other hand, the only statistically significant finding between the youngest age group and the others was made for the second follow-up year, while the difference for the whole follow-up period did not approach even marginal significance.

A similar *gradually declining tendency* in the number of in-patient days from the second follow-up year onwards was noted for the variables reflecting *marital status* and *separation from the primary family* at the time of the basic examination: the groups of unmarried and non-separated patients had significantly higher numbers of in-patient days mainly during the second and third follow-up years, but no longer during the last two follow-up years.

A similar tendency towards uniformity was also noted in the group of patients *lacking a stable heterosexual identity* at the time of the basic examination. An opposite tendency was found among the *typical schizophrenic patients with alcohol problems at the time of the basic examination*: they had a marginally significantly greater need for hospital treatment than the others only during the last follow-up year.

The connections between the number of in-patient days and such clinical background variables as the duration of symptoms prior to admission and their acute

Table 88. Number of in-patient days during the whole follow-up period. Effect of background and/or treatment variables (logistic regression analysis

Explaining variables	risk	p
All patients		
Neuroleptic treatment:		
more than average	4.26	.000
Unemployed	2.37	.053
Group of regressive disintegration	2.64	.038
Typical schizophrenics		
Neuroleptic treatment:		
more than average	3.80	.001
Unemployed	2.50	.016
Not separated from primary family	1.80	.092

or slow onset were unexpectedly small. Neither of them had a statistically significant connection with the number of in-patient days in either the whole series or the group of typical schizophrenics. The social groups of both the parents and the patients also lacked any connections with the number of in-patient days. Willingness to receive treatment, admission on the basis of judicial sanctions and negative attitude towards at least one mode of treatment did not affect the number of days spent in hospital, and the same was also true of insightfulness at the stage of the basic examination.

For the *logistic regression analysis*, the series of patients was divided dichotomously into two groups: those having more than 200 days and those having less. The variables explaining the total number of in-patient days during the follow-up period are shown in Table 88.

The first explaining variable in both the whole series and the group of typical schizophrenics is the amount of medication, the second explaining variable in both groups is unemployment at the time of the basic examination. The number of unemployed patients at that time was relatively the same in the diagnostic category of typical schizophrenics and the ego-dynamic group of regressive disintegration as outside these groups. The effect of the unemployment variable must hence be interpreted completely as a psychosocial factor.

6.5.2 Patients Treated in Hospital During the Last Two Follow-up Years

The *group of typical schizophrenics* as well as the ego-dynamic *group of regressive disintegration continued to be highly significantly overrepresented among the patients who were hospitalized at least once during the last two follow-up years*. Of the 31 patients of this kind, 27 were typical schizophrenics, 18 of them being regressively disintegrated, 7 suffering from paranoid disintegration and 2 from acute disintegration.

As regards the treatment variables, the patients with more-than-average medication had a significant connection with hospital treatment. The *group of psychotherapy cases* had a marginally significant connection ($p = .097$) with the lack of need for hospital treatment during the last two years in the group of typical schizophrenics.

Table 89. Patients with hospital treatments during the last two follow-up years. Effect of background and/or treatment variables (logistic regression analysis)

Explaining variables	risk	p
All patients		
Neuroleptic treatment: more than average	14.69	.000
Group of regressive disintegration	3.42	.023
Typical schizophrenics		
Neuroleptic treatment: more than average	6.81	.000
First unit of treatment (Clinic of Psychiatry/open care and Kupittaa Hospital)	2.25	.036

Of the psychotherapy cases included in our diagnostic nuclear group, 13 (40.6 %) had been in hospital, while 19 had not; the corresponding figures for the other patients in the nuclear group were 14 (63.6 %) and 9. None of the other psychotherapy variables was connected with this prognostic variable even at a marginal level.

The first treatment unit, on the other hand, had an almost significant connection with need for hospital treatment during the last two follow-up years in the whole series ($p = .024$) as well as in the group of typical schizophrenics ($p = .022$). The patients admitted into the Clinic of Psychiatry were in the best position: only 12 of all patients and 9 (32.1 %) of typical schizophrenics had been in hospital during the last two years, while the corresponding figures for the patients admitted via the out-patient units were 7 (41.2 %) and 7 (63.6 %) and for the patients first admitted into the Kupittaa Hospital 12 (52.2 %) and 11 (73.3 %).

Of the other background variables, only 6 were statistically connected with this prognostic variable. Clearly the most conspicuous of these was the more favourable position of *women* than that of men ($p = .009$ in the whole series, $p = .006$ in the group of typical schizophrenics). Of the patients who needed hospital treatment, 9 were female (7 typical schizophrenics) and 22 male (20). The other variables predicting a smaller need for hospital treatment during the last two follow-up years were short duration of the illness prior to the first admission, acute onset of symptoms, presence of hostile relatives, unemployment problems and reserved or suspicious contact upon admission.

In the *logistic regression analysis*, the amount of neuroleptic medication is again the first explaining variable, nor is the second position of the group of the regressive disintegration in the whole series in any way unexpected. What is interesting is that the effect of the first unit of therapy now emerges as the second explaining variable in the group of typical schizophrenics in such a way that the psychotherapeutically oriented wards of the Clinic of Psychiatry correlate with a small need for hospital treatment during the latter part of the follow-up period, while the patients first admitted into the Kupittaa Hospital or an out-patient unit are in a less favourable position.

6.5.3 Summary and Discussion

The duration and number of in-patient episodes during the follow-up period in our series were already dealt with in Chapter 5.1.1. We will here summarize the most important findings on that as well as the most central findings of the present chapter where the in-patient periods and the factors contributing to them were examined as a prognostic dimension.

During the five-year follow-up period, the average number of *in-patient days* per patient in our whole series was 193.16, the corresponding figure in the diagnostic nuclear category being 266.02 days. This means that the patients spent an average of 10.58 % of the five-year period following their admission in hospital in the whole series and 14.51 % in the group of typical schizophrenics. This figure was notably higher during the first follow-up year, 20.6 % in the whole series, ranging quite evenly within 7–8.5 % during the period between the two-year and five-year follow-up examinations. The use of the day hospital was scant relative to this: an average of 27.32 days were spent in day hospital by the patients of the whole series during the entire follow-up period, the corresponding figure in the group of typical schizophrenics being 35.18 days. There were 12 patients who were not in-patients of a psychiatric hospital at any stage of their therapy, though three of them were in day hospital. 32 patients were in hospital once, 21 patients twice and 6 patients at least ten times. The duration of in-patient periods was clearly greater in the male group (13.8 % of the follow-up period) than in the female group (9.1 %).

At the end of the follow-up period 8 patients were in hospital, which corresponds to the average of the last follow-up years. Of these, *only two patients could be classified as institutionalized chronic inmates,* and only one of them was in hospital throughout the last follow-up year. Altogether 4 patients had been in hospital for more than two years during the follow-up period.

The figures do not differ from the results of the other follow-up studies of schizophrenic patients carried out in Helsinki and Turku. The patients first admitted into hospital in 1950 in Helsinki studied by Achté et al. (Niskanen and Achté 1972, Achté et al. 1980) had admittedly spent in hospital 18.35 % of the five-year follow-up period following their admission, and the patients admitted in 1960 had spent 18.18 % of that period in hospital, the percentages of surviving patients in hospital at the end of the follow-up period being 22.9 % and 14.7 % respectively. However, in the group admitted in 1965 the average proportion of in-patient periods of the five-year follow-up was only 11.6 % and 10.6 % of the surviving patients were in hospital at the end of the follow-up period. The corresponding in-patient figures for the population admitted in 1970 have not been reported, but the number of patients in hospital at the end of the five-year follow-up period had further decreased, being 6.3 % of the survivors.

In the series of patients of the schizophrenia group admitted during 1965–1967 studied by Salokangas (1978) the average percentage of in-patient days was 8.4 % of the 7½-year follow-up period; at the end of the follow-up period, 7.7 % of the surviving patients were in hospital. The corresponding figures in the group admitted in 1969 (Salokangas 1984) were 12.02 % in-patient days during the eight-year follow-up period and 11.4 % of the surviving patients in hospital at the end of the follow-up. It is notable that our series differed from these in that it also included patients admitted via the out-patient system of mental health care. We should therefore add 12 % to each of our figures in order to make them comparable with the findings reported by Achté et al. and Salokangas. It can be postulated, on the other hand, that, owing to the poorly developed out-patient care in Finland in the 1960's, part of the patients who now remained out-patients would most probably have been hospitalized at the early years of the Turku project, which serves to minimize the difference between the different populations in this respect.

Most of the works carried out elsewhere have shown the need of schizophrenic patients for hospital therapy to be greater than was the case in these Finnish investigations. Hence, Lassenius et al. (1973) reported the need of schizophrenic patients admitted during 1959–1960 in Sweden for hospital therapy to be about 30 % among the male and about 10 % among the female patients during the follow-up of 10 years. The first admission schizophrenics followed up by von Sivers (1983) for an average of nine years spent an average of 13.7 % of that period in hospital, and 13 % of them were in-patients at the end of the follow-up, the percentage being again clearly higher for male (17 %) than for female patients (9 %). Of the schizophrenic patients followed up by Harrow et al. (1978) for 2.7 years, 19 % were in hospital at the end of the follow-up. The average in-patient period of the first admission schizophrenic patients of 1963–1975 followed up by Bland et al. (1978) for more than ten years was 13.3 % of the follow-up period.

In the series of schizophrenic patients first admitted in the early 1950's followed up by Brown et al. (1966), the need for hospital therapy was less than 10 % in a hospital with intensive out-patient care, but 25 % in areas where the out-patient system was less effective. About 7 % of all patients in this series were in hospital for the entire follow-up period. In Gam's (1980) Danish material 15 % of the men and 9 % of the women were in hospital at the end of the study; and the patients spent an average of 418 days in hospital during the 5 follow-up years. The best results were presented by American Davis et al. (1972) for a study carried out in the late 1960's, where the goal was particularly to prevent hospitalization: during the five-year follow-up period, the patients spent 7–10 % of the time in hospital.

In our own work, the *need of typical schizophrenics for hospital treatment was highly significantly greater than the corresponding need of the other patients, but only from the third follow-up year onwards*; prior to that there was no statistically significant difference. For the *logistic regression analyses* we divided the patients dichotomously into two groups: the ones whose total sum of in-patient days was more than 200 and the ones who had spent less than 200 days in hospital. The first variables explaining the number of in-patient days in both the whole series and the nuclear group were more-than-average neuroleptic medication and unemployment at the time of the basic examination. The third explaining variable was inclusion in the group of regressive disintegration in the whole series and lack of separation from the primary family at the time of admission in the group of typical schizophrenics – a background variable which also emerged in the analysis of the decrease of nuclear symptoms during the follow-up.

Inclusion in the group of psychotherapy cases did not diminish the total number of in-patient days, although a slight tendency to such development appeared in the series towards the end of the follow-up. This was clearly connected to the fact that most of the in-patient days during the latter part of the follow-up belonged to a few patients, and that such patients in need of long-term hospital treatment were seen both among the psychotherapy patients and outside this group. It was interesting to observe, however, that the *first unit of treatment had a definite effect on the need for hospital treatment during the follow-up*. The patients who started their treatment on the psychotherapeutically oriented wards of the Clinic of Psychiatry had a clearly longer first in-patient episode and a longer average in-patient period during the first year than the patients first admitted into more conventional hospital wards, but when the development of the patients in this respect was followed up on the basis of the first unit of treatment, the situation changed as soon as the second year of follow-up to be favourable for the patients treated on psychotherapeutically oriented wards. During the latter part of the follow-up, the average need for hospital treatment among these patients was smaller than the corresponding need of either patients treated on conventional wards or in out-patient units (see Fig. 4. in Chapter 5.1.1.2.).

This finding was confirmed when we found out *which of our patients also needed hospital treatment, even for a short period, during the last two follow-up years*. There were 31 such patients, and 27 of them were typical schizophrenics. Inclusion in the group of psychotherapy cases had a marginally significant connection with the lack of need for hospital treatment in the group of typical schizophrenic patients. The significance increased when the patients were again divided according to the first unit of treatment: of the 59 patients who started their treatment in the Clinic of Psychiatry (including the 5 admitted into the day hospital), 21.8 % had in-patient periods during the fourth and fifth follow-up years in the whole series and 32.1 % in the nuclear group, the corresponding figures being 52.2 % and 73.3 % for the patients who started their therapy on conventional wards and 41.2 % and 63.6 % for those who were first treated in an out-patient unit. In the group of typical schizophrenic patients, this background variable was one of the two variables explaining the need for hospital treatment during the last two follow-up years after more-than-average neuroleptic medication, which was again most clearly connected with the need for hospital therapy both in this group and in the whole series.

As we already pointed out before in Chapter 5.1.1.2., the patients admitted into the two hospitals in this area did not differ as regards the severity of their primary disturbance, whereas they did differ as to their social background, which was poorer on an average among the patients first admitted into conventional wards. The latter group also included relatively more men than the patients admitted into wards working as psychotherapeutic communities. These differences did not, however, explain the effect of the first therapeutic unit on this prognostic variable. The results of the logistic regression analysis therefore confirm that a *first in-patient period aiming at a therapeutic contact with both the patient and his family on a long-term basis had the effect of diminishing the subsequent need for in-patient treatment in our series*.

The difference in the need for hospital treatment between male and female patients appeared uniform throughout the follow-up period. It is interesting that the initially greater number of in-patient days among the youngest age group levelled off during the follow-up years: although the difference compared with the two oldest age groups was statistically significant for the whole follow-up period, it gradually lost its significance by the last follow-up year, nor was there any significant difference observable in the number of patients in need of hospital treatment during the last two follow-up years. A parallel development was seen in the background variables for marital status and separation from the primary family. Whether the relative decrease in the need for hospital treatment by the young unmarried patients was due to the fact that many of them were psychotherapy patients remains to be found out conclusively by the future follow-up examination. An opposite tendency to an increased need for hospital treatment compared with other patients was seen among the patients with alcohol or other addiction problems at the time of the basic examination.

Background variables pertaining to social groups had no effect on the need for hospital treatment in our series. The family variables again presented a sign of a poor prognosis: the finding of hostile or poorly understanding relatives at the basic examination stage was now connected with the need for hospital treatment during the last two follow-up years in the group of typical schizophrenics.

6.6 Development of Families and Family Relationships

6.6.1 Psychic Health of Family Members

The follow-up observations revealed no great changes in the state of psychic health of the patients' family members. We only became aware of one transient psychotic disorder that had developed during the follow-up period in a close relative (a spouse) of one of our patients. The spouses had started couple therapy even prior to this, and the husband's psychotic condition thereby passed without hospitalization. The daughter of the psychotic couple in our series was hospitalized for a short period because of a "puberty crisis".

At least 10 relatives of the patients started psychiatric out-patient therapy of their own during the follow-up. These therapies were often associated with our family-oriented therapeutic approach and do not necessarily reflect any real deterioration of the relatives' psychic health: in some cases rather the opposite may be true, at least as far as increased insight into one's problems is concerned.

The case of the parents of a young female patient with borderline schizophrenia who was given intensive individual therapy can be considered typical. Both suffered from notable anxiety because of their daughter's illness and her living habits. The mother resorted heavily to the specialized nurse of our team, visiting her almost regularly to discuss her problems. The problems pertained to the daughter, but also to the patient's father who had alcohol problems and a tendency to paranoid reactions. At a later stage, when the daughter had gained independence and her state of health had improved, the parents together consulted an A-clinic to get couple therapy.

On the basis of our experience, we concluded by postulating that *our family therapy and the support given the patients' family members in many cases prevented the aggravation of the relatives' anxiety and other psychic strains and disorders.* Many of them had reached the "limit of their tolerance". Even so, it is difficult to postulate whether our family-oriented approach was, in some cases, able to prevent a suicide that would otherwise have been committed or the onset of a psychosis.

The relatives of our patients that *died of somatic diseases* during the five-year follow-up included two mothers, six fathers and at least two siblings. No deaths occurred in the secondary families.

6.6.2 Follow-up of the Marital Relationships

During the first two follow-up years, the *divorces* of 8 patients separated at the time of the basic examination were confirmed; the remaining one patient in this group also continued to live separate from the spouse. New separations took place in the case of 7 other patients, whereas 3 patients *got married*, none of them having been married before.

During the three latter follow-up years, 4 patients *divorced*, including 2 who had got married during the previous follow-up period. Six patients *got married*, in addition to which one couple who had separated during the previous follow-up period had resumed cohabitation. Two of the patients who now got married had been married before.

At the end of the five-year follow-up period, 24 of the 95 patients included in the study were married. The number of separated or divorced patients had gone up to 22, and there was one widow and 48 unmarried patients. The number of separated or divorced patients had hence increased, while the number of unmarried and married subjects had somewhat decreased compared with the basic examination. It is interesting, however, that a relatively high number of new marriages had been entered, particularly during the latter follow-up period between the two- and five-year examinations. 2 of the new married patients were included in the group of typical schizophrenia.

New babies had been born to 2 patients during the first follow-up period and to 9 during the following three years. With the exception of one, these patients were married, and 4 of the babies were born into marriages entered during the follow-up period. The number of children in our series had thus come up to a total of 70.

Can we infer anything from *the effect of couple therapies* by observing the development of the patient's marital situations? Of the 28 patients who were married at the time of the basic examination, 14 were given couple therapy, while the other 14 were not. 11 couple therapies were started during the first two follow-up years (and, with the exception of one, also concluded during that period), whereas 3 were undertaken during the latter follow-up period.

Our estimates concerning the relationships between the spouses in these 28 cases at the times of the basic examination and the two follow-up examinations are shown in Table 90.

The figures indicate that the relationship between the spouses was conflict-ridden in most cases in our series at the time of the basic examination. A majority of the couple therapies were undertaken in these cases. Of the 6 patients whose relationships with their spouses were described as harmonious, only one was given couple therapy.

No marked changes are to be seen during the follow-up in the development of the marriages of the patients given and not given couple therapy. A few more separations and/or divorces took place in the group not given couple therapy, and a slight tendency towards better even in the harmonious relationships was seen in the group given couple therapy, while a corresponding unfavourable tendency was seen in the group not given couple therapy. The Figures do not, however, justify any further conclusions.

When we analyzed the connections between the prognostic development of our married patients and the inclusion in or exclusion from the group given couple therapy, we found no statistical connections. The patients given couple therapy showed, however, more favourable development than the others on most variables. The

Table 90. Development of the marital relationships of the patients who were married at the time of the basic examinations in the groups given and not given couple therapy

Quality of the relationship	Number of patients		
	Basic examination	Two-year follow-up	Five-year follow-up
Given couple therapy			
Relationship			
harmonious	1	2	2
conflict-ridden	13	9	8
broken	–	3	4
Not given couple therapy			
Relationship			
harmonious	5	4	3
conflict-ridden	9	5	5
broken	–	5	5
not known	–	–	1

difference came closest to statistical significance in an analysis of the decrease of the nuclear symptoms of schizophrenia ($p = .11$). These analyses were made difficult by the small number of the cases.

As regards the *new marriages*, the relationship of the spouses at the time of the two-year follow-up examination was estimated as harmonious in 1 case, conflict-ridden in 1 case and already broken in 1 case. By the time of the five-year follow-up examination, even the marriage that had been assessed as "harmonious" had broken up, while the one described as "conflict-ridden" had become harmonious. In all of the six new marriages entered during the period between the two-year and five-year follow-up examinations, the relationship between the spouses was found to be harmonious at the time of the five-year follow-up examination, but the follow-up of the marriage was too short to justify any more far-reaching conlusions.

6.7 Effects of Psychotherapy and Medication on Prognosis: Statistical Analysis

It has been pointed out in several connections before that the patients given psychotherapy had better prognostic development than the others. Statistically, this was shown by cross-tabulations and, at some points, by the factors explaining the prognosis in the logistic regression analyses. It was, however, impossible to take into account the selective factors contributing to the inclusion in or exclusion from the group of psychotherapy cases in these analyses.

The most significant of these factors for each prognostic variable are the background variables which emerged as explaining variables in the logistic regression analyses. *Statistical analysis provides a better view of the effect of psychotherapy alone independent of the selective factors, when the effect of the background variables explaining the prognosis is kept constant*, i.e. their effect on the prognosis/change of the prognosis is taken into account, and the effects of psychotherapy are only examined thereafter.

But not even this analysis gives completely exact information on the effect of therapy, because the factors influencing the selection are so numerous. 45 different background variables were discriminated after the basic examination. *We could, however, pick out the background variables most markedly connected to the patient's favourable prognostic development, noting that once the effect of these explaining variables had been taken into account, the other background variables were no longer of any significant influence.*

6.7.1 Inclusion in the Group of Psychotherapy Cases and Medication

The variable to be primarily examined in the new analysis was *inclusion in the group of psychotherapy cases*, because this variable provides information on the effect of our global, case-specifically indicated therapeutic approach as a whole. This variable was also easier to analyze statistically than the other psychotherapy variables because of its uniform distribution (follow-up data on 54 psychotherapy cases and 41 patients not given psychotherapy).

The second treatment variable to be analyzed was *more-/less-than-average medication* during the follow-up period. In the previous analyses this variable emerged at several points as an explaining variable in such a way that the patients given more-than-average amount of neuroleptics had a less optimistic prognosis than the patients given less-than-average medication. This effect can be postulated to be due to the greater need for medication of the patients who were primarily more ill or had otherwise a poorer starting-point. But was this so? Or can our finding be interpreted as suggesting that continued neuroleptic medication had adverse effects on the patients' prognosis?

We will analyze separately the effects of case-specifically indicated psychotherapy during the follow-up period (inclusion in the group of psychotherapy cases) and *the amount of medication on the prognosis/change of prognosis, when the background factors affecting it most strongly have been kept constant, i.e. their effect on the prognosis/change of prognosis has been taken into account.* For this purpose, logistic regression analysis was applied to find among the clinical and psychosocial background variables the factors which had the most conspicuous statistical effect on the prognostic variable in question. After this, the theory of log-linear models was applied to examine the partial connection between the treatment variables, called *psychotherapy* and *medication* below, and the prognostic/prognostic change variable in question, after the background variables important for the prognosis had been kept constant. – Since in the logistic regression analyses presented in the Chapters 6.2.–6.5., when explaining the good prognosis/prognostic change, the different groups of variables (clinical background variables, psychosocial background variables, treatment variables) were considered of completely equal value, and now the background variables most strongly connected with the prognosis/change of prognosis were first sought out without treatment variables, it may be that the best background variables of the previous logistic regression analyses are not completely identical with the constant background variables here presented. This was the case in e.g. the analysis of the factors contributing to the decrease of nuclear symptoms, where the explaining background variable of lack of separation from the primary family was replaced by the variable of serious personality disorder of the mother.

Owing to the small number of cases, the analyses of the whole series only include four variables at the most: two background variables + prognosis/change of prognosis + one treatment variable (psychotherapy or medication) *or* one background factor + prognosis/change of prognosis + two treatment variables (psychotherapy and medication). *The analyses of typical schizophrenic patients included three variables at the most:* one background variable + prognosis/change of prognosis + one treatment variable (psychotherapy or medication) *or* prognosis/change of prognosis + two treatment variables (psychotherapy and medication). If the analyses revealed a combined effect of more than two variables, statistical examination was continued (a combined effect of this kind was only noted in the analysis of the connection between inclusion in the psychotherapy cases and the global prognosis, cf. 6.7.3.).

The purpose of including both of the treatment variables in the analysis was to ensure that one of the treatment variables does not explain the effect of the other, i.e. when both were included in the analysis, one of them was the constant factor.

One central variable from each sub-area of the prognostic examination was selected as a prognostic variable: decrease of the nuclear symptoms of schizophrenia (clinical prognosis), increase of insight (psychodynamic prognosis), maintenance of working capacity (psychosocial prognosis), and in-patient episodes during the last two follow-up years (prognosis for the need of hospital treatment).The results are shown in theTables 91–98.

The analysis was carried out, as previously, separately in the whole series and in the group of typical schizophrenias.

When the background factors are kept constant in the whole series, neither psychotherapy, nor medication have any statistically significant connection with the *decrease of the nuclear symptoms of schizophrenia* during the five-year follow-up period

Table 91. Statistical significance (p) of the connection of inclusion in the group of psychotherapy cases and medication with the *decrease of nuclear symptoms* (decrease/no decrease), when the background variables most significantly explaining the decrease of nuclear symptoms are kept constant. *Whole series*

Constant background variables	Treatment variable	N	p
Diagnosis of typical schizophrenia (no/yes) and disorder of mother's personality (no/yes) at the time of the basic examination	medication	55	.643
Same as above	psychotherapy	55	.245
Diagnosis of typical schizophrenia (no/yes) at the time of the basic examination	medication	74	.501
	psychotherapy		.083(+)
Disorder of mother's personality (no/yes) at the time of the basic examination	medication	55	.199
	psychotherapy		.375

In this and the following tables a (+) sign after the p-value indicates a positive connection between the treatment and the prognostic variables, a (–) sign a negative connection.

Table 92. Statistical significance (p) of the connection of inclusion in the group of psychotherapy cases and medication with the *decrease of nuclear symptoms* (decrease/no decrease), when the background factors most significantly explaining the decrease of nuclear symptoms are kept constant. *Typical schizophrenic patients*

Constant background variables	Treatment	N	p
Previous psychiatric treatment (no/yes) prior to the basic examination	medication	47	.535
Same as above	psychotherapy	47	.024$^{(+)}$
Mother's personality disturbed (no/yes) at the time of the basic examination	medication	34	.550
Same as above	psychotherapy	34	.099$^{(+)}$
--	{ medication	47	.463
	psychotherapy		.031$^{(+)}$

(Table 91). Psychotherapy does correlate marginally significantly with a good prognosis, when the effects of the diagnosis of typical schizophrenia and medication are kept constant, but the significance disappears, when we take into account the personality disorder of the patient's mother: the mothers of the psychotherapy patients were not equally often seriously disturbed as were the mothers of the other patients (35 % vs. 62 %), which means that the starting-points in this respect were better in the psychotherapy cases than in the others. In the case of the patients with psychoses of the schizophrenia group whose mothers had serious personality disorders, a sufficient psychotherapy could not be accomplished as often as in other cases.

When we analyze separately the *typical schizophrenic patients* (Table 92), *the situation appears altered: inclusion in the group of psychotherapy cases and the decrease of nuclear symptoms show an almost significant positive connection* when we take into account the patient's previous treatment (p = .024) and the amount of the patient's medication (p = .031), and a *marginally significant connection* when we further take into account the severity of the mother's personality disorder (p = .099). The effects of the inclusion in the group of psychotherapy cases hence appear more significant in the group of typical schizophrenics than in the whole series, and the favourable effect of psychotherapy on the decrease of the nuclear symptoms of schizophrenia in this group does not seem to be explained by the other factors. Since, however, our series is very small here (34–47 cases), the conclusions, if any, should be drawn with caution. The amount of medication was not statistically connected with the decrease of nuclear symptoms in the diagnostic category of typical schizophrenics, either.

Table 93 shows that the positive connection between inclusion in the group of psychotherapy cases and the *increase of insight* among the patients of our whole series *continues to remain clearly significant* even when the other variables are kept constant. The amount of medication received by the patient, on the other hand, is not significantly connected with the increase of insight despite the fact that the connection between less-than-average medication and the increase of insight approaches marginal significance in some analyses. On the basis of the analysis, we can assume that *psychotherapy contributes significantly to the increase of insight*, but we cannot claim that abundant medication as such diminishes the patient's ability to see his problems and symptoms as part of himself and to endeavour to solve them.

Table 93. Statistical significance (p) of the connection of inclusion in the group of psychotherapy cases and medication with *increase of insight* (increase/no increase), when the background factors most significantly explaining the increase of insight are kept constant. *Whole series*

Constant background variables	Treatment	N	p
Tendency to alcohol or other addiction problems at the time of the basic examination (no/yes) and abnormal social background (yes/no)	medication	92	.133
Same as above	psychotherapy	92	$.002^{(+)}$
Tendency to alcohol or other addiction problems at the time of the basic examination (no/yes)	medication	92	.225
	psychotherapy		$.004^{(+)}$
Abnormal social background (yes/no)	medication	92	.111
	psychotherapy		$.002^{(+)}$

In the *group of typical schizophrenic patients* (Table 94), the *significant positive connection between inclusion in the group of psychotherapy cases and the increase of insight is at least of the same order* as in the whole series. The amount of *medication now also has a marginally significant connection* with the increase of insight: the patients with less-than-average medication have been able to increase their insight more often than the patients with more-than-average medication. This connection might be postulated to be explained by the primarily poor condition of the patients with abundant medication. We were not, however, able to find in our series any background factor measured at the time of the basic examination which would have explained this connection.

The *maintenance of working capacity* (Table 95) seems to be strongly connected with the medication given to the patient. The patients on *more-than-average medication* were *highly significantly more often incapacitated* at the time of the five-year follow-up than the other patients. This connection was not explained by the more frequent unemployment and/or lack of occupational identity, which were baseline characteristics in the group given more-than-average medication. The connection between inclusion in the group of psychotherapy cases and the maintenance of working capacity, which was almost significant in the cross-tabulation, is, however, explained by the fact that the patients given psychotherapy were less often unemployed at the basic examination stage than the others (13 % vs. 32 %). Even so, the analysis did suggest that *inclusion in the group of psychotherapy cases helped the patients who had a stable*

Table 94. Statistical significance (p) of the connection of inclusion in the group of psychotherapy cases and medication with the *increase of insight* (increase/no increase), when the background factors most significantly explaining the increase of insight has been kept constant. *Typical schizophrenic patients*

Constant background variables	Treatment	N	p
Tendency to alcohol or other addiction at the basic examination stage (no/yes)	medication	54	$.089^{(-)}$
Same as above	psychotherapy	54	$.001^{(+)}$
--	medication	54	$.085^{(-)}$
	psychotherapy		$.002^{(+)}$

Table 95. Statistical significance (p) of the connection of inclusion in the group of psychotherapy cases and medication with *working capacity* (normal/declined) in the five-year follow-up, when the background factors most significantly explaining the maintenance of working capacity have been kept constant. *Whole series*

Constant background factors	Treatment	N	p
Unemployment (no/yes) and occupational identity (stable/unstable) at the time of the basic examination	medication	95	.000$^{(-)}$
Same as above	psychotherapy	95	.148
Unemployment at the basic examination stage (no/yes)	medication	95	.000$^{(-)}$
	psychotherapy		.202
Occupational identity at the time of the basic examination (stable/unstable)	medication	95	.000$^{(-)}$
	psychotherapy		.052$^{(+)}$

occupational identity at the basic examination stage to retain their working capacity. It should be pointed out that the analysis did not pertain to the change that had taken place during the five follow-up years, but to the patient's working capacity as measured in the five-year follow-up examination.

The clinical background variables did not appear to have any effect on the maintenance of working capacity, that could have made them constant background variables even when the logistic regression analysis was carried out on the basis of the background variables alone.

In the group of *typical schizophrenic patients* (Table 96), we *can see both the negative effect of medication and the positive effect of inclusion in the group of psychotherapy cases on the maintenance of working capacity.* None of the three variables explaining the maintenance of working capacity seem to explain the *significant connection* between the two treatment variables and the maintenance of working capacity. Here, too, we must point out that the variable labelled "working capacity" does not describe the change that has taken place during the five years (as was the case with nuclear symptoms and insight), but rather refers to the patient's condition

Table 96. Statistical significance (p) of the connection of inclusion in the group of psychotherapy cases and medication with *working capacity* (normal/declined) in the five-year follow-up, when the background factors most significantly explaining the maintenance of working capacity have been kept constant. *Typical schizophrenic patients*

Constant background variables	Treatment	N	p
Tendency to alcohol or other addiction at the time of the basic examination (no/yes)	medication	54	.001$^{(-)}$
Same as above	psychotherapy	54	.005$^{(+)}$
Sex (female/male)	medication	54	.001$^{(-)}$
Same as above	psychotherapy	54	.003$^{(+)}$
Unemployment at the basic examination stage (no/yes)	medication	54	.001$^{(-)}$
Same as above	psychotherapy	54	.005$^{(+)}$
--	medication	54	.000$^{(-)}$
	psychotherapy		.007$^{(+)}$

Table 97. Statistical significance (p) of the connection of inclusion in the group of psychotherapy cases and medication with *in-patient episodes during the last two follow-up years* (no/yes), when the background factors most significantly explaining the in-patient episodes have been kept constant. *Whole series*

Constant background variables	Treatment	N	p
Inclusion in the ego-dynamic group of regressive disintegration (no/yes) and quality of the contact made by the patient (not suspicious or reserved/ suspicious or reserved) at the basic examination stage	medication	95	.000$^{(-)}$
Same as above	psychotherapy	95	.083$^{(+)}$
Inclusion in the ego-dynamic group of regressive disintegration at the basic examination stage (no/yes)	{ medication psychotherapy	95	.000$^{(-)}$ .183
Quality of the contact made by the patient at the basic examination stage (not suspicious or reserved/suspicious or reserved)	{ medication psychotherapy	95	.000$^{(-)}$ .821

at the time of the five-year follow-up. It is not probable, however, that the result would have changed if the working capacity prior to the patients' admission had been determined at the time of the basic examination. This seems to be suggested by e.g. the fact that unemployment as a baseline characteristic no longer explains the effect of the treatment variables in this analysis.

Table 97 shows that more-than-average medication is highly significantly connected with *in-patient treatment during the last two follow-up years* in the whole series. *The patients given more-than-average medication during the follow-up period had to resort to psychiatric hospital treatment during the last two follow-up years* despite the two background variables most conspicuously explaining the need for in-patient treatment, inclusion in the ego-dynamic group of regressive disintegration and/or the quality of the contact made by the patient at the examination stage. Inclusion in the group of psychotherapy cases was marginally connected with avoidance of in-patient episodes when the aforesaid two background variables were kept constant, but the connection disappeared when the amount of medication was also kept constant.

Table 98. Statistical significance (p) of the connection of inclusion in the group of psychotherapy cases and medication with *in-patient episodes during the last two follow-up years* (no/yes), when the background factors most significantly explaining the in-patient episodes have been kept constant. *Typical schizophrenic patients*

Constant background variables	Treatment	N	p
Regressive ego disintegration at the time of the basic examination (no/yes)	medication	54	.000$^{(-)}$
Same as above	psychotherapy	54	.010$^{(+)}$
Sex (female/male)	medication	54	.000$^{(-)}$
Same as above	psychotherapy	54	.172
First therapeutic unit (Clinic of Psychiatry or day hospital/Kupittaa Hospital our out-patient care)	medication	54	.000$^{(-)}$
Same as above	psychotherapy	54	.289
--	{ medication psychotherapy	54	.000$^{(-)}$ .342

The connection of more-than-average medication with in-patient episodes during the last two follow-up years is highly significant even in the group of typical schizophrenic patients (Table 98). None of the three background variables included in the table alone explained this connection. In a separate cross-tabulation, inclusion in the group of psychotherapy cases was marginally significantly connected with avoidance of hospitalization during the last two follow-up years. The connection became almost significant when the inclusion in or exclusion from the ego-dynamic group of regressive disintegration was kept constant in the group of typical schizophrenics. When the other two background variables included in the analysis were kept constant, the statistical connection between avoidance of hospitalization and inclusion in the group of psychotherapy cases disappeared. A larger proportion of female patients than of males were psychotherapy cases (67 % vs. 53 %), and female patients were hospitalized less often during the last two follow-up years than males (29 % vs. 67 %). The patients who started their therapy in the Clinic of Psychiatry were more often psychotherapy cases than those who were first admitted into the Kupittaa Hospital or out-patient care (71 % vs. 46 %), and the patients first admitted into the Clinic were less often in-patients during the last two follow-up years than the corresponding patients of the Kupittaa Hospital and the out-patient units (32 % vs. 69 %). Also, when the amount of medication was kept constant, the statistical connection between the psychotherapy cases and the avoidance of in-patient treatment lost its significance.

The fact that the first unit of therapy explained the connection between inclusion in the group of psychotherapy cases and the need for in-patient treatment during the last two follow-up years shows that although the patients first admitted into the Clinic of Psychiatry became psychotherapy cases more often, inclusion in the group of psychotherapy cases as such was not sufficient to explain the lesser need for in-patient treatment, but the explanation of the connection (also) required the other background variables affecting the selection of the first unit of therapy and the other effects of the in-patient episode in the first unit of therapy.

6.7.2 Intensive Individual Therapy and Treatment in a Psychotherapeutic Community

Similar analyses were also made on the connections between intensive individual therapy and intensive therapy or intervention in crisis in a psychotherapeutic community on the one hand and the prognosis of our patients on the other. The prognostic variables and the constant background variables were the same as in the analyses presented above, and the effects of more-than-average or less-than-average medication were also taken into account in the same way.

Cross-tabulation had shown that *intensive individual therapy* and *the decrease of nuclear symptoms* were almost significantly connected in the whole series. When, however, two background variables, inclusion in the group of typical schizophrenia and severity of the mother's personality disorder, were kept constant, the connection lost its significance ($p = .174$) and was mainly explained by the smaller number of mothers whose personality was seriously disturbed in the group of patients given intensive individual therapy compared with the other patients (29 % vs. 53 %). When the analysis was restricted to the *typical schizophrenic patients*, the connection between intensive individual therapy and the decrease of nuclear symptoms came very close to marginal statistical significance (when the background variable of previous psychiatric treatment was kept constant, $p = .109$; when the background variable of the severity of mother's personality disorder was kept constant, $p = .113$; when the medication variable was kept constant, $p = .077$). The patients given intensive individual therapy hence did not differ significantly from the rest of the series even in this analysis. The reliability of the analysis was again diminished by the small cell frequencies.

The connection between the *increase of insight* and *intensive individual therapy* was *at least almost significant in the whole series* and *clearly significant in the group of typical schizophrenic patients* even after the explaining background variables and the medication variable were kept constant. The negative connection between more-than-average medication and the increase of insight was also marginally significant in the analysis of the group of typical schizophrenic patients both when the explaining background variable (no tendency to alcohol or other addiction as a baseline characteristic) was kept constant and when the variable of intensive individual therapy was kept constant.

Individual therapy was not statistically significantly connected with the *maintenance of working capacity* in the whole series even in cross-tabulation, and the situation was not altered after the central background variables were kept constant. The *almost significant positive connection seen at this point in the group of typical schizophrenics, however, remained at least marginally significant* even after the background variables had been kept constant. The connection between more-than-average medication and the loss of working capacity emerged highly significant in these analyses, as it also did in the previous ones.

In-patient episoded during the last two follow-up years were not connected with intensive individual therapy either in the whole series or in the group of typical schizophrenics.

After corresponding analyses, *intensive therapy or intervention in crisis in a psychotherapeutic community* turned out to have two statistical connections with the good prognostic development of the patients, both when the analysis was restricted to *the group of typical schizophrenic patients*. The connection with the *increase of insight* was statistically almost significant and that with the *maintenance of working capacity* marginally significant. Neither positive nor negative connections were found for the other sub-areas of prognosis examined.

6.7.3 Global Prognostic Assessment According to Strauss and Carpenter Outcome Scale

In order to investigate the prognosis of our patients and the factors influencing it from a global point of view, *we included in the five-year follow-up examination an assessment of the prognosis of our patients using the outcome scale presented by Strauss and Carpenter* (1972). The prognosis is there divided into the following four items:

1. Duration of nonhospitalization for psychiatric disorder
   4. Not in hospital in past year.
   3. Hospitalized less than three months in past year.
   2. Hospitalized three to six months in past year.

1. Hospitalized over six months, up to nine months in past year.
0. Hospitalized more than nine months in past year.

2. Social contacts (do not include meetings with friends at work or "over the back fence").
4. Meets with friends on average at least once a week.
3. Meets with friends two to three times a month.
2. Meets with friends about once a month.

Include all acquaintances

1. Does not meet with friends except "over the back fence", at work or at school.
0. Does not meet with friends at all under any conditions.

3. Usefully employed (include work as housewife, student. Exclude time in hospital.).
4. "Employed" continuously.
3. "Employed" more than half year but less than continuously.
2. "Employed" part-time or full-time about half of the time in the past year.
1. "Employed" less than half of the time in the past year.
0. No useful work.

4. Absence of symptoms (in past month).
4. No signs or symptoms.
3. Slight signs and symptoms most of the time, or moderate signs and symptoms on rare occasions.
2. Moderate signs and symptoms some of the time.
1. Severe signs and symptoms some of the time, or moderate signs and symptoms continuously.
0. Continuous and severe signs and symptoms.

All these variables are rated on a 5-point scale where 0 is the negative and 4 the positive pole. The scores can be summed into a total outcome score with a maximum of 16 points and a minimum of 0 points.

The first three variables are defined on the basis of the situation that prevailed during the year preceding the follow-up examination, while the last, i.e. the one pertaining to symptoms, is defined on the basis of the situation of the preceding month. The rating scales have been made as concrete and easily reproducible as possible. The inter-rater reliability reported by Strauss and Carpenter themselves was quite high (for all variables $p < .001$, $r = .087 - 0.96$). Our team felt the scales to be easy to use, because their assessments were based on concrete criteria. We took the variable pertaining to symptoms to refer to psychotic symptoms in particular. It seems that the Strauss and Carpenter outcome scale has already been used in prognostic studies (e.g. Harrow et al. 1978, Sjöström 1982, McGlashan 1984). In theTables 99-100 below we will present the findings of our own followup examination, which can then be compared with the results obtained by the other investigators who have used the same scale.

The mean total outcome score was 11.19 in the whole series and 9.81 in the group of typical schizophrenics. The corresponding figures in the group of psychotherapy cases were 11.55 and 10.65 and for those among the patients who were not psychotherapy cases 10.69 and 8.50. The difference between the psychotherapy cases and the other patients was not statistically significant in the whole series, but was almost significant in the group of typical schizophrenic patients (t-test: $p < .05$). The total outcome score of

Table 99. Distribution of the patients on the Strauss and Carpenter prognostic outcome rating scales in the five-year follow-up examination. *Whole series*. The figures are percentages

Prognostic item	Outcome scores					
	4	3	2	1	0	Mean
Time in hospital	72	18	6	0	4	3.53
Social contacts	19	18	35	25	3	2.24
Employment	44	4	3	12	36	2.09
Symptoms	58	31	0	9	2	3.33

Table 100. Distribution of the patients on the Strauss and Carpenter prognostic outcome rating scales in the five-year follow-up examination. *Typical schizophrenic patients*. The figures are percentages

Prognostic item	Outcome scores					
	4	3	2	1	0	Mean
Time in hospital	60	22	11	–	6	3.33
Social contacts	15	14	35	31	6	2.00
Employment	31	6	2	11	50	1.57
Symptoms	36	45	0	17	4	2.91

the patients given intensive individual therapy was 12.46 in the whole series and 12.43 in the group of typical schizophrenic patients (the difference in comparison with the other patients was now marginally significant in the whole series and significant in the group of typical schizophrenics).

Strauss and Carpenter (1972) reported corresponding findings from an investigation based on a two-year follow-up of the U.S. series of the WHO International Pilot Study of Schizophrenia.

The total outcome score was 10.86. The outcome scores they reported for hospital treatment and the occurrence of symptoms were lower than the scores we obtained both in our whole series and in the group of typical schizophrenics, whereas their findings on employment and social contacts were more favourable than ours. In a 2.7-year follow-up study conducted by Harrow et al. (1978) the total outcome score was 9.70. Both of these series consisted of recently admitted patients, though not quite exclusively first admissions. In the Chestnut Lodge follow-up study (Mc Glashan 1984), where the patient series largely consisted of chronic patients, the schizophrenia cohort scored 6.5. on the same scale. In Sjöström's (1982) study of patients treated by Barbro Sandin (cf. Ch.2.3.1.) the total outcome score was about 12 for the probands and less than 8 for the controls.

In our series we also analyzed the connections of the clinical and psychosocial background variables defined in the basic examination as well as the treatment variables with the global prognosis determined by means of the Strauss and Carpenter outcome rating scale by dividing the patients into two groups: those with a high total outcome score (12 or more, 53 patients in the whole series, 22 in the group of typical schizophrenics) and those with a low total outcome score (11 or less; 42 patients in the whole series and 31 in the group of typical schizophrenics).

The statistical connections with a high global outcome score that emerged are shown in Appendices 7 and 8.

Of the *clinical variables*, exclusion from the groups of typical schizphrenia and regressive disintegration had the highest connections with the global prognostic assessments (both, $p < .01$) in the whole series. The group of regressive disintegration, however, lost its connection with poor global prognosis when the analysis was restricted in the group of typical schizophrenia. The *psychosocial variables* of sex and unemployment had also clearly significant connections with this global assessment, as they had had in many of the sub-areas of the prognosis, but the *favourable significance of empathic relatives appeared notably more conspicuous* in this global examination than it has been before. The second family variable, i.e. the disturbance of the mother's personality, also had strong connections with the global prognosis.

Of the *treatment variables*, the one pertaining to medication appears the most central: the connection between more-than-average neuroleptic medication and poor prognosis was highly significant in the whole series and almost equally significant in the group of typical schizophrenics. At least the former of these connections could be assumed to be explained largely by patient-specific background variables. The same is also true of the marginal statistical connection between family therapy and poorer-than-average prognosis in the whole series. Intensive individual therapy only came close to marginal statistical significance in its connection with good global prognosis in the whole series, but reached this connection at a significant level in the group of typical schizophrenics. In that group, inclusion in the group of psychotherapy cases also had a marginally significant positive connection with higher-than-average outcome score.

In the *logistic regression analysis* (Table 101) the first three explaining variables were the same in the whole series and in the group of typical schizophrenics, being even in the same order of importance: a *good global prognosis* was connected with *less-than-average neuroleptic medication* during the follow-up period, the *presence of empathic*

Table 101. Global prognosis of the patients according to the score of multidimensional Strauss – Carpenter criteria: influence of background and/or treatment variables

Explaining variables	R	p
All patients		
Neuroleptic treatment: less than average	3.00	0.000
Empathic relatives: yes/no	2.11	0.000
Sex: female	1.69	0.013
Not unemployed	2.73	0.022
Typical schizophrenics		
Neuroleptic treatment: less than average	2.81	0.000
Empathic relatives	2.68	0.006
Sex: female	2.80	0.015
Intensive individual therapy	2.32	0.034

relatives in the patient's family at the time of the basic examination and the *female sex*. The fourth explaining variable in whole series was the patient's *not being unemployed* at the time of admission, while in the group or typical schizophrenias the fourth variable was *intensive individual therapy.* The clinical background variables dropped out in this analysis.

The connections between the treatment variables and the global prognosis were therafter examined, keeping the background variables most significantly explaining the prognosis constant in the same way as in the Chapters 6.7.1. and 6.7.2. The background variables that were kept constant in the analyses of both the whole series and the typical schizophrenic patients were the presence of an empathic relative at the basic examination stage and the patient's sex. The results for inclusion in the group of psychotherapy cases and the amount of medication are shown in the Tables 102 and 103.

Table 102. Statistical significance (p) of the connection of inclusion in the group of psychotherapy cases and medication with higher-than-average total outcome score according to Strauss and Carpenter multidimensional criteria, when the background factors most significantly explaining the outcome score have been kept constant. *Whole series*

Constant background variables	Treatment	N	p
Empathic relatives at the basic examination stage (yes/no) and sex (female/male)	medication	82	$.000^{(-)}$
Same as above	psychotherapy	84	.869
Empathic relatives at the basic examination stage (yes/no)	{ medication	82	$.000^{(-)}$
	psychotherapy		.562
Sex (female/male)	{ medication	94	$.000^{(-)}$
	psychotherapy		.988

Table 103. Statistical connection of inclusion in the group of psychotherapy cases and medication (p) with higher-than-average total outcome score according to Strauss and Carpenter multidimensional criteria, when the background factors most significantly explaining the outcome score have been kept constant. *Typical schizophrenics*

Constant background variables	Treatment	N	p
Empathic relatives at the basic examination stage (yes/no) and sex (female/male)	medication	47	$.000^{(-)}$
Same as above	psychotherapy	47	$.068^{(+)}$
Sex (female/male)	medication	53	$.006^{(-)}$
Same as above	psychotherapy	53	.134
--	{ medication	53	$.003^{(-)}$
	psychotherapy		.210

Both in the whole series and in the group of typical schizophrenics *medication retains its connection with the total outcome score in such a way that the patients with less medication have a better prognosis* than the patients with more medication. The finding remains highly significant in the whole series and clearly significant in the group of typical schizophrenics. *Inclusion in the group of psychotherapy cases* and high total outcome score, however, do not correlate in the whole series. A more detailed analysis revealed, however, that when the patient did not have empathic relatives and received more-than-average medication, the psychotherapy cases, in comparison with the patients excluded from this group, had a positive connection with a high Strauss-Carpenter total outcome score ($p = .063$). The patients on less heavy medication showed no corresponding connection.

In the analysis of typical schizophrenic patients, inclusion in the group of psychotherapy cases retained its marginally significant connection with the high total outcome score when the background variable of empathic relatives was kept constant, but lost its significance when the sex variable was kept constant. Female patients had a better global prognosis than the male patients and the connection between inclusion in the psychotherapy group and the global prognosis was explained by the sex. A similar finding was made when the medication variable was kept constant: the total outcome score of the patients on less-than-average medication was better than that of the patients on more-than-average medication, and the connection between psychotherapy and the total outcome score was explained by the medication.

Since the variables explaining the total outcome score lacked any clinical variables, despite the fact that they were significantly connected with it in the cross-tabulation, we further made a separate analysis of whether the clinical background variable that had the most significant connection with the global prognosis in the whole series, i.e. inclusion in the ego-dynamic group of regressive disintegration, explained the connection between the amount of medication and the poor global prognosis.

The result could be interpreted in such a way that the low outcome score was only connected to more-than-average medication and not at all to the patient's inclusion in the ego-dynamic group of regressive disintegration at the time of admission. The reliability of the analysis, however, was diminished by the very small size of the cell frequencies.

Direct cross-tabulation of *intensive individual therapy* and high Strauss-Carpenter total outcome scores did not yield statistically significant findings in the whole series, and the situation did not change when the most significant background variables were kept constant. The connections did, however, come very close to marginal significance ($p = .103$) when the constant background variable was the presence or lack of empathic relatives and the medication variable was also kept constant. *In the group of typical schizophrenic patients*, where intensive individual therapy had emerged as an explaining background variable, *the connection between intensive individual therapy and high total outcome scores remained almost significant when the significant background variables were kept constant* (when the presence or lack of empathic relatives was kept constant, $p = .013$; when the patient's sex was kept constant, $p = .023$) and after the medication variable was kept constant ($p = .032$). *Intensive therapy or intervention in crisis in a therapeutic community* was not connected with the assessment of the global prognosis.

6.7.4 Summary and Discussion

As a summary of the statistical analyses presented in this chapter, we can say that the *effects of psychotherapy were most undisputable on the increase of insight*. Both in the whole series and in the group of typical schizophrenics the increase of insight was clearly significantly more common among the patients classified as psychotherapy cases than among the other patients, when the explaining background variables and the medication variable were kept constant. In the group of typical schizophrenics, intensive individual therapy also had a clearly significant connection and intensive therapy or intervention in crisis in a psychotherapeutic community an almost significant connection with the increase of insight after the variables were kept constant.

The connection between the *decrease of nuclear symptoms and inclusion in the group of psychotherapy cases also remained at least marginally significant in the group of typical schizophrenic patients*. The connection between *intensive individual* therapy and the decrease of nuclear symptoms also came close to significance of this level in this group. An analysis of the whole series revealed no statistically significant connections after the background variables were kept constant. Although intensive individual therapy had previously (cf. 6.2.2.) emerged as one variable explaining the decrease of nuclear symptoms in a logistic regression analysis of both background and treatment variables in the whole series, the effect of this mode of treatment was explained in the new analysis by the better background of the patients with regard to the severity of the mother's disturbance. This finding can also be interpreted as suggesting that it was more difficult to establish long-term psychotherapeutic relationships with patients whose mothers had severe ego disorders than with patients whose mothers were healthier.

The favourable effects on the *maintenance of working capacity were also obvious in particularly the group of typical schizophrenias* after the background variables were kept constant. The connection between *inclusion in the group of psychotherapy cases* and optimistic prognosis remained significant in that group and both *individual therapy* and *intensive treatment or intervention in crisis in a psychotherapeutic community* had a marginally significant connection with the maintenance or working capacity. In our whole series inclusion in the psychotherapy cases had previously turned out to be significantly connected with the maintenance of working capacity, which connection now disappeared when one background factor of the basic examination stage, namely unemployment, was kept constant. Nevertheless, the analysis suggested that inclusion in the group of psychotherapy cases helped the patients with a stabilized occupational identity at the basic examination stage to retain their working capacity.

The marginal connection with inclusion in the group of psychotherapy cases noted in the cross-tabulation of *the need for hospital treatment during the last two follow-up years* remained after the two most significant background variables – inclusion in the ego-dynamic group of regressive disintegration; quality of the contact established with the patient in the basic examination – were kept constant, but lost its significance when the medication variable was kept constant. Among the typical schizophrenic patients the decrease of the need for hospital treatment in the group of psychotherapy cases was explained by two background factors, the first unit of therapy and the patient's sex, which were differently weighted in and outside the group of psychotherapy cases.

A corresponding connection between factors affecting the prognosis was also noted when *the global prognostic score* was examined with the Strauss and Carpenter outcome scale. In cross-tabulation, inclusion in the group of psychotherapy cases was not connected with higher outcome scores in the whole series, though a marginally significant connection emerged in the group of typical schizophrenic patients. The latter connection persisted when one of the most significant background factors, the presence or lack of empathic relatives, was kept constant, but disappeared when the other, the patient's sex, was kept constant. Female patients had a clearly better global prognosis than males, and the connection between inclusion in the group of psychotherapy cases and the global prognosis was explained by the patient's sex. *Intensive individual therapy,* on the other hand, which had emerged as a variable explaining good prognosis in the logistic regression analysis in the *group of typical schizophrenics*, retained its connection with high total outcome score as almost significant even after the aforesaid background variables (as well as the medication variable) were kept constant. No corresponding statistically significant finding was made in the whole series.

After the background variables were kept constant, *the amount of medication* was no longer connected with the decrease of nuclear symptoms. The connection between the increase of insight and less-than-average medication remained marginally significant in the group' of typical schizophrenics, but did not emerge in the whole series. *The connection between more-than-average medication during the follow-up period and pessimistic prognosis*, on the other hand, *remained highly significant with two prognostic variables, maintenance of working capacity and the need for hospital treatment during the last two follow-up years*, even when the explaining background variables were kept constant. The background variables for working capacity were psychosocial, while the variables for the hospital episodes of the last two years also included the patient's inclusion in or exclusion from the ego-dynamic group of regressive disintegration. Medication also had a *parallel connection with the total outcome score* despite the background variables that were kept constant, the connection being highly significant in the whole series and clearly significant even in the group of typical schizophrenic patients.

The negative connection between more-than-average neuroleptic medication and the patient's poor prognosis should not, despite the results of these statistical analyses, be interpreted in a very straightforward manner, but *should rather be seen as related to the effects of the therapeutic approach as a whole.* We will return to this question at the end of the Chapter 6.8.

6.8 Prognosis and the Factors Affecting It: Summary and Discussion

The summaries of the findings on our patients' prognoses and the factors affecting them were already presented for the different sub-areas of prognosis at the end of the Chapters 6.2.-6.5. and 6.7. Below, we will review these findings from a global point of view, attaching special attention to the predictive significance of the different background factors and the conclusions relevant for the development of the therapy of patients of the schizophrenia group.

Before we are proceeding, however, it should be pointed out once again that our findings should not be generalized to pertain to the overall effects of the psychotherapeutic approach. Since the foundation of the Clinic of Psychiatry in 1967 (cf. Ch. 1) the psychotherapeutic approach gained ground in this hospital and gradually also in the out-patient system, while the approach of the other hospital, the Kupittaa Hospital, remained pharmacologically oriented and even lost its contact with the psychotherapeutic ways of thinking which were already emerging during the mid-60's when the "university wards" were located in the premises of the Kupittaa Hospital. The first unit of treatment was the most significant variable explaining selection in the group of psychotherapy cases in both our entire series and the group of typical schizophrenic patients and the second variable explaining selection for more-than-average medication during the follow-up period in the whole patient series. The discrepancy between the predominantly psychotherapeutically and predominantly psychopharmacologically oriented treatment approaches thus became particularly poignant and our results should be perceived from this point ot view.

6.8.1 Comparison of the Different Sub-Areas of Prognosis

The notion that *our therapeutic outcome was good with regard to the disappearance of symptoms and the decrease of the need for hospital treatment, but less optimistic for the working capacity and the patients' social development* received support when we compared above the distribution of our patients on the different items of Strauss and Carpenter's outcome scale with the findings presented by the authors for their own series (1972). The facts that the findings reported by Strauss and Carpenter were made in a two-year follow-up examination, while ours were made in a five-year follow-up examination, and that the patient populations were even otherwise slightly different do not constitute a source of error when we are comparing the findings on the different subareas of prognosis with each other.

A parallel conclusion can be made when our findings are compared with the results obtained by Salokangas (1977, 1978) in a series of patients admitted in Turku ten years previously, whose follow-up examination was carried out 7½ years after the admission: our own findings are somewhat better as regards the patients' clinical condition, more or less similar as regards the in-patient treatment (the results reported by Salokangas on this item were quite good), but slightly poorer as regards the maintenance of working capacity and the pensions. The comparison of social relationships is difficult because of a lack of uniform criteria. We can more adequately compare our findings with the results reported by Salokangas as soon as the follow-up period is the same, i.e. when the results of the eight-year follow-up examination to be undertaken on our series are known.

The relative difference between the clinical and psychosocial prognoses in our patient population is probably explained, in part, by the employment situation that deteriorated during 1973–1974 and has remained poorer ever since. The unemployment percentages of the working-age Turku population were about 1 %, or even less, in the late 1960's and the early 1970's, while the corresponding percentage after 1976 has been 4 – 8 %. The economico-social trend prevailing in Finland has also impeded the development of the rehabilitation of patients with psychosis for work, which rehabilitation was even otherwise lagging behind in Turku compared with many other mental health districts of Finland.

The effects of the psychosocial factors on the development of the working capacity of our patients are also reflected in the fact that the maintenance of working capacity was explained particularly by psychosocial, not by clinical background variables in the logistic regression analyses. The typically schizophrenic patients had a notably more pessimistic clinical prognosis than the rest of the series, while the difference in the psychosocial prognosis, though existent, was clearly smaller.

Although there was a significant connection between the clinical prognostic variables and the maintenance of working capacity in the group of typical schizophrenics neither the disappearance of psychotic symptoms nor the decrease of nuclear symptoms had any statistically significant connection with being on pension after five years or avoidance of such pension. This confirms our previous assumptions concerning the factors affecting disability pensions.

In a society burdened by unemployment, individuals suffering from psychoses of the schizophrenia group are in a particularly difficult position, and the patients with the least advantageous psychosocial starting-points fare even worse than the others. The institutions of society have "blessed" the situation by favouring a practice whereby prolonged disability pension is a better alternative for these patients than unemployment benefit, even when there is a change toward better taking place in the patient's condition. The high-standard social security in itself provides the patients with adequate consolation and support. This trend is clearly illustrated by the fact that although obvious progress had taken place in the overall clinical status of the patients as well as in their interpersonal relations and grip on life during the period between the two-year and five-year follow-up examinations, the number of individuals on disability pension had further increased. *Active enhancement of the rehabilitative functions* seems highly justified in the light of these observations.

When our findings are compared with the results reported by Strauss and Carpenter, the difference most difficult to explain is the one seen in the development of the social relations. It could have been expected that the development of the clinical condition and the social relations would have been mutually dependent, which would also have been observable in the comparison. It is possible that, despite our effort to the contrary, our assessment criteria at this point were not completely identical with those of the original team. Cultural difference may also serve as a partial explanation. It must be admitted, nevertheless, that the findings on the development of the interpersonal relations of our patients outside their primary families for example were partly quite negative. They also indicate that the *field of social relations*, apart from the development of psychotherapeutic activities, *is in need of increased supportive functions to help the patients* (clubs, friend services, etc.). It was encouraging to find out that the interpersonal relations of the patients had improved during the period between the two-year and five-year follow-up examinations. This was partly also reflected by the marriages of some patients towards the end of the follow-up period.

Despite the differences noted in the patients' development between the different sub-areas of prognosis, the *findings on the different prognostic sub-areas made in the five-year follow-up examination were quite notably interrelated*. The connections between the prognostic variables are presented in *Appendix 10*.

The connections between the prognostic variables on the one hand and the emphatic importance of certain background variables in certain sub-areas of the prognosis on the other confirm the notion expressed by e.g. Strauss and Carpenter (1977) according to which the different *sub-areas of the prognosis of schizophrenia are mutually related, but each of them is additionally influenced by background factors more "specific" to each sub-area*. From the viewpoint of the development of the treatment and rehabilitation, it is necessary to approach the prognosis from several different directions, not focussing on the patient's clinical condition alone.

6.8.2 Patient-Specific Background Factors As Predictors of the Prognosis

We will now discuss in a summary fashion the predictive effect of the different background variables on the prognosis and point out the sub-areas of prognosis where the effect was particularly pronounced (to the extent of being an explaining background variable).

The statistical connections between the most central prognostic variables with the background variables are presented in Appendices 7 and 8. The scales of assessment are shown in Appendix 4 for the prognostic variables.

As regards the different *diagnostic categories* of our series, the patients considered *typically schizophrenic* in accordance with the Nordic tradition developed by Langfeldt et al. (1952), had *clearly less optimistic prognosis* than the other patients of the schizophrenic group despite the fact that the effect of psychotherapy on the prognosis of these patients was at least equally obvious as the corresponding effect on the prognosis of the other patients. It should be underlined that while making the diagnoses (3.1.2.), we deemed it important to take into account not only the presence or non-presence of the "typical" symptoms, but also the duration of them defined rather on the basis of the stabilization of the symptoms as preliminary established parts of the personality functions than on the basis of merely temporal criteria.

The inclusion in the group of typical schizophrenic patients emerged as the variable most conspicuously explaining the prognosis in our series, as a negative factor, particularly for the clinical prognostic variables of disappearance of psychotic symptoms and decrease of nuclear symptoms. In addition to this, inclusion in this group emerged as a variable explaining the prognosis as regards the new *psychosocial* prognostic variable, the loss or maintenance of the grip on life. The nuclear group also had highly significant connections with the two prognostic variables pertaining to in-patient treatment. As regards the development of insight, on the other hand, the typical schizophrenic patients did not differ from the rest of the series. The other *psychodynamic* variables measuring the changes that took place during the follow-up period gave rise to an interesting observation: *progressive changes were roughly equal in frequency in the group of typical schizophrenic patients and in the rest of the series, while regressive changes were much more numerous in the group of typical schizophrenics*. The same was also true of the achievement or loss of occupational identity during the follow-up period. Case-specific analysis revealed a clear connection between the progress of development and psychotherapy, particularly intensive individual therapy.

Of the other, numerically quite small diagnostic categories, only the category of *schizo-affective psychoses* emerged as an explaining variable for one psychodynamic prognostic variable: the increase of interpersonal relationships during the follow-up period. Otherwise, the prognoses of these diagnostic categories did not differ notably from each other. Slight psychotic symptoms at the end of the five-year follow-up period were only seen in a couple of patients diagnosed as borderline schizophrenias, while in-patient episodes diminished slightly more rapidly in this group than in the group of schizophreniform psychoses and schizo-affective psychoses.

The *ego-dynamic groups* did not emerge equally conspicuously in the study of the prognosis as in the selection for treatments. The *group of regressively disintegrated patients* was one variable explaining both the total number of in-patient days during the follow-up period and the patient-specific hospital admissions during the last two follow-up years in the whole series. Pensions were significantly more frequent in this group than in the others, while psychotic symptoms at the end of the follow-up period were slightly more numerous in the group of paranoid disintegration. This can be taken as one indication of the favourable effects of psychotherapy on this group of patients, which was also suggested by some of the other findings. Of the 12 patients who definitely lacked psychotic symptoms at the end of the follow-up period, but had been classified into the group of regressive disintegration in the basic examination, 11 belonged to the group of psychotherapy cases.

As it was to be expected, the ego-dynamic groups of imminent disintegration and acute disintegration had the best prognoses.

Of the other clinical background variables, the *slow onset of symptoms* was of explaining significance for the finding on the presence of psychotic symptoms even after the follow-up period. This was true of both the whole series and the group of typical schizophrenias. In addition, this background variable emerged as a factor explaining the regression of psychosexual development in the whole series, and it also had connections with some other prognostic variables, e.g. the loss of the grip on life and the loss or working capacity. These connections were, however, notably weaker than the connections of the inclusion in the group of typical schizophrenia.

The division of the patients on the basis of whether the *psychotic symptoms* had *lasted* for more or less than a month prior to admission turned out a less significant background variable. Although this variable also had connections with the prognosis, they were relatively weak, and this background variable did not emerge as an explaining variable at any point.

Of the other psychiatric symptoms noted at the basic examination stage, the presence of *alcohol or other addiction problems* had the greatest significance for the prognosis. This background variable emerged as an explaining variable in the whole series at four points: inhibiting the increase of insight and the increase of the number of interpersonal relationships, retarding psychosexual development, and increasing the number of patients granted a pension. The effects were thus most notable on the psychosocial and psychodynamic dimensions. The alcohol problems noted at the time of admission (other addiction problems were exceptions) also had a statistical connection with the number of in-patient days during the last follow-up year.

Although *neurotic symptoms* were connected with a good outcome development at some points, particularly in the field of clinical prognostic variables, they did not have the significance of an explaining variable. The same was also true of *depressive symptoms*. The presence of *acting-out symptoms,* on the other hand, had such significance in the whole series as preventing the decrease of suicidal tendencies. The patients with acting-out tendencies who were difficult to involve in long-term psychotherapy – as it was pointed out in Chapter 5 – also had clearly more in-patient days than was the average in the series.

The *degree of insight* and the *patient's mode of contact* upon admission did not turn out background variables significant for the prognosis despite the fact that they, similarly to depressive symptoms, had explaining connections with the selection for psychotherapies. The same was also true of *admission on the basis of judicial sanctions*, whose only explaining connection with the prognostic variables was positive: it was connected with the decrease of suicidal tendencies in the group of typical schizophrenic patients. The connection is explained by the fact that the suicidal tendencies upon admission were connected with admission on the basis of sanctions. The administrative procedure was, generally speaking, due more to the patient's contemporay condition than to the severity of his disease in the long run: as we remember, these patients were most numerous in the group of schizophreniform psychoses.

The assessment of the *patient's reluctance to be admitted for treatment* made independently of the judicial sanctions also had an explaining connection with only one prognostic variable: regressive development in the psychologic separation from the primary family. Initial refusal of treatment had hardly any connections with the prognosis, nor had violence or suicidal tendencies present as baseline characteristics.

The significance of the psychosocial background variables for the prognosis turned out to be *quite great* in the present work. They had more explaining significance for the psychodynamic and psychosocial development of the patients than had the clinical background variables, and some of them emerged as explaining factors even in the analysis of the patients' clinical development and the factors contributing to their need for hospital treatment.

The *social group* of the patient and his primary family had hardly any significance for the outcome development, and the patient's *basic education* also emerged as an explaining variable at only one point: higher basic education was connected with the maintenance of working capacity in both the whole series and the group of typical schizophrenics. *The prognosis was*, however, *extensively influenced by the patient's sex, the factors associated with his family environment and his employment situation at the time of admission.*

The significance of sex, i. e. the better outcome of female patients compared with males, was obvious on all the prognostic dimensions. The difference was smallest in the clinical prognosis.

Apart from explaining the *global prognosis* and the decrease of *suicidal tendencies,* the patient's sex emerged as an explaining variable in the whole series for *the progress of psychosexual development and the progress of separation from the primary family as well as the maintenance of the working capacity.* The findings were similar in the group of typical schizophrenic patients. *A fourfold number of female patients compared with males were able to work at the end of the follow-up period in the group diagnosed as typically schizophrenic*. The difference was also significant in many other analyses of psychosocial and psychodynamic prognostic variables.

Above (6.4.4.), some factors associated with the *social roles* of women and men were suggested as possibly explaining the difference in the prognosis between the sexes. At least in our own series, we must further add the *greater willingness of women to receive treatment in comparison with males*, which was also clearly emphasized in our observations on the implementation of psychotherapeutic treatments. Ultimately, this is probably a matter of the greater liability of women to rely on other people in general, which may be especially conspicuous in the Finnish cultural environment: the accepted ego ideal of the man does not easily permit any strong expressions of emotions or admission of being dependent on others. In our series the effect of this factor was certainly twofold: the female patients resorted more to their fellow-people even outside the therapies than the males, and they also found it easier to consult therapist than the males did and they experienced they derived more benefit from the therapies. As it was pointed out in Chapter 5, male sex was one of the variables explaining exclusion of the patients from the group of psychotherapy cases and, in the group of typical schizophrenics, of the amount of neuroleptic medication, which was greater among the male patients.

The patient's *age group* only emerged as an explaining variable once in our analyses: suicidal tendencies decreased more in the younger age group than in the older. Otherwise, the age groups only had very few significant connections with our prognostic variables even in the group of typical schizophrenic patients. The only clearly significant statistical connection was noted for the total number of in-patient days during the follow-up period, which was greater in the youngest age group because of a few patients in need of prolonged in-patient episodes. But not even a marginal connection was seen in the analysis of the patients in hospital treatment during the last two follow-up years. We consider it probable that these findings also are related to our psychotherapeutic approach, which included slightly more young patients than old ones in the scope of the most active functions.

The significance of *marital status* for the prognosis also proved to be relatively small in this work. Being unmarried at the time of the basic examination (in contrast to being married or divorced) emerged as an explaining variable at one point: regression of the psychosexual development during the follow-up period.

The significance of the background variables associated with the primary family was notable in several sub-areas of the prognosis, their mutual weighting being variable. *Lack of psychologic separation from the primary family* as a baseline characteristic appeared to have a *particular effect on the clinical prognosis*: it explained the poor outcome concerning the decrease of nuclear symptoms both in the whole series and in the group of typical schizophrenics and also the total number of in-patient days in the latter group. *Mother's personality disorder graver than neurosis* emerged as an explaining variable in the *regression of occupational identity and of the quality of the interpersonal relationships outside the primary family,* being also almost significantly connected with the diminished decrease of nuclear symptoms as well as with the loss of working capacity and being granted a disability pension. The severity of the *father's personality disorder* was of lesser effect. Lack of serious personality disorder in the father did, however, explain the progressive development of the psychosexual identity among our patients (especially female ones).

Findings of *a close relative with an empathic attitude* towards the patient at the time of the basic examination (either a parent or a spouse) *seemed to have a lesser effect on the clinical prognosis, but an extremely marked effect on some sub-areas of the psychodynamic and psychosocial prognosis*. This background variable emerged as an explaining variable in both the whole series and the group of typical schizophrenics as regards *avoidance of disability pension* and the *good global prognostic assessment* based on Strauss and Carpenter's total outcome score, in addition to which it explained the *improvement of the quality of the interpersonal relationships outside the* primary family in the whole series and *the maintenance of the grip on life* in the group of typical schizophrenics. A *hostile or poorly understanding attitude of the relatives,* in turn, had a corresponding negative effect on all these sub-areas, which emerged as an explaining variable in the analysis of the *working capacity* in the whole series at the end of the follow-up period. This was all the more conspicuous, as we noted in Chapter 4 that these relatives were relatively most frequent in the group of borderline schizophrenias, where the prognosis was good.

Abnormality of the social life course of the patient's primary family (which was, however, quite complex as a background variable) had a positive explaining significance for two psychodynamic prognostic variables: increase of insight and avoidance of regression of the process of separation from the primary family.

Our findings hence confirm that the *significance of the psychologic factors involved in the family environment for the prognosis of the patients of the schizophrenia group is quite notable*. This can be interpreted quite straightforwardly, especially as regards the relatives' attitudes: empathic attitudes also include understanding of the patients developmental needs and thereby serve to support even the developmental process taking place in psychotherapy. The interpretation of the significance of the mother's personality disorder is naturally more difficult, because it is also possible to suggest the importance of genetic factors and not only factors pertaining to the psychology of the family environment. The recent findings have not, however, suggested that disorders of the psychotic level in the patient's parents or in his family in general would have any significant effect of the prognosis of schizophrenia (e.g. Bleuler 1972). We have given particular attention to the phenomenon that personality disorders more serious than neurosis, which generally affect the ego functions, usually occur parallel to an increased need for dependence and transactional defence mechanisms (Räkköläinen and Alanen 1982), resulting in mutual, often quite rigid entanglements, which contribute to increased difficulty of the patient's development of individuation both prepsychotically and during the psychotherapy given to him. We had several examples of this in our series, precisely in the families where the parents had serious personality disorders.

According to our observations, the *patient-specific psychodynamic background variables* had clearly fewer connections with the prognosis than the family-specific ones. Some of them emerged as explaining variables in the psychodynamic prognosis: *a lack of stable heterosexual identity* as a baseline characteristic in relation to an increase of the number of interpersonal relationships during the follow-up period in the group of typical schizophrenic patients, a *tendency to avoid aggressions* in relation to qualitative improvement of the interpersonal relationships in the whole series, and a *lack of interpersonal relationships outside the primary family* in relation to the stabilization of occupational identity during the follow-up period in the whole series. The connections appear ostensibly paradoxical, but are explained by the fact that progressive development in these prognostic variables was particularly notable among the patients with poor starting-points who were given intensive psychotherapeutic treatment.

The patient's *being unemployed at the time of admission turned out a very significant background factor for his subsequent psychosocial prognosis*: both in the whole series and in the group of typical schizophrenics, this variable had marked statistical connection with *working incapacity, loss of the grip on life*, and *being on disability pension* at the end of the five-year follow-up period. In the case of the first two of these items, unemployement as a baseline characteristic emerged as a background factor explaining the poor prognosis in the whole series, in the case of the loss of the grip also in the group of typical schizophrenics. The same was also true of the *number of in-patient days* during the follow-up period as well as Strauss and Carpenter's *total outcome score* in the whole series. This background variable was also almost significantly connected with the persistence of the psychotic symptoms.

The patient's employment status at the time of admission had no connections with either the clinical categories or the ego-dynamic groups in the total series or the group of typical schizophrenics, though it had an almost significant connection with the slow onset of the symptoms, the presence of acting-out symptoms and the lack of depressive symptoms. Unemployment had the most marked connection ($p = .006$ in the whole series, $p = .015$ in the group of typical schizophrenics) with a low educational level and a nearly similar connection with the patient's social group. What further attracts attention is the almost significant connection between unemployment and the presence of hostile or poorly understanding relatives.

The other background variable closely associated with working life, the *possession of a stable occupational identity,* was of positive explaining significance for the maintenance of working capacity and the grip on life in the whole series. It also had a statistically similar (almost significant) connection with avoidance of pension. In the group of typical schizophrenic patients this background variable did not emerge equally significantly.

In the psychodynamic prognosis, the occupational identity turned out particularly important for separation from the primary family. The finding is easy to understand: the achieved occupational identity and the ensuing possibility to find a job are one of the important prerequisites for gaining independence from entaglement in the primary family.

On the whole, these findings clearly indicate *how important it is, at the time of the initial examination already, to supplement the individual clinical and psychodynamic examination of the patient with an exploration of the patient's family-psychologic situation and his other important interactional relationships* – including the attitudes of the significant others towards the patient – *as well as his contemporary social situation.* In addition to being of predictive prognostic significance, as shown by our findings, this multiple approach is *essentially important for the case-specific planning of different therapeutic and rehabilitative measures* and for the consideration of the preconditions for carrying out these measures.

6.8.3 Conclusions of the Effect of Treatment

The connection between our treatment variables and the central prognostic variables have also been combined as a table in Appendix 9. In Ch. 6.7. we examined which statistical connections maintained their significance after the explaining background variables were kept constant for the four prognostic variables (decrease of nuclear symptoms, working capacity, increase of insight, inpatient episodes during the last two follow-up years).

Although the connections of the psychotherapy variables with prognostic variables were not as significant as those of the most influential background variables, the *conclusion that the implementation of the psychotherapeutic approach had favourable effects on the prognosis of the patients seems clearly justifiable in the light of these findings.* The significance of the therapies appears most clearly in our assessments of the *increase of the patient's insight,* but it is also quite obvious in the *maintenance of working capacity,* especially in the analyses of the typical schizophrenic patients. Suggestions of favourable effects were also obtained for the improvement of clinical symptoms.

It is interesting that *the effect of the global psychotherapeutic approach on the prognosis* did not, in the light of these statistical analyses, appear to be any lesser in the group of typical schizophrenic patients than in the rest of the series, rather on the contrary. This was certainly partly due to the fact that the prognosis of the patients excluded from the nuclear group was better even without therapy. In the group of typical schizophrenic patients one factor explaining the selection into the group of psychotherapy cases was the relatively acute onset of the symptoms, which is considered a favourable prognostic predictor. The claim that psychotherapy planned to meet the needs of the patients *also* improves the average prognosis of the patients with typical schizophrenia is, however, justified in the light of both our overall findings and the observations on the development of several individual patients in our series.

As regards the different modes of therapy, *the best experiences were obtained from intensive individual therapy on the one hand and from psychotherapeutic communities on the other.* Intensive individual therapy also emerged as a variable explaining the optimistic prognosis in several analyses: in the whole series it explained the decrease of nuclear symptoms, the prevention of the decrease of interpersonal relationships during the follow-up period, and the stabilization of the occupational identity, while in the group of typical schizophrenic patients it explained the increase of insight and the global prognosis calculated on the basis of Strauss and Carpenter's total outcome score. In the latter group the connection between intensive individual therapy and the increase of insight remained significant and the connection between intensive individual therapy and the global total outcome score almost significant even after the background variables were kept constant.

In this respect our findings clearly differ from the negative notions presented on the basis of some psychotherapeutic studies regarding the individual therapy of schizophrenia (May 1968, Grinspoon et al. 1972, cf. also Klerman's 1984 discussion of the results reported by Gunderson et al. 1984) although they are close to the experiences obtained from some other projects (Karon et al. 1972, Sjöström 1982, Furlan et al. 1985) as well as the experiences of other therapists of psychotic patients.

One reason for the difference between our own findings and the more negative findings of the other projects probably lies in the difference of the research designs. The patients given intensive individual therapy in our own series did not represent the schizophrenic population as a whole, but particularly the schizophrenic patients with better-than-average suitability to individual therapy. In a randomized series, the good results obtained with patients suited to this mode of therapy and the poor results obtained with non-suitable patients are intermixed, which hides the aforesaid good results. A strictly "controlled" research design also means that the therapy is carried out according to a certain pre-planned formula without any exceptions to the therapeutic plan and often probably without the kind of creative enthusiasm which is frequently very important in the treatment of precisely schizophrenic patients. The patients suited to individual therapy in our series were mainly patients who had a preliminary insight into their problems even initially and also had a motivation to establish a confidential long-term therapeutic relationship with the therapist. There were, however, also patients who were only gradually motivated to long-term treatment.

The treatments we call intensive individual therapies were carried out in about one fourth of our series, with typical schizophrenics numbering more or less the same as the other patients. The name may be partly misleading. As it was explained in the earlier chapters, these therapies consisted, first and foremost, of *empathic, reliable and supportive therapeutic relationships which did not aim at a profound analytic process although the goals of the therapy also included increase of the patient's comprehension of himself and his problems.* It was in precisely these therapies that many of our staff members without actual psychotherapeutic training achieved good results.

We would consider it of primary importance that at least the kind of "good" individual therapy patients described above could be guaranteed an opportunity to receive the therapy they are in need of notably more often than is the case now, even in the normal circumstances, i.e. within the community psychiatric health care system. This does not seem impossible from the viewpoint of the temporal resources. Although the number of sessions at the initial stages of the therapeutic process was often two or three per week, the average frequency of sessions thereafter was one per week for several years.

These experiences lead us to emphasize that *we should not underestimate the importance of individual therapies based on relatively infrequent sessions, but an empathic and confidential therapeutic relationship* for the treatment of psychotic patients. For the patient, a long-term, positive interactional relationship is important as a source of hope and it also serves especially to enhance his identification with the therapist. The significance of the therapeutic relationship as such as well as the personal properties of the therapist are especially important in this group of patients compared with the more technically oriented psychoanalytic therapies of neurotic patients. Therapeutic "holding" (Winnicott 1960, Salonen 1976), which satisfies empathically the patient's symbiotic needs, but also supports his growth into differentation forms the basis for such therapeutic relationships. Serious transference crises, which frequently result in a discontinuation of the therapy, are easier to avoid in this kind of therapy than in more intensive, psychoanalytically oriented therapies. In addition to the lesser intensity of the therapy, the therapist's role as a member of the therapeutic community and the family orientation of the treatment also often serve to diminish the possibility of a transference crisis: the therapist and/or the other members of the team have also established contacts with the patient's family milieu and may maintain these contacts during the course of the therapy, the patient being aware of it. There was also a statistical correlation between intensive individual therapy and support given to the patient's family at an almost significant level. We consider it possible that this family and milieu orientation supporting the individual therapies also served to diminish the suicidal risk among our patients.

But we should also ask how permanent the results of such therapies are. More than half of these treatments were still going on at the time of the five years follow-up. The continuation of therapeutic relationships can also be interpreted as an indication of a persistence of the dependency relationships. Without doubt, many of the patients experienced a growth of the resources of their personality through the kind of "transmuting internalization" described by Kohut (1977) as well as an increase of their ability to perceive connections between the present and the past and the possibility to analyze the conflicts between their own internal world and the external reality without disintegrating. But are the patients able to tolerate also the termination of the therapy, the discontinuation of the "holding"? In some terminated therapies it seemed that the patient had been able, with the help of the therapy, to create other significant interpersonal relationships, and the termination of the therapy coincided with their consolidation – e.g. marriage.

The infrequent individual therapies, which were numerically slightly fewer in our series than the intensive therapies and had even lower frequency of sessions, had a significantly poorer outcome than the intensive individual therapies. They did not generally involve a continuous therapeutic process, but merely consisted of an exclusively supportive therapeutic relationships or control of medication.

Further illustration for these questions will be received from the eight-year follow-up study, when the number of completed individual therapies will be higher than at the present.

In the light of our findings, the results of *family therapy* remained much poorer than the corresponding results of individual therapy, which is largely opposite to the notions presented in some recent reviews (Mosher and Keith 1980). It is therefore necessary to emphasize that our statistical findings on family therapy are not comparable with the findings on individual and community therapies. Since the family therapies carried out were fewer in number, we also had to include the less intensive family therapies, in order to get some idea of the outcome of this mode of treatment. As it was understood earlier, the educational prerequisites for family therapy were also clearly poorer in Turku at the beginning of the project than were the prerequisites for individual therapy. Moreover, the family therapies of primary families were carried out among very seriously ill patients. The results of couple therapies were better, but do not stand out in our statistical analysis.

Family therapy emerged as an explaining variable twice in our analyses contributing positively to the decrease of the suicidal tendencies and negatively to the progress of the separation from the primary family, in the whole series. It is questionable whether either of these findings would have persisted if the background variables had been kept constant for these prognostic variables, too.

Systematic training for family therapy in Finland was only started two or three years after the admission of our patients. The interest in system-centered family therapy has thereafter increased notably in Turku. As far as we know, the results have also improved, but they can only be reported in follow-up investigations of new patient series, which are being carried out.

As far as we can see, however, *it remains to be elucidated, how far it is possible by means of family therapy to influence serious schizophrenia based on a deep-rooted, long-term disorder of the personality development.* In most of the American and British studies reviewed in Chapter 2, the follow-up periods were relatively short and the goals of therapy mainly supportive, aiming at an out-patient status of the patient and a promotion of his rehabilitation. In this respect, the benefits of the psycho-educational family therapeutic approach (e.g. Anderson 1980, Falloon et al. 1982) are obvious and easy to understand. In Finland we have also previously obtained experiences of psychodynamic family therapies, which have resulted in a liberation of positive forces within the family and a consequent individuation and emancipation of the patient (Alanen 1972, 1976). This has generally been best possible in the families with the best motivation to analyze their problems, which include only a small portion of the primary families of seriously disturbed schizophrenic patients.

In rigid families with strong transactional defences (i.e. the kind of families that the primary families given intensive family therapy in our series generally were), resistance to change turned out an almost insurmountable obstacle for the development of such a process. A systemic strategic intervention is more effective in the homeostatically weighted structure of such families. The extent to which it is also possible to develop the patient's personality on a long-term basis within this system remains to be elucidated. We assume this to necessitate a developmental process based on a dyadic relationship, to which the patient arrested in his internal and interpersonal growth is able to transfer both his dependence and his need for growth. Optimally, a systemic family-therapeutic intervention should therefore be followed by a long-term individual-therapeutic process, for which the intervention has made way as regards both the patient and the other family members. It seems that *family-therapeutic intervention yields the most rapid and permanent results in both transactional development and clinical recovery in the crises of somewhat further individuated patients*, which include many of the psychoses of the schizophrenia group precipitated by conflicts of the marital relationships and/or other interpersonal relationships outside the primary family.

It may seem paradoxical in the light of the scantness of family-therapeutic success that *we consider one of the central conclusions of our experiences to be that the family-therapeutic activities should be strongly increased*. As far as we can see, the inadequate outcome in this field was not due to the family-therapeutic approach being wrong in itself, but to our inadequate command of this therapeutic mode. The "family nature" of psychoses of the schizophrenia group was clearly demonstrated by the exceedingly obvious connections between the family-dynamic background variables on the one hand and the selection for treatments and the patients' prognosis on the other.

Although our variable based on *treatment in a psychotherapeutic community* did not emerge as an explaining variable in any subarea of the prognosis, the community therapy variable also had a clear statistical connection with the increase of insight and the maintenance of working capacity, which retained its significance in the group of typical schizophrenics even after the background variables were kept constant. This is all the more conspicuous as (even among the typical schizophrenics) the patients selected for intensive treatment or intervention in crisis in a psychotherapeutic community were disturbed more seriously than the average. Even more conspicuous was that another variable, *the first treatment unit*, emerged as the explaining variable in the analysis of the factors which contributed to the patients' not needing in-patient treatment during the last two follow-up years, in such a way that patients first treated in the psychotherapeutically oriented hospital wards were less often in hospital treatment compared with the patients of the other hospital and even those first treated in the open care units.

Despite the criticism of the psychiatric hospital institution and the efforts to minimize the role of hospitals in psychiatric health care, we interpret our own experiences as indicating that the *ward communities with an open and empathic atmosphere are still of pivotal significance for the psychotherapeutic treatment of schizophrenic patients*. It is true, of course, that we have had our share of the risks of excessive hospital orientation. The follow-up study carried out by Salokangas (1983, 1985) on the patients of the schizophrenia group first admitted into the Turku Clinic of Psychiatry at the initial stages of its operation gave rise to the conclusion that long-term treatment in a psychotherapeutic community prognosticated a subsequent need for long-term in-patient episodes. The results of the present project were hence opposite in this respect: the shortcomings of the therapeutic approach had been overcome. Apart from the development of the out-patient activities, this was due to the emphatic recommendation that the therapeutic communities of the wards should not consider themselves self-sufficient, but extend their activities to the patients' living milieus outside hospital.

Ward communities with an open and warm atmosphere free from excessive hierarchy are needed by especially the most seriously disturbed patients, who largely lack the ability to make contacts and who also lack at this stage the motivation to therapy which is necessary for out-patient activities. In a psychotherapeutic community they have a possibility to overcome their need-fear dilemma and to establish a confidential relationship, wherein they are able to express their emotions more freely than previously.

Another group typically in need of long-term community therapy consisted of the patients whose interpersonal relationships or social situation involved particularly difficult problems, which had effected a catastrophic change in the previous situation. They need, for some time, a safe pivotal point for seeking new starting-points for their life. Cooperation with auxiliary forces found outside the hospital is particularly important for the solution of the problems of these patients.

The role of the *day hospital* in our community treatment remained relatively modest. The share of the day hospital activities has later increased in our therapeutic system. Good experiences have also been obtained in the Turku Clinic of Psychiatry during the past few years of an arrangement wherein a patient who begins his treatment on a closed ward later becomes a day patient of the same ward, continuing the therapeutic relationship initially started there. This has lead to a shortening of the in-patient periods.

The scantness of *rehabilitative activities* and the necessity to increase them were already referred to above while discussing the psychosocial background factors and prognosis of our patients. The better prognosis of our psychotherapy cases compared with the other patients was still, as a matter of fact, more notable in the maintenance of working capacity than in the disappearance of psychotic symptoms. There were, however, no significant differences with regard to the loss of the grip and the granting of pensions. It is probably in these latter findings that the lack of an adequate rehabilitative system to complement the psychotherapeutic activities is most obviously reflected.

The list of the *negative connections with the prognostic variables* that emerged as explaining variables for the *more-than-average neuroleptic medication* during the follow-up period is long. These prognostic variables in both the whole series and the group of typical schizophrenics included disability pensions, loss of the grip on life, total number of in-patient days during the follow-up period, in-patient episodes during the last two follow-up years, and the global prognosis based on Strauss and Carpenter's total outcome score, in addition to which some other variables emerged either in the whole series or in the group of typical schizophrenics. The focus hence lied on the psychosocial variables and the variables pertaining to hospital treatment, although the connections where global. The negative connections with *working capacity* as well as the connections with the *in-patient treatments during the last two follow-up years* remained clearly significant in our series even when the background variables most significantly explaining the prognosis were kept constant. The same was also true of the *total outcome score*. The only prognostic variable included in the analyses with constant background variables that lost its (even otherwise weak) connection with the medication variable was the decrease of nuclear symptoms.

The negative effect of the more-than-average medication on the patients' prognosis compared with lesser-than-average medication hence does not seem to be explained adequately by the assumption that the patients who were primarily more seriously ill and had otherwise poorer starting-points with regard to the background variables were selected for more-than-average medication. We interprete the findings presented in Chapter 6.7. in such a way that they should be seen as related to the effects of the therapeutic approach as a whole, not exclusively to the amount of neuroleptic medication. The boundary between the psychotherapeutic and psychopharmacologic therapeutic approaches was rather strict at the time of our project. The patients given predominantly psychotherapeutically oriented treatment had a better prognosis than the ones given predominantly psychopharmacologically oriented treatment.

At this point we should further emphasize the point already underlined in the discussion (5.6.) of Chapter 5: the more-than-average medication in our project refers, in fact, to dosage that is moderate at the most, though it may have lasted for several years. A majority of the patients on lesser-than-average neuroleptic medication were without medication for the last three follow-up years. The continuity of psychotherapeutic treatment and the decrease of medication were clearly connected. Neuroleptic medication with predominantly low doses supported the psychotherapeutic treatments initially (in many cases even later), but high-dose (= moderate) medication continued towards the end of the follow-up period had a marked connection with a poor prognosis, particularly psychosocially. Even if we find it obvious that the more abundant medication of the subsequent years was at this stage given to the patients in a poor condition – who were almost regularly left without psychotherapeutic treatments – we can say that the medication at least did not improve their prognosis compared with other patients. The notion that the patients with psychoses of the schizophrenia group should primarily be treated with long-term medication and that psychotherapeutic treatments would not be of any notable significance for them was not confirmed by our findings. According to our experience, such a notion is a scientific myth, which has been supported by investigations of inadequate relevance in some respects.

7 Development of Need-Specific Treatment of Schizophrenic Psychoses

7.1 Need-Specificity of Treatment As Concept

What kind of global model for the treatment of schizophrenia our experiences seem to suggest and what kind of therapeutic activities appear indicated for the different patient groups within this model?

While developing the treatment of psychoses of the schizophrenia group in accordance with the integrated concept of illness, we recognized the central position of the *concept of the need-specificity of treatment*. By this we mean a *therapeutic approach that has been planned and is implemented at the same time both globally,* integratively combining therapeutic activities based on the different models of illness (cf. Chapter 1.1.), and *in a manner that meets the needs of each patient as well as the people making up his personal interactional network.*

The characteristics of need-specific treatment include the following:

1. *The planning and implementation of both diagnostic work and therapy are typically global, flexible,* and – as long as the treatment is continued – *sufficiently intensive and active.* In practice, this also means that the *process nature of therapy is clearly perceived.*

2. *The therapeutic activities are case-specifically accordant with the needs identified on the basis of the patient's clinical status and his psychologic and social life situation.* When identifying these needs, the therapist should take into account, in addition to the patient's individual needs, the need for help of the *interactional network* of which the patient makes a part.

3. *The diagnosis and treatment are dominated by an explicit psychotherapeutic general approach striving towards psychologic understanding.*

4. *The different therapeutic activities are carried out integratively in such a way as to make them mutually supportive.* Their mutual weighting and sequential order are determined by the case-specific global therapeutic plan, which can be altered whenever therapeutic needs emerge which require such alteration. This means that particular attention should be given to integrative measures (especially to integrative case meetings, where the therapeutic plans are checked and, when necessary, revised, and which are attended by the patient himself, the people responsible for his therapy, and often also members of the patient's personal interactional network). This item also means that the dosage of medication is made accordant with the goals of the patient's therapy, and taking into account the strains he has to experience in his interactional relationships and life situation.

7.2 Implementation of Need-Specific Treatment in Our Project and the Factors Affecting It

In the follow-up examination we found out that the therapeutic approach with these characteristics had been achieved highly variably in our series. In order to elucidate the questions pertaining to the need-specificity of treatment and its achievement we divided the patients in each follow-up examination into four groups according to whether we considered the need-specificity of their treatment good, satisfactory, passable or poor. The following premises were used in this classification:

1. *Need-specificity of treatment good*. In these cases, both case-specific and global principles had been observed in the diagnosis of therapeutic needs and in the implementation of therapy. Both the individual-psychologic and the transactional models had been taken into account at the time of the examination already. This did not necessarily mean that the two approaches would have been observed as parallel and of equal weight in the treatment, but that the situation had been approached from both points of view, appraising the consequent needs for treatment. The therapeutic solutions thereafter made could hence represent either an individual-oriented or a family-oriented mode or both together.

The use of psychotherapeutic communities and the planning and administration of pharmacotherapy also served as parts of a global and long-term therapeutic plan. The therapeutic solutions were to show both long-term significance and realistic and flexible applicability as to be accordant with the process nature of therapy.

2. *Satisfactory need-specificity of treatment* was characterized by case-specifically planned treatment with a genuine psychotherapeutic approach, but lesser agreement with the integrated model of illness. This was shown by either inadequate mutual integration of the therapeutic activities or an excessively narrow scope of the treatment relative to the needs. The most common restriction was excessive individual orientation, which occasionally resulted in problems at more advanced stages of the treatment; e.g. the patient's development in individual-oriented therapy was arrested because of a resistance that emerged in the family system, but remained untreated. In these cases the individual-therapeutic relationship became – if seen from the transactional point of view – a static part of the pathologic total constellation. There were, however, also some patients who were given either treatment in a psychotherapeutic community or family-oriented therapy, but whose individual needs for development were largely ignored. The continuity between in-patient and out-patient therapies was often insufficient, which was mostly due to the self-sufficient attitude of the hospital staff. Some patients classified into the group of good need-specificity in the two-year follow-up examination had to be classified into the group of satisfactory need-specificity at the time of the five-year examination, because the implementation of their therapies had lost its intensity and/or flexibility, becoming a routine procedure and a fully integrated part of the homeostatic standstill that had developed around the patient's situation. These cases revealed empathically the consequences of the discontinuation of integrative therapy-planning meetings.

3. *Passable need-specificity of treatment* in comparison with the above group, was characterized in most cases by a lack of psychotherapeutically oriented approach

despite the notable therapeutic activity seen occasionally. In most of these cases the biomedical model was observed too one-sidedly. The group further included patients who had been in hospital for long periods, but whose therapy had given hardly any attention to the patient's interpersonal life-field outside the hospital. In the cases of this group where a psychotherapeutic approach had been used, the therapeutic attitude was mostly characterized by formal routine and lack of sufficient intensity, in a couple of cases also by a non-realistic involvement in the patient's problems which was based on sub-conscious motives.

4. *The group of poor need-specificity of treatment* consisted of patients who had, practically speaking, remained without any therapy or whose therapy had been planned with very short-term goals. There seemed to have been hardly any understanding attitude towards the patient as a human being and his life situation in these cases, and the therapeutic solutions had been mostly administrative, having often been restricted to the most necessary minimum. The typical modes of treatment included, for example, prompt "intervention" in acute psychosis by means of medication or electroshock treatment without planning for any further measures or showing any interest in the patient's life.

Some support was given to the relatives even in this group, but they consisted of contacts separate from the rest of the treatment and initiated by the relatives.

A summary of the assessments made in the follow-up examinations is shown in Table 104.

Table 104. The team's assessments of the need-specificity of treatment at the time of the follow-up examinations. The figures are percentages

Follow-up period	N	Good	Satis-factory	Passable	Poor
0–2 years	100	30	29	15	26
2–5 years	69	17	22	35	26
0–5 years	96	23	32	25	19

As is shown by the Table, assessments of the need-specificity of treatment at the time of the five-year follow-up examination were made separately for the latter follow-up period and the whole five-year follow-up period. The latter assessment was made on 96 patients (the treatment of one of the 5 patients "lost" to the five-year follow-up had been terminated prior to the two-year follow-up and was assessed accordingly). The assessment concerning the last three follow-up years only covered the patients whose therapy had been continued throughout this period and for whom it was possible to make such an estimate.

According to the assessments, the treatment during the first two follow-up years was at least satisfactorily need-specific in about 60 % of the cases, the corresponding percentage during the latter three follow-up years being 40 % of the patients who still continued to receive treatment. The need-specificity of treatment hence showed a relative decline during the latter follow-up years. In practice, this was most clearly shown by the fact that the treatment of many patients became increasingly routine-like and lost its sufficient intensity. *With regard to the entire follow-up period, however, the need-specificity of treatment appeared good or satisfactory in 55 % of the cases*. Slightly less than one fourth of the patients belonged to the best group with good need-specificity.

The relationship between the psychotherapeutic modes of treatment and the groups of need-specificity is shown in Table 105. The percentages show the portion of patients in each group of need-specificity receiving the kinds of treatment specified in the Table.

Table 105. Implementation of psychotherapeutic treatments in the different need-specificity groups. The figures show the percentage of the implementation of treatment in each group

Mode of therapy	Need-specificity group			
	Good N = 22	Satisfactory N = 31	Passable N = 24	Poor N = 19
Initial intervention in crisis	41	39	21	5
Individual therapy:				
intensive	55	39	8	0
less intensive	27	39	29	26
Family therapy:				
intensive	45	13	4	0
less intensive	14	13	8	0
Supportive contact with family member(s)	55	39	29	37
Group therapy:				
intensive	0	0	4	0
less intensive	0	0	4	0
Psychotherapeutic community:				
intensive	45	32	17	0
less intensive	23	10	29	11
intervention in crisis	55	23	4	0
Intensive treatment or intervention in crisis in a psychotherapeutic community	82	52	21	0
Psychotherapy case	100	81	29	0

There was a strong positive connection between intensive psychotherapeutic treatments and good need-specificity. This is particularly conspicuous in the categories of intensive family therapy and intensive treatment or intervention in crisis in a psychotherapeutic community. The distribution of the less intensive treatments was more uniform, though showing a slight tendency to concentrate on the classes of better need-specificity. The same is also true of supportive contacts with family members.

The table also clearly indicates the connection between the group of psychotherapy cases and good or satisfactory need-specificity of treatment. Even so, some psychotherapy cases were also included in the group of passable need-specificity, while the group of satisfactory need-specificity includes some less seriously ill patients with short-term therapy who did not belong to the group of psychotherapy cases.

Good or satisfactory need-specificity of treatment correlated highly significantly with all the background variables based on the psychotherapeutic treatments described in Chapter 6 (intensive individual therapy, intensive or less intensive family therapy, intensive therapy or intervention in crisis in a therapeutic community, inclusion in the group of psychotherapy cases), the X^2 values being 19.8, 13.5, 27.2 and 50.6 in the aforesaid order.

The total amounts of *neuroleptic medication* consumed during the five-year follow-up period by the patients classified into the different need-specificity groups are shown in Table 106.

Table 106. Amount of neuroleptic medication during the five-year follow-up period in the different need-specificity groups. The figures are percentages

Need-specificity group	Amount of neuroleptic medication	
	more than average	less than average
Good	36	64
Satisfactory	39	61
Passable	61	39
Poor	68	32

More-than-average medication was hence typical of the groups with poor achievement of need-specificity, whereas less-than-average medication was typically given to the groups with better need-specificity. Our treatment variable demonstrating the amount of neuroleptic medication hence had an inverse connection with good or satisfactory need-specificity approaching the level of clear significance ($X^2 = 6.6$, $p = .010$).

In principle, the concept of need-specificity should be widened so as to include not only the quantity but also the quality of the neuroleptic treatment applicated, possibly defined on the ground of the patients' biological – if also clinical and environmental – situation. The studies of Rappaport et al (1978), and Carpenter et al (1977) referred at the end of Chapter 2, already pointed out that there may be groups of patients for whom the drug treatment is not indicated at all. A more differentiated discussion of these questions, however, goes beyond our abilities. We may also refer to Wyatt et al (1982), who, summarizing their review on the biological studies of the etiology of schizophrenia, conclude: "With our paucity of knowledge and working tools, necessity dictates that we continue to treat the full spectrum of patients similarly". Concerning the psychotherapeutic and psychosocial modes of treatment, we no more can agree with this.

The patient-specific factors contributing to the implementation of need-specific treatment were in our study analyzed by determining the connections *between the better-than-average* (good or satisfactory) *or poorer-than-average* (passable or poor) *need-specificity and the clinical and psychosocial background variables of our series.*

The background variables included two which correlated with good or satisfactory need-specificity of treatment at a highly significant level in the whole series: *female sex* ($p = .0004$) and *presence of depressive symptoms* ($p = .0009$). Two background variables had an almost significant connection: exclusion from the group of unemployed patients at the time of admission ($p = .023$) and lack of serious personality disorder of the patient's mother ($p = .042$). Marginally significant connections were noted for several background variables: acute onset of illness, voluntary admission for treatment, lack of refusal of any mode of treatment, baseline contacts that were not reserved or suspicious, exclusion from the group of schizophreniform psychoses and the ego-dynamic group of paranoid disintegration, inclusion in the ego-dynamic group of acute disintegration, better-than-average basic education, and psychologic separation from the primary family by the time of admission.

A separate analysis of our group of typical schizophrenic patients showed that better-than-average need-specificity was again connected significantly with the presence of depressive symptoms ($p = .007$) and almost significantly with an acute onset of symptoms ($p = .012$), female sex ($p = .013$) and a lack of alcohol problems ($p = .028$). This analysis did not reveal background variables with marginally significant connections.

In addition to these background variables, we must also bear in mind the influence of the *first unit of therapy* on the subsequent nature of the treatment: in the whole series, the two best need-specificity groups included 65 % of the patients first admitted into an out-patient unit, 64 % of those first admitted into wards of the Clinic of Psychiatry or the day hospital, and 29 % of those first admitted into the Kupittaa Hospital. The corresponding figures in the group of typical schizophrenics were 55 %, 61 % and 33 %, respectively. The first therapeutic unit and the better-than-average need-specificity of treatment had a clear statistical connection in the whole series ($p = .012$). In the group of typical schizophrenics this effect remained below the level of statistical significance.

Female patients were clearly more numerous in the group first admitted into the Clinic of Psychiatry than in the group who started their treatment in the Kupittaa Hospital. But when the patients' sex or the first unit of therapy was kept constant, it turned out that the sex variable correlated more strongly with the need-specificity groups.

The patient' primary insightfulness had no statistical connection with better-than-average need-specificity of treatment, although this connection approached marginal significance in the whole series ($p = .11$). The same was also true of such background variables as admission on the basis of judicial sanctions and the patient's and his parents' social group. Nor were the relatives' empathic or hostile attitudes significant: the notable effects they seemed to have on the patients' prognosis must hence be concluded as being independent of the therapy given.

7.3 Need-Specificity and Prognosis of Treatment

The analysis of the connections between the prognostic variables and the need-specificity of treatment is particularly significant as confirming our definition of the need-specificity of treatment and the assessments concerning it. If there is a definite connection between the prognostic development of the patients and the need-specificity of treatment classified as satisfactory or better, the justification of our concept receives support. Admittedly, there is a danger of subjectivity in this comparison despite our effort to keep the outcome of treatment separate from our assessments of need-specificity; this is shown by e.g. the fact that the prognostically favourable schizophreniform psychoses were inversely connected with better-than-average need-specificity of treatment.

Table 107. Connection between the patient's prognosis and good or satisfactory need-specificity of treatment. The p-values indicate the statistical significance of a positive connection

Prognostic variable	Connection with achieved need-specificity	
	Whole series	Typical schizophrenia
Disappearance of psychotic symptoms	p = .002	p = .001
Decrease of the number of nuclear symptoms	p = .039	p = .058
Progress of psychosexual development	n. s.	p = .022
Progress of psychologic separation from primary family	n. s.	n. s.
Increase of the number of interpersonal relationships	p = .011	p = .005
Improvement of the quality of interpersonal relationships	n. s.	p = .032
Improvement of insight	p = .014	p = .0008
Maintenance of working capacity	p = .0007	p = .0000
Not on pension	p = .003	p = .013
Progressive development of occupational identity	n. s.	p = .072
Maintenance of grip	p = .0006	p = .003
Number of in-patient days during the follow-up period	n. s.	n. s.
No in-patient episodes during the last two follow-up years	p = .059	p = .029

n. s. = not significant

The statistical connections between the most central prognostic variables and good or satisfactory need-specificity of treatment are shown in Table 107.

We can see that *there is a clear connection between better-than-average need-specificity of treatment and the patient's favourable prognosis* in the case of nearly all prognostic variables. Exceptions to this rule are the total number of in-patient days during the follow-up period and the progress of the psychologic separation from the primary family, two prognostic variables which were also minimally influenced by the psychotherapeutic treatments. As regards hospital treatment, there is, however, a connection between need-specific treatment and avoidance of in-patient episodes during the last two follow-up years.

The connections between the need-specificity of treatment and the patient's prognosis are almost regularly conspicuous in the group of typical schizophrenic patients compared with the total series, which is shown by e.g. the marginally or more significant connections of some prognostic variables which lacked any statistical connections in the whole series. The patients of the nuclear group did not, however, differ from the rest of the series with regard to the degree of need-specificity of treatment; need-specificity was good or satisfactory in 52 % of the cases and passable or poor in 48 %.

The statistical connections with working capacity as well as maintenance of the grip on life were statistically highly significant, and the connection with the disappearance of psychotic symptoms was of nearly the same order. In the group of typical schizophrenic patients, the improvement of insight and the increase of the number of interpersonal relationships outside the primary family were also clearly significantly connected with good or satisfactory need-specificity of treatment. *The findings hence support our notions of the need-specificity of the treatment of patients of the schizophrenia group and the criteria we set for it.*

7.4 Indications of Psychotherapeutic Treatments: Five Patient Groups Differentiated on the Basis of Primary Therapeutic Concern

Using our concept of need-specific treatment, we made a retrograde assessment in the five-year follow-up examination to point out the kind of psychotherapeutic treatment or combination of treatments that would have been best suited to each patient. Apart from the experiences obtained from our research series, our classification was also influenced by the experiences we later obtained from especially system-oriented family therapy, as we further developed our therapeutic approach.

We ended up by *differentiating between five groups according to which mode of treatment makes up the primary therapeutic concern in each.* We simultaneously endeavoured to find out the background variables with which each of these groups was connected in our series, and how far each of these five therapeutic orientations had been pursued.

The groups were roughly of equal size: they all comprised about 20 patients. Two patients were left out of these groups. They both had an exceedingly negative attitude towards any therapeutic activities requiring cooperation. They both belonged to the ego-dynamic group of paranoid disintegration and, diagnostically, one of them had schizophreniform psychosis and the other typical schizophrenia. With the exception of brief hospitalization, they had refused treatment, but had managed moderately well socially, though the patient who belonged to the nuclear group was living in extreme isolation. We considered it appropriate that they were left to manage on their own.

The other 98 patients were classified into the following five groups.

7.4.1 Primary Treatment Long-Term Individual Therapy

The primary treatment of the patients in this group consisted of *long-term individual therapy supplemented, when necessary, by supportive contacts with the patient's family.* Some patients begin their therapy directly as out-patients, while the others are initially given in-patient therapy in a psychotherapeutic community. In most cases the therapeutic relationships persist for years. When the therapy is given in a community psychiatric setting, the frequency of the therapeutic visits is first 2 – 3 per week, but later – in a majority of the cases – one per week, and ultimately even less than that. If crises occur, the frequency of sessions must be temporarily increased. Most of the patients need *low-dose* (50 – 150 mg chlorpromazine equivalent per day) *neuroleptic treatment during the first few years of the therapy* to promote their social coping. The medication is discontinued while the psychotherapy is still being continued.

In our retrograde assessment of indications, this group came to include 18 patients. Of these, 17 were unmarried. The other two characteristics that were clearly significant were the lack of violence and the lack of acting-out tendencies. Slightly more than half of these patients lacked an established heterosexual identity, but the connection between this background variable and the group was only marginally significant.

Of the diagnostic categories, borderline schizophrenias were statistically most notable in this group of indications (p = .031), though only 7 of the patients belonged to this category. There were 8 patients with typical schizophrenia, 2 with schizophreniform psychosis and 1 with schizo-affective psychosis. As regards the ego-dynamic groups, an almost significant connection emerged for the group of imminent disintegration into which the aforesaid patients with borderline schizophrenia belonged. There were 6 patients with regressive disintegration, but none with paranoid disintegration.

Of the social baseline characteristics, the lack of unemployment emerged (p = .014), while the background variable for education level remained below marginal significance and the factors pertaining to social groups and family environment turned out non-significant. It was somewhat unexpected that the presence of at least some insight into one's own problems remained statistically non-significant. Despite this, the group included relatively more patients classified as insightful in the basic examination (12 out of 18) than the other groups. The patients' mode of contact was not statistically significant for selection into the group either, nor were the patient's sex and age, although the youngest age-group and the female patients (11) were slightly over-represented.

According to the logistic regression analysis, selection into the group was explained, first and foremost, by unmarried status and additionally by scantness of acting-out tendencies.

Summarizing these findings, we can say that long-term individual therapy as the primary mode of treatment appears to be best suited to patients who are *unmarried* and who *lack any tendency to acting-out behaviour and violent expression of aggressions.* The bonds to the primary family are less marked than in group 3. *The group includes both patients with relatively minor disturbance classified as borderline schizophrenias and patients who are initially quite seriously psychotic and regressive.* Although the degree of primary insightfullness did not emerge as a statistically significant factor, it is, similarly as the patient's overall motivation to the therapeutic relationship, significant for selection into this group in practice. We might here refer to the term "helping alliance", the patient-therapist relationship characterized by confidential commitment, which, according to Luborsky et al. (1980), begins to develop after 3-5 sessions. Our Miss L (cf. Ch. 5.2.2.) serves as an example of the patients in this indication group; her "helping alliance" was only established at the second attempt at individual therapy.

7.4.2 Primary Treatment Couple Therapy Or Conjoint Therapy of the Patient's Procreated Family

A conjoint treatment of the secondary family is indicated for patients whose illness began while they were married or lived with a long-term partner, *provided that the patient's problems are clearly associated with the interactional relationships within this family system*. If the patient has *children*, it is important to involve them in the therapy whenever the therapeutic approach is based on systemic intervention. *Less experienced therapists succeed better with couple therapy* not attended by the children, but questions and problems pertaining to the children should, nevertheless, be discussed.

The treatment is *generally shorter in duration* than in the first group, and is best accomplished by a *pair of therapists or a team*. The need for medication is case-specific, often initially obvious, but of short duration. The same also applies to in-patient treatment, which must be carried out in accordance with the principles set for intervention in crisis in a psychotherapeutic community.

The obviously important background variables included marital status (only one of our patients was unmarried), established heterosexual identity (in all cases) and psychologic separation from the primary family (only 3 patients lacked this characteristic). The two oldest age-groups were almost significantly overrepresented in comparison with the youngest group, as was also the greater proportion of females among our married patients. What was more unexpected was that a significant portion of these patients lacked any social abnormality of their primary family background ($p = .004$). Only one patient was unemployed.

The group included 20 patients. Fourteen of them were *typically schizophrenic*, which slightly exceeded the average proportion of this diagnostic category among our married patients. Borderline schizophrenias, on the other hand, only numbered one. Of the ego-dynamic groups, the group of paranoid disintegration with 7 patients ($p = .048$) and the group of acute disintegration with 8 patients (non-significant) were most numerously represented. Compared with the rest of the series, the illness had marginally significantly often begun suddenly and lasted for less than one month prior to the admission. The patients had been violent almost significantly more often than the others (9 cases, $p = .039$), which was also manifested as a high frequency of aggressive behaviour after the admission. As regards the other symptoms, the lack of neurotic symptoms was marginally significant. Lack of insight was almost marginally significantly more frequent among these patients than in the rest of the series. Hostile or poorly understanding relatives were less common than the average ($p = .047$).

The *logistic regression analysis* brought out three background factors explaining the formation of this group of indications: *at least ostensibly successful separation from the primary family, lack of social abnormality in the primary family*, and *sudden onset of the psychotic symptoms*.

As far as we can see, *couple therapy or conjoint therapy of the patient's procreated family is the most optimal mode of psychotherapeutic treatment for about 2/3 of the patients whose psychosis of the schizophrenia group begun while they were married or living with a long-term partner.* This is associated with the central importance of the problems of the marital relationships, which are often based on ambivalent dependence, for the onset and prognosis of the psychosis in these cases. *Many – perhaps 20 – 30 % – of the patients would further benefit from individual therapy following couple therapy*; in some cases such therapy might also be beneficial for their spouses. Initial introduction of individual therapy may result in unnecessary setbacks particularly if the patient's partner has not been taken into account at all when beginning the therapy. In the light of both the notions based on our series and our subsequent experiences, we consider many of the patients in this group the most optimal target group for family therapy among psychoses of the schizophrenia group. The couple therapy of Mr. P and his wife (Ch. 5.2.3.) can be taken as an example of this.

7.4.3 Primary Treatment Conjoint Therapy of the Patient's Family of Orientation

The primary treatment consists of *family therapy of the patient's nuclear family* (the patient, his parents, his siblings living at home and the possible other family members) *in the form of conjoint sessions*. We consider a conjoint session of this kind diagnostically necessary for the beginning of the treatment of all new schizophrenic patients who live with their parents or are otherwise non-separated from their primary families. Whether the treatment is continued as conjoint family therapy depends on the psychologic situation of the family. The subsequent experiences have clearly shown us that the *treatment in these cases is best accomplished as systemic intervention by a team*.

It is also necessary to create *a personal contact with the patient* at the time of the diagnostic examination already. To support the patient's and the family's motivation to treatment (and often also to improve the patient's clinical condition), it is *frequently necessary to begin the treatment in a psychotherapeutic community on a hospital or day hospital ward*. The contact with the patient is established through a personal nurse, separately from the family therapy, but yeat integrating the different therapeutic relationships. In out-patient care the need for the two modes of treatment must be assessed case-specifically. Our general rule is that the *treatment of a patient who is enmeshed with the family through mutual interactional bonds is best started as family therapy, but should be continued as individual therapy* as soon as the family therapy has created the necessary premises for it. The latter treatment is often long in duration and is occasionally aided by family meetings held from time to time or support given to the other family members during the patient's process of individual therapy. It is recommendable in these cases that the family therapists and the persons who support the family are different members of the same therapeutic team as the individual therapist, though it may also be beneficial for the individual therapist to participate in the family-therapeutic team.

The significance of *medication* is usually somewhat greater than in the former group. The dosage is determined on the basis of both the patient's clinical status and the family-dynamic situation.

In our retrograde assessment this group came to include 22 patients. Their common characteristics are illustrated by four closely connected psychosocial background variables which correlated highly significantly or significantly with the group: unmarried status (all but one patient), non-separation from the primary family (all but 2 patients), lack of stabilized heterosexual identity (15 patients) and inclusion in the youngest age group (13). Almost significant connections were noted for avoidance of aggression, unemployment, the fact that the patient did not primarily refuse any mode of treatment, and lack of empathic relatives. Of the clinical background variables, the following had a connection of the same level: inclusion in the ego-dynamic group of regressive disintegration, slow onset of the illness, previous psychiatric treatment given to the patient (i.e. either as a child or outside the public psychiatric system), and exclusion from the ego-dynamic group of acute disintegration. The group included 14 patients with typical schizophrenia, while another large portion consisted of borderline schizophrenias (6 patients). The remaining two had had schizo-affective psychosis; no patients with schizophreniform psychosis were included in the group. The patients lacked insight marginally significantly more often than the rest of our series.

On the basis of the *logistic regression analysis*, *non-separation from the primary family* and *exclusion from the ego-dynamic group of acute disintegration* explained family therapy of the primary family being the primary therapeutic concern.

Summarizing, we can say that *this group included young-patients enmeshed in their primary families, most of whom were seriously* ill. There were, however, also a few borderline schizophrenias. The onset of the illness had been slow; the *long history of the disturbance of several patients* is also reflected by their previous treatments. Deficiencies in the process of development of the patients' personalities and the structure of their ego functions were clearly most notable in this group.

Successful treatment of these patients is exceedingly difficult without taking into account the family environment. In our own series this was shown quite clearly by some patients classified into this group of indication in the retrograde assessment, who had primarily been receiving intensive individual therapy, which had come into a standstill because family-oriented treatment had been ignored. In these cases the patient's age was certainly not always crucial: there was, for example, a man over 30 with a strongly symbiotic relationship with his mother, whose only contact outside the primary family at the end of our follow-up period was the contact with the therapist. Active family dynamic intervention is necessary to solve a cul-de-sac situation of this kind for the very reason that the interdependence is mutual and both of the individuals need support to be able to detach themselves. As the experiences obtained from our series indicated, the results are not easy to reach even then. It is therefore necessary to have a team well acquainted with family-therapeutic strategies.

It is an altogether different matter, however, that we are not inclined to believe that the defects and delays in the patient's development are corrected spontaneously through detachment from pathologic interactional relationships by means of family therapy. The dependence should be re-channeled into the individual-therapeutic relationship, where the patient is continuously supported in his process of growth and development, and which helps him gradually to increase his interpersonal relationships. After-care of this kind would also have been appropriate for Miss R, whom we described as an example of family therapy of the primary family (5.2.3.).

7.4.4 Primary Treatment Flexible Family- and Environment-Oriented Intervention in Crisis

The primary treatment in this group of patients consists of *flexible intervention in crisis*, which is *short in duration and usually family- and environment-oriented*. This means that the patient's family situation is explored in an active and pre-planned manner, taking contacts with the patient's family members, significant others, employer, etc. The patient himself participates in the meetings thus arranged. Their central goal is to explore extensively the patient's life situation and to help him achieve more balance in his life. The therapeutic work may often take place in *out-patient units*, but it is occasionally necessary to resort to *short-term in-patient treatment* because of either the patient's acute symptoms or reasons involved in his life situation. *If other, more regular, psychotherapeutic treatments are needed, they are only instituted after this intervention in crisis*.

The patients to be indicated into this group numbered 19. They had a highly significant statistical connection *with the presence of acting-out behaviour* on the one hand and with *the patients' exclusion from the group of typical schizophrenias* on the other (there were only 3 patients from the diagnostic nuclear category). These two background variables also emerged as the explaining variables in the *logistic regression analysis*.

A clearly significant connection was noted for the lack of patients classified into the ego-dynamic group of regressive disintegration, the overrepresentation of patients classified into the ego-dynamic group of acute disintegration and the group of schizo-affective psychoses, and the tendency to impulsive aggressiveness. Married and divorced patients were clearly more numerous in this group than unmarried ones. Apart from the schizo-affective psychoses, there were also almost significantly more schizophreniform psychoses than was the average in the series. The establishment of heterosexual identity and the number of interpersonal relationships outside the primary family also came to this level. These patients further had empathic relatives almost significantly more often than the average, whereas serious personality disorders of the mother and the father were marginally significantly less frequent than among the other patients.

We hence get an idea of *relatively mildly disturbed (not typically schizophrenic), but impulsive patients with acting-out tendencies*. This agrees well with the finding that the psychosis of these patients had been precipitated by conflict situations evolving in externally contradictory interpersonal relationships more often than was the case otherwise. They were most commonly associated with marital and/or dating relationships, but often also involved the primary family.

A good example of the latter was Miss T, a young female patient who was admitted because of intense psychotic panic and whose condition was classified as borderline schizophrenia. Her life over the past few years had been coloured by conflicts characterized by serious emotional ambivalence and masochistic embitterment towards her parents, especially the stern and strict father. She lived now at home, now with some of her male or female friends, and consumed alcohol in increasing amounts.

Having recovered from her panic – where the central feature was a fear of an anonymous killer – Miss T was adviced to consult an individual therapist. She got some support from it, but discontinued the therapy halfway through ("perhaps I didn't quite understand it or else I just didn't stand it"). The follow-up examinations showed that the previous conflicts persisted as both a defiant and simultaneously dependent relationship with the home and sadomasochistic relationships with men. It was psychodynamically interesting that the previous anxiety symptoms of the fantasy level had been, as it were, replaced by real interpersonal life situations: when Miss T. was asked whether she still had the kind of fears of men she used to have, she replied she was so used to violence and threats in her concrete life that she had no fantasy fears any more. Her male friend at that time – married man – had been in prison for assault and was in the habit of "showing the knife" and threatening and battering our patient. At the same time Miss T's previous suicidal thoughts had been replaced by self-destructiveness of the entire life course and the associated possibility of an early death either through the effects of alcohol or as a consequence of the violence of her male friend.

Family-oriented intervention in crisis would not be easy in this case, but, if successful, might open up possibilities for a different development. Admission of the patient into treatment would have provided the only possibility for this.

Some patients of this group would also be in need of regular individual or family therapy (either of the primary or the secondary family) after the initial intervention in crisis to organize and stabilize the situation.

7.4.5 Primary Treatment Extensive Support to the Patient to Help Him Cope in His Social Environment

The primary therapeutic concern in these cases consists of *extensive activities on both the patient and his closest interactional network and social environment, whose purpose is to support the patient socially and to help him to cope better with his environment.* Various rehabilitative measures should make up an essential part of these activities. All these activities, however, should be based on a confidential contact with the patient, which only makes it possible to help him in a long-term supportive manner. Discussions attended by the patient and the people living close to him are also an important part of the therapeutic process.

The patients belonging to this group are often relatively seriously ill, while they also have serious social problems. It is therefore often easier to commence long-term therapeutic activities on a hospital ward than to do it in an out-patient unit. *The treatment requires team work, whose internal integration is important.* Social support often remains the central part of the treatment, but more specific therapies can be introduced later on in some cases. The significance of *neuroleptic medication* is often greater than in the groups described above, but it should not be essentially important.

In practice, the kind of treatment described here probably covers quite a notable portion of the patients with serious schizophrenia in most community psychiatric systems. In our own retrograde examination this group was not larger than the others; it came to include 19 patients. Of these, 16 belonged to the group of typical schizophrenica and one into each of the other diagnostic categories. The high number of the patients of the nuclear group was also statistically significantly characteristic of this group of indications. The other baseline characteristics of this level were the patient's refusal of some mode of treatment suggested to him at the initial stage and the numerical scantness of his interpersonal relationships outside the primary family. Inclusion in the ego-dynamic group of regressive disintegration had an almost significant connection with this group, as had also unemployment, low social group of the parents, and short duration or lability of the interpersonal relationships outside the primary family. Patients from the group of paranoid disintegration were only slightly more numerous than the average, and the same was also true of such background variables as admission on the basis of judicial sanctions, duration and slow onset of the illness, and the presence of alcohol problems. The patient's own social group and educational level did not differ from the rest of the series. There were 12 male patients and 7 female patients in this group.

In the *logistic regression analysis,* inclusion in this group was explained by *inclusion in the group of typical schizophrenics* and initial *refusal of some mode of treatment.*

One should not think, however, that the treatment of these patients within the scope of the psychotherapeutic approach would be impossible. As an example of this, we might describe the married couple who were both our patients.

After a stormy marriage of more than 10 years, the spouses A tried to divorce. Mr. A. a 40-year-old carpenter, was, however, hospitalized relatively soon afterwards because of paranoid schizophrenia. He had been suffering for a long time from jealousy delusions pertaining to his wife and hypochondriac symptoms based partly on problems of the sexual functioning. He now believed he had been sterilized under narcosis and also felt the smell of death and thought he was being eavesdropped.

Mrs A, who came from exceedingly poor social conditions and was also slightly deficient intellectually, was hospitalized five months later. She was brought into hospital by the welfare police after the home situation had become so difficult that she was unable to manage there any longer. Upon admission she was openly psychotic, incoherent and regressive, with numerous delusions of being poisoned, etc.

Both of these patients developed a relationship with their personal nurses during their in-patient periods. When Mrs. A was admitted and Mr. A re-admitted they were given couple therapy.

Attempts to live together supported by therapy resulted in rehospitalizations, however. Mr. A was thereafter an in-patient of a psychotherapeutic community, making the decisive step towards final divorce, which was followed by serious attempts to return to working life. He then continued the supported contact with the former family therapist now working with out-patients. Mrs. A fared worse, at first, clinging to her illegitimate adolescent daughter, who was also treated and even briefly hospitalized because of a "character disorder". Mrs. A, who actually never had been self-supportive, was pensioned; she as well as her daughter gradually developed separate out-patient therapeutic contacts. The couple's legitimate child, a boy aged then, was taken care of by Mr. A's mother during the most disordered months of the failing marriage, but returned to the father later on.

The follow-up examinations indicated that the development of both of our patients involved both progress and setbacks. Mr. A has been continuing his infrequent therapeutic contacts, but has not been able to avoid brief hospitalizations. They have been partly due to problems of both the social environment and the interactional relationships: he has been temporarily unemployed, he has moved several times, and his previous sexual problems have resulted in conflicts and feelings of being rejected in his relationships with the female sex. Even so, he continues to live with his son and is again working temporarily. He still has hypochondriac and paranoid symptoms that can be classified as being of borderline severity, occasionally even psychotic. He does not want any medication, because he believes it to cause impotence.

Mrs. A was also re-hospitalized twice owing to e.g. auditory hallucinations. At the time of the five-year follow-up examination, however, her situation was relatively stable: she now lives as a pensioner with a male partner, keeping house for him, though more or less isolated otherwise. She also continues visiting the mental health office and has no manifest psychotic symptoms. The daughter, with whom the patient occasionally had struggles associated with the daughter's attempted separation, had grown up and moved away from her mother.

This group consists thus of a number of *seriously ill patients, who usually also have serious social problems. The possibilities of psychotherapeutic treatment are often restricted by a negative attitude towards treatment.* The primary mode of therapy consists of team work by the therapeutic staff particularly in the field of social support and rehabilitation. Yet even some of these patients may later be motivated to psychotherapeutic treatment given as individual, family or group therapy.

7.4.6 Discussion

The mutual sequential integration of these five groups differentiated on the ground of the primary therapeutic concern is graphically presented in Fig. 7.

The arrows in Fig. 7 indicate the shifts of primary therapeutic concern during the treatment. When needed, they almost regularly *are directed towards more specific or individual-centered therapeutic modes.* According to this rule, it is always recommendable to *begin the treatment of a new patient of the schizophrenia group with a family- and/or environmental-centered investigation* (already including therapeutic

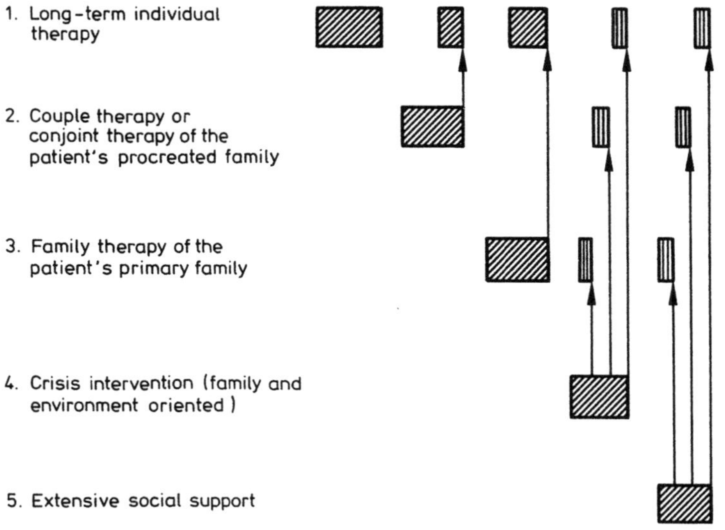

Fig. 7. The sequential integration of treatment in the patient groups differentiated according to the primary therapeutic concern

viewpoints), and decide accordingly whether a shift to a more individual-centered emphasis is indicated even from the beginning or (possibly) later on.

It should be emphasized that the primary treatment does not necessarily exclude other therapeutic activities possibly needed simultaneously but indicate the dominating treatment mode.

The summary in the Table 108 indicates *how well or poorly need-specificity was achieved for our patients classified in retrospect into the classes described above.*

Table 108. Achievement of need-specificity in the indication categories defined in retrospect. The figures are percentages

Primary therapeutic concern	Achieved need-specificity			
	Good	Satisfactory	Passable	Poor
1. Individual therapy	44	33	11	11
2. Couple therapy	33	39	11	17
3. Family therapy of primary family	0	46	36	18
4. Intervention in crisis	6	44	33	17
5. Extensive social support	39	0	28	33

The table indicates that treatment with good or moderate need-specificity was clearly most common – more than 70 % – in the first and second indication categories, where the primary therapeutic concern was long-term individual therapy and couple therapy (or family therapy of the secondary family). Need-specificity was also relatively often good in the group of extensive social support, where, however, more than half of the patients received passable or poorly need-specific treatment. In the groups of family therapy of the primary family and intervention in crisis, in turn, good need-specificity was rare, while satisfactory need-specificity was relatively common, about half of the patients being classified into the categories of passable or poor need-specificity. Compared with the categories of individual and couple therapy, the lack of treatments classifiable as having good need-specificity in these two groups reflects our qualitative criteria: although family therapies of primary families and interventions in crisis were carried out in these series, we considered their manner of implementation to be based on less global premises or being otherwise incomplete. The figures hence clearly reflect the shortcomings and developmental challenges we have already referred to while discussing the therapeutic approach above.

7.5 Prerequisites for Developing Need-Specific Treatment

We will finally discuss, more or less in general, *the properties we consider the development of the need-specific treatment of schizophrenic patients to require of the structure and internal dynamics of the therapeutic system.*

The treatment of patients of the schizophrenia group is mainly carried out within the public psychiatric health care system of society. This will also be the case in the future. The treatment of a schizophrenic patient can seldom be ascribed to a single doctor or therapist. Most patients must be treated, at least initially, both in hospital and in out-patient care, and different methods of treatment must be combined as adequately as possible to meet the needs of each individual patient. This means that the therapeutic staff should have versatile knowledge, a capacity to creative empathy, flexibility, practical realism and the courage to cast off the blinders of theory. The ability to cooperate with others is of particularly great importance. This ability is needed both within the system of psychiatric health care and outside it, for functions not part of the system of psychiatric health care – basic health care, social welfare – are also important for the treatment and rehabilitation of many patients.

It has been a relatively common notion in community psychiatry that an extensive and sufficiently intensive psychotherapeutic approach is not possible to carry out in the treatment of schizophrenic patients within the community-psychiatric framework owing to a lack of the qualitative and quantitative resources required by this approach.

We disagree with these opinions, as did Ugelstad (1979). In our own series, where the diagnostic spectrum of the schizophrenia group was fairly extensive, we could respond at least satisfactorily to the therapeutic needs of more than 50 % of our patients. The ones who remained outside this line of demarcation included patients of the kind who are never easy to involve in a psychotherapeutic relationship, though there were also some for whom psychotherapeutic treatment with better need-speficity would have been clearly indicated. Apart from the contribution of one team member liberated from her regular duties in research and therapeutic work, our project was in no way a "separate" effort in the normal work of the Turku Mental Health District, but was intentionally merged into the regular mental health district functions.

The preliminary results obtained from the state-wide project to develop the treatment and rehabilitation of schizophrenic patients in Finland (Alanen and Montell

1984, National Board of Health 1985) also run counter to the claim that the psychotherapeutically oriented approach would not be possible in "ordinary" mental health districts – it is, as long as the other preconditions for this exist.

What are these preconditions then?

As regards the *quantitative resources*, we can agree with the norms set by the Finnish National Board of Health as objectives in our country: the number of psychiatric outpatient staff per 10 000 inhabitants must be 3.5 at least, and the number of staff on actively functioning psychiatric hospital wards must be 1.0 – 1.5 per patient. These norms are notably higher than was the practice in the Turku Mental Health District during the years 1976 – 1977 and still is.

The qualitative resources and viewpoints can be divided into two parts: *the development of the theoretical notions concerning the principles of therapy* and *the questions pertaining to the training of the therapeutic staff and the improvement of their psychotherapeutic skills.*

The model of our therapeutic functions is essentially based on a consistent notion of the need-specific treatment of schizophrenic patients (7.1.), whose theoretical starting-point consists of acceptance of the integrated model of illness. It is characterized by a psychotherapeutic basic attitude towards the patient and his illness and an awareness of the dependence between the etiology as well as the contemporary state of the illness and the patient's transactional relationships. Our model thus combines the individual psychologic and transactional models of schizophrenia presented in Chapter 1. The biomedical model of illness is also included in our integrated notion.

As it has been apparent, we appreciate neuroleptic medication within our therapeutic approach, but consider it a part of globally planned treatment which is designed to support the psychotherapeutic approach. Our findings on the psychosocial prognosis further confirms that one of the important points governing both the theory and practice of the approach should consist of appreciation of the patient as a member of the community and attention given to his psychosocial rehabilitation from the beginning.

One essential prerequisite for the implementation of need-specific treatment is that *management* – especially the medical management, but also, to a sufficient degree, the politico-administrative management – *has internalized the notion of treating schizophrenia in accordance with the integrated model of illness*, and are hence committed to promote and support its development in the field or unit of health care they are responsible for. If the management are not committed to this goal, global implementation of the therapeutic approach is impossible and the position of psychotherapeutically oriented staff is difficult.

However, the psychotherapy of schizophrenic patients generally does not succeed if carried out upon "order", but requires personal devotion. It is therefore also necessary to create *an atmosphere where psychotherapeutic functions can be carried out on a uniform and extensive basis.* To create such an atmosphere, it is necessary that both the management and the staff work actively towards this goal.

In the Turku Clinic of Psychiatry, the creation of the atmosphere has been improved in certain respects by the adoption of the principle of co-determination, or "hospital democracy". Through common meetings, and occasionally through a staff committee elected internally by the members of the working community, the staff and their representatives find it possible to have their say on the problems of the working conditions.

Even so, it has probably been of greater significance for the creation of the psychotherapeutic atmosphere that *the different members of the community show interest in and appreciation of each other's work*. When such interest and appreciation is shared by the whole staff, it is not difficult to stimulate the psychotherapeutic activities and to create a therapeutic atmosphere: a majority of the staff feel that their work is made more meaningful and rewarding by the implementation of the psychotherapeutic relationships and the supervision given for them. But it should be realized that we also need staff members not equally well motivated to personal psychotherapeutic work, who, nevertheless, bring an important contribution to the functions of the psychotherapeutic community in other ways (being secure mother or father figures on the ward, conducting sporting and other activities, etc).

As regards training, the *development of extensive on-the-job training and a system of supervision and consultation for the therapeutic staff* is of primary importance. The individuals who have received psychoanalytic training and family-therapist training are in a key position here. It is important, however, that they have experience of the psychotherapy of psychotic patients in particular. Whenever there are no such individuals available in the therapeutic system, it would be useful to employ outside instructors to give regular supervision and arrange seminars. This effort would best be organized so as to give the most experienced members of the existing staff an opportunity to work gradually parallel to the outside instructors and under their guidance, giving supervision to the other staff members. According to our own experience, even many staff members lacking psychotherapeutic special training not only doctors and psychologists, but also specialized nurses and social workers – gradually acquire, on the basis of the experience they have under such guidance and instruction, the competence to act as supervisors, though this also depends on their personal inclinations.

The supervision and on-the-job training must simultaneously serve *the whole working unit* – the ward community or out-patient team. The psychotherapeutic treatment of the schizophrenic patient and/ or his family is equally much dependent on the therapist's supervision and the support given by the larger working community. Without this support, the therapy is often very difficult and the chances of success are few. This also restricts the use of outside psychiatrists of psychologists through "purchased services" in these cases, although it is advisable in some selected cases to use such outside therapists to supplement the existing resources. A central question of contemporary importance in our country is the *arrangement of psychotherapeutic training for the psychiatric health care personnel*. Such training should aim at being multioccupational (physicians, psychologists, nurses and social workers) and versatile: capacities would be needed for both individual, family, group and community therapies. It is further important that the supervision included in the training should be focussed on the therapeutic relationships that the therapists are actually carrying out in their work and that are need-specific in it. The tradition of psychoanalytic training has generally focussed on less serious disorders, especially neuroses. It has been pointed out above that the psychotherapy of psychoses requires partly different capacities from those needed in the psychotherapy of neuroses. The therapy of psychotic patients often provokes more anxiety, crises are common, and the therapist's own personality is there subject to more tumultuous influences; also, the therapist's empathy and occasionally common sense as well as his supportiveness are more important than his technico-interpretative contribution.

In the development of the psychiatric treatment organization, the focus globally lies on the *development of sectorized district psychiatry.* In this system, districts with populations of 100000 – 500000 (in Finland, an upper limit of 180000 has been proposed) with uniform management and some shared functional units are divided into *smaller catchment areas,* to which most of the practical functions are delegated. This permits a shift from institution- or unit-specific responsibility to regional responsibility, which combines out-patient care, semi-out-patient care and in-patient care within the same catchment area.

This organization has several advantages in the development of the treatment of psychotic patients. The significance of out-patient care is emphasized, and the continuity of the therapeutic relationships between the in-patient and out-patient units can be guaranteed better than at the present. Family-oriented activities are facilitated, as the services come closer to the population; this is important particularly in sparsely populated areas. The regional cooperation with the basic health care and the social welfare, which is important for the development of particularly rehabilitation, also becomes easier and more natural, as do probably also the other contacts between the psychiatric health care system and the surrounding population. Sectorized district psychiatry is, without doubt, the organization model of future psychiatry; yet the planning of this model should naturally not be strictly formal, but should always take into account the local special conditions and strive to correct the defects that emerge when the therapeutic practice is being developed.

From the viewpoint of our psychotherapeutic approach, we wish to emphasize particularly *how important it is to maintain the qualitative standard of the work, even when the functions are regionally differentiated.* This must be borne in mind especially in the development of the training and supervision system: more extensive, district-level models are needed for that. Psychotherapeutic knowhow must be distributed into the smaller catchment areas along with the delegation of functions, and this should be the responsibility of the integrative management of the district. The minimal objective is that *all the small catchment areas have some staff familiar with psychotherapeutic work,* and that all the *psychiatric teams have the possibility of receiving supervision.* The importance of *rehabilitative activities* even in the group of first-admission schizophrenics was confirmed by the finding made in the state-wide developmental program (Salokangas and Räkköläinen 1985, National Board of Health 1985), which shows that more than 50 % of the new patients admitted already had a need for rehabilitation. The need for rehabilitation in our own series was more or less of the same order in both the two-year and the five-year follow-up examinations. The most prominent needs appeared to be the needs for supervision in finding a job and other matters associated with rehabilitation for work as well as the needs for occupational guidance and occupational or re-training. The other important rehabilitative functions include the aid and support to some patient's lodging problems as well as to their possibilities for social relations (clubs, friend services, etc.).

The necessary rehabilitative activities should be integrated in the psychotherapeutic measures for the schizophrenic patients much more effectively than was done in our own series, as they constitute an important part of the global treatment. This also requires support from the social institutions outside the psychiatric health care system as well as changes in attitude that make this support possible.

The summary of this chapter is presented in 8.5.

8 Towards Need-Specific Treatment of Schizophrenic Psychoses: Summary

8.1 Goals of the Study and Methodologic Planning

The present monograph includes the findings from a study of *action research* type, whose purpose is to *develop the treatment of patients of the schizophrenia group within the system of community psychiatry* on the basis of an *integrated illness model* of schizophrenia.

The development of the treatment of schizophrenic patients seems to have suffered greatly from the lack of an integrated approach which strives to combine the biomedical, individual-psychologic and transactional concepts of illness as a basis for the treatment as well as the social support of the patient in his living milieu. Our own approach focusses on the development of *psychotherapeutic* and *family-oriented* treatments, where the deficiencies have generally been greatest.

The studies of the effects of psychotherapy on schizophrenia have generally dealt with the application of a certain mode/modes of psychotherapeutic treatment to an unselected patient population, which has been compared with a similar control sample. The mode of treatment under study has been applied unflexibly in accordance with a pre-made plan.

Our own developmental project differs from these method-oriented works. Our purpose is to develop the treatment in a *case-specific manner* which is determined by the needs of the patient and his closest human interactional network. The patient series consists of 100 successive patients aged 16 – 45 years, who were admitted for treatment for the first time for a disorder included in the schizophrenic group within a single community psychiatric catchment area, the Mental Health District of Turku, Finland, during 19 months in 1976 – 77. These patients were subjected to a comprehensive individual- and family-oriented psychiatric basic examination, on the basis of which case-specific therapeutic plans were established. Similar follow-up examinations were carried out 2 and 5 years later. The psychiatric examinations were complemented by a psychologic examination, which was not, however, of equal importance for the planning of the therapies.

The limits of the schizophrenia group were defined relatively widely, which we considered appropriate for our developmental objectives. In accordance with the Nordic tradition created by Langfeldt et al. (1952), however, we distinguished among our 100 patients a nuclear group of 56 typical schizophrenic patients which was analyzed separately from the whole series. The other diagnostic categories were schizophreniform psychosis, schizo-affective psychosis and borderline schizophrenia.

As far as possible, the research functions were integrated as part of the normal activities of the Mental Health District. This meant that each therapeutic unit assumed responsibility for the treatments carried out there. We realized quite soon that not all of the treatments were implemented in accordance with our plans, but were influenced by several selective factors emanating from among both the therapeutic staff and the patients. This is what always happens in the field: the question of what kind of patients are given psychotherapeutic treatment and what kind of patients are not is also a highly relevant object of study.

The most central objectives of our project were as follows:

1. *How widely* were we able to carry out the different activities included in our global approach, and *what kind of patients* did we treat?
2. *What effects* did the therapeutic orientation on the whole and the different therapeutic activities involved in it have on the prognoses of the patients?
3. What experiences did we have concerning *the indications* for the different therapeutic activities? What was the *global model of therapeutic activities* we ultimately constructed and what kind of resources are ultimately required for its optimal implementation?

As a prognostic investigation, our project naturally has certain weaknesses compared with the method-oriented works referred to above. The examination of the effects of the psychotherapeutically oriented approach was to some extent made possible by the fact that not all of the patients were given treatment of this kind, partly because the whole district was not committed to this principle: while the wards of the university hospital where most of the research was carried out functioned as "psychotherapeutic communities" (Alanen 1975), the wards of the other hospital of the district functioned along more conventional lines, focussing on psychopharmacologic treatment. The most important starting-point for the investigation of the psychotherapeutic global orientation in the series was, however, the group of psychotherapy cases differentiated from the other patients. This group accounted for slightly more than half of the series, whose prognosis could be compared with the prognosis of the other patients in the follow-up examination.

The out-patient units of the district were psychotherapeutically oriented, and the development of their activities was emphasized strongly.

The two-year follow-up examination consisted of follow-up by the present team and a corresponding examination by an independent psychiatric examiner not familiar with the patients in advance. The mutual correlation between the assessments made by the team and by the independent examiner was of the order of 0.5 – 0.7. The prognostic assessments made by the independent psychiatrist were clearly more optimistic on an average than the assessments made by the team, particularly notably so in the clinical evaluations. This was most crucially due to the fact that the team members had been familiar with the patients for a longer period and had information on them from sources other than the single patient interview, on which the independent examiner had to base her assessments. The independent examination was not repeated at the time of the five-year follow-up, because we did not deem it essential for providing additional information to meet our goals.

Painstaking attention, however, was attached to the *statistical evaluation of the factors that affected both the implementation of the therapies and the prognoses*. This was done in the five-year follow-up examination, whose results constitute the foundation for the main part of the monograph.

On the basis of the psychiatric basic examination, 45 clinical and psychosocial background variables were constructed, whose connections with the implementation of the therapies during the five-year follow-up period were analyzed by means of cross-tabulation and the X^2-test as well as *stepwise logistic regression analysis* (Breslow and Day, 1980). The latter method is a statistical multivariate method suited to the analysis of the mutual relations between categorical variables when one of the variables is a dichotomous response and the others are factors or explaining variables, which may be categorical and/or numerical. In this way it was possible to *find out which background factors explained both the inclusion in the group of psychotherapy cases and the use of the most important modes of treatment* (including psychopharmacologic treatment).

The prognosis was also analyzed multidimensionally on the basis of the five-year follow-up findings. The logistic regression analysis included among the factors or explaining variables not only background variables, but also variables constructed on the basis of the implementation of the treatments. In addition to this, *the connections between the central modes of therapy and the prognosis were analyzed when the connections between the explaining background variables and the prognostic findings had been kept constant.* The *theory of log-linear models* (Bishop et al. 1975) was applied. For these analyses, 4 prognostic variables representing different areas of the prognosis were selected (decrease of the nuclear symptoms of schizophrenia during the follow-up period, increase of the insight shown by the patients into the connection between their illness and their problems, the patients' working capacity at the end of the follow-up period, and avoidance of hospitalization during the last two years of follow-up). It was thus possible, independently of the background variables most strongly influencing the prognosis, to have an idea of the effects of inclusion in the group of psychotherapy cases, more-than-average or less-than-average neuroleptic medication, and intensive individual therapy as well as treatment in a psychotherapeutic community on the prognosis.

8.2 Findings of the Initial Psychiatric Examination

The extensive, psychodynamically oriented exploration of the clinical and psychosocial baseline characteristics of the patients carried out at the time of the psychiatric basic examination confirmed our notion that the *onset of the illness was significantly due to disorders of their individual-psychologic development and the interactional relationships within their family milieu as well as their psychosocial problems.* The different diagnostic categories did not differ notably as to the family background, but attention was attracted to the high frequency of deviant external structure of the patient's childhood family in the category of schizophreniform psychoses and the high frequency of "poorly understanding" or "hostile" relatives in the category of borderline schizophrenias.

As an innovative grouping, we proposed *differentiation of the psychoses of the schizophrenic type according to the nature of ego dysfunctions.* Particular attention was given to the level and orientation of the dynamically meaningful defensive functions associated with the onset of the illness. This *ego-dynamic classification* consisted of 4 groups: imminent disintegration, acute disintegration, regressive disintegration and paranoid disintegration. These ego-dynamic groups were more clearly related to the various psychotherapeutic modes of treatment than were the diagnostic subcategories. This grouping was clearly helpful in determining the need-specific therapeutic requirements of the patients of the schizophrenia group.

8.3 Implementation of Treatments

We were moderately satisfied with the number of psychotherapeutic treatments implemented during the course of the project, although the optimal extent and intensity seeing to the needs of the patients and their families was not yeat reached. The findings clearly indicate that the *qualitative resources are more crucial than the quantitative resources* in the development of the psychotherapeutic treatment of patients of the schizophrenia group. One prerequisite for increasing the extent of therapeutic activities is extensive participation of staff from the different occupational groups in the therapies, which is made possible by intensive on-the-job training and supervision of the therapeutic relationships. When given supervision, even therapists lacking actual psychotherapeutic training achieved quite good results.

Of the different modes of therapy, initial intervention in crisis, individual therapy and treatment in a psychotherapeutic community were the ones implemented most adequately. The role of actual family therapy remained less significant, while support given to the family members turned out more adequate. This also served to support the individual therapies. Group therapies were implemented infrequently, but various group functions were of considerable significance for treatment in a psychotherapeutic community. The development of rehabilitative functions in the district was badly delayed.

On the basis of the implementation of intensive or otherwise sufficient therapies, we were able to distinguish from among our 100 patients *a group of 56 psychotherapy cases*, whose prognosis was compared with the prognosis of the other patients in the follow-up examination. About 80 per cent of the out-patient psychotherapies were accomplished in the frame of the public health care system, 20 per cent in the private sector.

The most basic variable explaining selection into the group of psychotherapy cases was the first treatment unit. The group of psychotherapy cases included notably more patients with disturbances of more-than-average severity classified into the group of regressive ego disintegration. The patients of the group of psychotherapy cases had also, however, some background variables favourable for the prognosis and the treatment, including the patients' motivation to treatment and his tendency to symbiotic reliance as well as, in the group of typical schizophrenic patients, the relatively acute onset of the psychosis.

The relative frequency of typical schizophrenic patients was more or less the same in both the group of psychotherapy cases and among the patients excluded from this group.

Several other patients also received less intensive psychotherapeutic treatment. Among the 20 patients *not given any mode of psychotherapy requiring personal participation,* the most notable characteristics were a lack of depressive symptoms and lower-than-average basic education. Men were nearly four times as numerous as women among these patients most difficult to motivate to psychotherapeutic treatment. The typical schizophrenic patients were especially often characterized by inclusion in the ego-dynamic group of paranoid disintegration, a tendency to alcohol or other addiction, and problems of employment.

Intensive individual therapy, which was assumed to have been pursued regularly for at least two years and consisted of a minimum of 80 psychotherapeutic sessions, was given to 26 patients, of whom 14 were typically schizophrenic. The most important background variables explaining selection into this group were the patient's preliminary insight into the connection between the illness and the problems and a lack of acting-out behaviour. The onset of the illness was acute more often than was ordinarily the case, and the mother's personality was significantly less often severely, i.e. more seriously than neurotic, disordered than in the group of patients not given this mode of therapy, the latter feature being especially notable in the group of typical schizophrenics.

It was in precisely this mode of therapy that many therapists lacking actual psychotherapeutic training, but given supervision, achieved quite good outcomes. An empathic and confidential therapeutic relationship, which is also essentially contributed to by the therapist's personality, is especially important in the psychotherapy of psychoses as compared with the more technically oriented psychoanalytic therapies of neurotic patients. Our findings indicate that we should not underestimate the importance of long-term individual therapies based on relatively infrequent sessions. Although these therapies do not reach as deep down as the more intensive, psychoanalytically oriented therapies, many of the patients do, however, experience a growth of the resources of their personality – we here refer to the "transmuting internalization" described by Kohut (1977). Serious transference crises are easier to avoid. It would be highly desirable that the patients with the aforesaid baseline characterictics could be guaranteed, much more often than is the case at the present, an opportunity to receive this kind of therapy within the scope of the community psychiatric health care system. However, a continuing therapeutic process is less likely to happen if the frequency of sessions is less than one session a week.

The experiences obtained from *family therapy* were most favourable as regards the couple therapies of the patients who were married at the time of the onset of their illness. The outcome of conjoint family therapies of primary families was quite unsatisfactory in our series, which was due to the lack of training on the one hand and the severity of the disturbance of the patients and families selected for therapy on the other. We cannot consider our findings to give an adequate view on family therapy in schizophrenia. This was also demonstrated by the more optimistic results obtained in Turku later on, when training in family therapy had been developed.

We had previously become aware of the disadvantages of excessive hospital orientation and therefore did our best in the present project to promote the psychotherapeutic activities carried out on an out-patient basis. Our findings revealed, nevertheless, that *a psychotherapeutically oriented ward commmunity* continues to be of crucial importance for the treatment of particularly the most seriously disturbed first-admission patients of the schizophrenia group. Many of these patients are only able after a relatively long in-patient period to establish a lasting therapeutic contact. It is also important to make a contact with the families and even otherwise extend the ward functions outside the hospital: one essentially important task of the in-patient treatment of schizophrenic patients is to arrange the continuation of their treatment within the out-patient system.

We were able in this investigation to compare patients who received their first treatment on psychotherapeutically oriented hospital wards and patients whose in-patient treatment was more conventional, aiming at rapid discharge. Although the patients of the former group were in hospital almost twice as long as the patients of the latter group during the first in-patient period, the patients treated in psychotherapeutic communities turned out to have a clearly lesser need for in-patient treatment than the others from the second follow-up year onwards.

Of our 100 patients, 98 received *neuroleptic medication* at some state of their therapy mostly in low or moderate doses.

The explaining factors influencing the selection of the patients for more-than-average medication during the whole follow-up period were inclusion in the ego-dynamic group of regressive disintegration, the first treatment unit and the presence of hostile or poorly understanding relatives; in the group of typical schizophrenic patients the male sex also emerged as one of the explaining variables.

Medication in low or moderate doses at the initial stages of the treatment provided definite support for the psychotherapy, and during the first two follow-up years there was even a positive statistical connection between the continuity of medication and psychotherapy. During the last three follow-up years, however, the connection between the inclusion in the group of psychotherapy cases and the amount of medication given to the patient was negative. Only one of the 11 patients whose average dose of neuroleptic medication during the last three follow-up years corresponded to more than 300 mg of chlorpromazine daily belonged to the group of psychotherapy cases, while the remaining 10 patients were outside this group.

The *psychologic basic examination* confirmed the significance of the patients' individual personality factors and their attitudes towards treatment for the selection into the different modes of treatment. The selection for predominantly psychotherapeutic or predominantly pharmacotherapeutic treatment was also, according to this part of our study, influenced by patient-specific psychodynamic characteristics. Some results of the psychologic examinations will be published separately.

8.4 Prognosis and Factors Contributing to It

Individual- and family-specific follow-up examinations were carried out 2 and 5 years after the patients' admission. They also included data acquired from the National Pensions Institute concerning the disability pensions granted to the patients on the basis of their illness, review of the patients' case histories in the different therapeutic units, and inquiries presented to the therapists. The prognosis was investigated multidimensionally, including both the clinical, psychodynamic and psychosocial variables and the prognostic variables pertaining to the in-patient treatment.

Adequate data were obtained on 97 patients in the two-year follow-up examination and on 92 – 95 in the five-year follow-up, depending on the prognostic dimension defined. Three of the patients had committed suicide, all during the first follow-up period.

Compared with the other recent follow-up studies of schizophrenic patients, the *clinical prognosis of our patients can be considered quite good*: 70 per cent of the entire patient population and 50 per cent of the typical schizophrenics had no manifest psychotic symptoms at the end of the five-year follow-up period. The same also applies to the patients' need for hospital treatment during the follow-up period. During the 2nd – 5th follow-up years, 7 – 8.5 per cent of the patients were in hospital daily. However, only two of the patients could be regarded as institutionalized chronic patients at the end of the follow-up period, while altogether four patients had been in-patients for more than two years during the follow-up period. The day hospital was not used much, and its use was almost completely restricted to the first few follow-up years.

The patients' psychosocial prognosis was clearly less optimistic than their clinical prognosis, which we interpreted as being a consequence of the poor employment situation and the current pension policy on the one hand and the inadequate supply of rehabilitation on the other. The subjects fully able to work at the end of the follow-up period accounted for 43 per cent of our patient population (33 per cent of the typical schizophrenics); 41 per cent were on disability pension (56 per cent of the typical schizophrenic patients). The psychodynamic prognostic assessments of the patients' psychosexual development and the development of their interpersonal relationships indicated that a definite deterioration on an average had taken place in these respects during the first two follow-up years, while some progress had taken place during the last three follow-up years; there were, however, also patients whose development had been clearly progressive compared with the initial situation.

Our results clearly confirm the notion put forward by e.g. Strauss and Carpenter (1977) suggesting that the *different sub-areas of the prognosis of schizophrenia are related, but that they are further influenced by background factors "more specific" to each area*. The clinical background variables were most clearly connected with the clinical prognostic findings. Both the psychodynamic and the psychosocial developments of the patients, however, were influenced more by the psychosocial than the clinical background variables. Hence the two background variables explaining most clearly the maintenance of working capacity by the patients in the whole series were that the patient was employed and had a stabilized occupational identity at the time of admission. Disability pension was most distinctly explained by more-than-average medication during the follow-up period and the baseline characteristic of a lack of an empathic parent or spouse and the presence of alcohol or other addiction problems. The connection between being granted a pension and the persistence of psychotic symptoms was highly significant in the whole series in the five-year follow-up examination, but not even marginally significant in the group of typical schizophrenics.

We presented a new psychosocial prognostic variable of *maintenance or loss of the grip* in the efforts to reach the goals and modes of satisfaction ordinarily associated with adult life. The definition was mainly based on the notions obtained of the patients's subjective attitudes through empathic observation: attention was also given to the patient's thoughts concerning his future, not only his topical situation. By the time of the five-year follow-up examination, 30 per cent of the patients turned out to have lost their grip: these patients were characterized by more-than-average neuroleptic medication during the follow-up period and unfavourable baseline characteristics in the background variables pertaining to occupational life.

As an example of how the psychosocial background variables influenced the patient's psychodynamic development, we might mention that favourable development of the psychosexual identity had been particularly common among female patients whose fathers did not have seriously disturbed personality, and that the lack of stabilized occupational identity at the time of the basic examination was the most important explaining variable for regression of psychologic separation from the primary family.

The patients diagnosed as *typical schizophrenics* in this work had a clearly less optimistic prognosis than the other patients of the schizophrenia group. The difference was particularly notable in the clinical prognostic variables and the patients' need for in-patient treatment during the follow-up period. The difference in the psychosocial prognosis was smaller. Regression of the psychodynamic development was also more common among the patients of the nuclear group, but progress – generally in the psychotherapy cases – was more or less equally frequent as in other cases in our series.

The *ego-dynamic groups* also had connections with the prognosis, although these connections were not equally emphatic as the ones noted for selection into the different groups of treatment. The prognosis was most pessimistic – as it was to be expected – in the group of regressive disintegration, which differed from the other groups particularly as regards the greater need for in-patient treatment. The frequency of psychotic symptoms at the end of the follow-up period, however, was no greater in this group than in the group of paranoid disintegration, and our findings also suggested that psychotherapy had a favourable influence on part of the patients in this group.

Female patients had a notably better prognosis than males. This was especially conspicuous in the psychosocial and psychodynamic prognostic variables. The number of patients fully able to work in the group of typical schizophrenics was fourfold among the females compared with the males. One reason for this gender difference in the prognosis was probably the greater willingness of females to receive therapy, which was noted in our findings on the implementation of the psychotherapeutic treatments.

As regards *the psychosocial background factors*, the patient's social group had hardly any effect on the outcome development, and the patient's basic education was similarly of relatively minor importance. The patient's *employment status* at the time of admission, however, turned out to be a predictive background variable explaining quite significantly the subsequent prognosis, especially as regards the psychosocial aspects, but also the number of in-patient days during the follow-up period. Stabilized occupational identity at the time of admission also emerged as a factor explaining the psychosocial prognosis, especially in the whole patient population, but not in the separate analysis of the typical schizophrenic patients.

The predictive prognostic significance of *psychologic factors associated with the family milieu* was quite conspicuous. Family-centred background variables had notably more connections with the outcome than did the individual psychodynamic background variables. The lack of psychologic separation from the primary family as a baseline characteristic influenced particularly the clinical prognosis. Disturbance of the mother's personality graver than neurosis, which we found to be also connected with increasing difficulty of the implementation of psychotherapeutic treatments, was a pessimistic prognostic predictor for primarily the psychosocial prognosis, but also the clinical prognosis. We suggest that this often is due to particularly entangling transactional defence mechanisms (Räkköläinen and Alanen 1982) typical to disordered parental personalities.

The findings deemed most astonishing by the team were the assessments of the relatives' attitudes made at the time of the basic examination. An empathic attitude shown by one of the patient's close relatives (parents or spouse) towards the patient emerged as an explaining variable in several areas of the psychodynamic and psychosocial prognosis. Correspondingly, the presence of a hostile or poorly understanding relative had negative connections with the subsequent prognosis, and this background factor was also a variable explaining crucially the more-than-average medication given to the patient during the follow-up period.

We interpret the conspicuous emergence of the family variables in our analysis as an indication for increasing family-therapeutic activities in our further development of the treatment of schizophrenic patients.

The conclusions that the *implementation of the psychotherapeutic approach had favourable effects on the prognosis of our patients seems clearly justifiable in the light of our statistical analyses*. The effect of the therapies was equally obvious in both the group of typical schizophrenics and the rest of the patient population. Three variables constructed on the basis of the implementation of the therapies – inclusion in the group of psychotherapy cases, intensive individual therapy, and intensive treatment or intervention in crisis in a psychotherapeutic community retained a significant connection with the most central prognostic variables even after the background variables explaining them most strongly were kept constant. The most intensive connection emerged, as it was to be expected, for *the increase of insight*: all the aforesaid three treatment variables retained their connection with a favourable development of this variable at a significant or almost significant level even after the background variables were kept constant, though the connection of the psychotherapeutic community variable was only restricted to the diagnostic nuclear category.

But the connection with *the maintenance of full working capacity* in precisely the group of typical schizophrenics remained significant for the psychotherapy cases and marginally significant for the patients given intensive individual therapy, as for the patients given treatment in a psychotherapeutic community, even after the explaining background variables were kept constant. The connection of the psychotherapy cases with a clinical prognostic variable, the *decrease of the nuclear symptoms of schizophrenia* during the follow-up period, also remained at least marginally significant in the nuclear diagnostic group after the background variables were kept constant. In the case of intensive individual therapy, this connection, which had been almost significant in the previous analysis in both the whole series and the group of typical schizophrenics, lost its marginal significance after the background variables were kept constant.

The favourable effects of intensive individual therapy on particularly the psychodynamic development of the patients were still visible in many different ways.

The decrease of *the total number of in-patient days* during the follow-up period was not significantly affected by the psychotherapeutic treatments. One reason for this was that a relatively small group of patients was responsible for the bulk of hospital days during the later follow-up years, and we also had a couple of patients of this kind among our psychotherapy cases. When the need for in-patient treatment was followed up from one year to another, the patients of the psychotherapy group, at any rate, show a slight declining overall tendency compared with the other patients. An interesting finding was made when it was found out which of the patients in the series had been *hospitalized for even a short period during the last two follow-up years*: the first unit of treatment turned out to be an explaining variable in particularly the group of typical schizophrenic patients in such a way that the patients initially treated on psychotherapeutically oriented wards were now in hospital clearly less often than the patients who started their treatment either as out-patients or more conventional hospital wards. The finding thus confirmed the aforesaid observation that a first in-patient period aiming at a therapeutic contact with the patient on a long-term basis had the effect of diminishing the subsequent need for in-patient treatment.

More-than-average neuroleptic medication given to the patient throughout the five-year follow-up period was notably connected with a pessimistic prognosis in our analyses, which was especially conspicuous in the psychosocial prognostic variables and those pertaining to the in-patient episodes. When evaluating this finding, it is good to emphasize that the more-than-average medication in our series refers, in fact, to dosage that is no more than moderate, though it may have lasted for several years. Most of the patients given less-than-average neuroleptic medication were without any neuroleptic medication for the last three follow-up years.

It seems a plausible assumption that these negative effects to the patients' prognosis would be explained by the selection of more abundant medication for the patients who were even primarily more seriously ill or have otherwise poorer starting-points as regards their background factors. Our analysis after the background variables were kept constant indicated that this interpretation is not sufficient: the connection between medication and the pessimistic prognosis remained highly significant with both the maintenance of working capacity and the need for hospital treatment during the last two follow-up years, even when the explaining background variables were kept constant. More-than-average neuroleptic medication also had a marginally significant negative connection with the increase of insight in the group of typical schizophrenics. However, the negative connection of the same level previously noted for the decrease of the nuclear symptoms in the whole series lost its significance when the background variables were kept constant.

We interpret these findings primarily as being related to the effects of the therapeutic approach as a whole, not as being connected directly to the amount of neuroleptic medication. *Psychotherapeutic treatments had a diminishing effect on the need for medication particularly towards the end of the follow-up period, and the patients given predominantly psychotherapeutically oriented treatment had a better-prognosis than the ones given predominantly psychopharmacologically oriented treatment.* Medication may have had directly adverse effects on the psychosocial prognosis of some patients.

The analysis we made in the five-year follow-up examination using the four-dimensional outcome scale developed by Strauss and Carpenter (1972) can be considered a summary of the factors contributing to the prognosis of our patients. According to the measure constructed of this scale, *a good global prognosis* in the whole series was explained by less-than-average neuroleptic medication during the entire follow-up period, female sex, and two baseline characteristics: the presence of empathic relatives in the patient's nearest family network and the patient's not being unemployed at the time of admission. In the group of typical schizophrenic patients the first three explaining variables were the same, the fourth variable being intensive individual therapy. The connections of the aforesaid treatment variables with the global outcome score remained significant even when the significant background variables were kept constant.

8.5 Development of Need-Specific Treatment of Schizophrenic Psychoses

There exists an obvious contradiction between the favourable experiences and notions held by several therapists concerning the psychotherapeutic treatment of schizophrenia on the one hand and the less optimistic results reported in a number of controlled investigations on the other.

The findings of our present project provide one explanation for this contradiction. One of our starting-points was that, for an optimal outcome, we need to apply the psychotherapeutic approach differently in the case of different patients of the schizophrenia group. Our experiences confirmed this assumption as being valid. They simultaneously support the conclusion that investigations where a single psychotherapeutic mode of treatment is applied rigidly in an unselected patient sample are, indeed, unable to give a sufficiently good idea of the opportunities of psychotherapeutic treatment in this group of patients on the whole.

While we were developing the therapeutic activities in accordance with the integrated illness model of schizophrenic disorders, we recognized the central position of the *concept of the need-specificity of treatment*. By this we mean *a therapeutic approach which is at the same time both global, combining integratively different therapeutic activities, and individually planned, striving to meet the needs of each patient in a case-specific manner.* This also means that the patient's psychologic and social situation is taken into account and the therapeutic needs are met that, undifferentiated from the patient, are involved in the network of his closest interpersonal relationships, primarily in his family system.

A therapeutic approach of this kind also means that the *process nature of therapy* is clearly perceived. Need-specific treatment does not refer to treatment which proceeds routinely in accordance with a pre-determined plan, but (rather) to treatment that follows therapeutic plans flexibly and can be altered whenever therapeutic needs emerge which require such alteration.

The most central criteria of need-specific treatment are the following:

1. The planning and implementation of both diagnostic work and therapy are typically global, flexible, and – as long as the treatment is continued – sufficiently intensive and active.
2. The therapeutic activities are case-specifically accordant with the needs identified on the basis of the patient's clinical status and his psychologic and social life situation, which are examined in both an individually oriented and a family-oriented way.
3. The diagnosis and treatment are dominated by an explicit psychotherapeutic general approach striving towards psychologic understanding.
4. The different therapeutic activities (including drug treatments) are carried out integratively in such a way as to make them mutually supportive. Their mutual weighing and sequential order are determined by this.

According to our retrograde assessment, the need-specificity of treatment in our project was good or satisfactory in 55 per cent of the cases and passable or poor in 45 per cent. The patients' prognosis had a clearly significant and extensive connection with this.

On the basis of both our present project and partly our subsequent experiences, we constructed *5 indication categories differentiated on the basis of the primary therapeutic concern*. A retrograde assessment of our own project showed that the number of patients classified into each group was more or less equal.

Long-term individual therapy as the primary treatment appears to be best suited to patients who are unmarried and lack any tendency to acting-out behaviour. The group includes both borderline schizophrenic patients and regressively disintegrated typically schizophrenic patients. The patient's willingness to receive treatment and his primary insightfullness are also significant, although the latter factor was not equally important in our retrograde definition of the indication as it was in our group of accomplished intensive individual therapies. The treatment is facilitated by the contact established initially with the patient's family, which, when necessary, can be continued throughout the individual therapy, the patient being aware of this.

Conjoint therapy of the patient's procreated family or couple therapy of the patient and his or her spouse is indicated for about two thirds of the patients who were married at the time of the onset of illness (or had been living for a long time with the same partner). The indication required that the problems resulting in the onset of the illness are clearly related to the interactional relationships within the family system. The treatment is of shorter duration than in the first group and is best accomplished by a pair of therapists or a team. Perhaps 20 – 30 per cent of these patients would further benefit from individual therapy following couple therapy.

Conjoint therapy of the patient's family of orientation is a necessary initial part of the therapy for the patients who are enmeshed with their families through excessive and mutual interactional bonds. Most of these patients are seriously ill, and the deficiencies of the personality development are most notable in this group. In addition to the regressively disintegrated patients, the group also includes some borderline schizophrenics. It is nearly always best to start the therapy while the patient is receiving treatment in a psychotherapeutic community, preferably through a systemic intervention by a family-therapeutic team. The family therapy is optimally followed by a long-term individual therapy, to which the patient's dependent needs are re-channeled and where the process of his growth and development are further supported.

A flexible family- and environmentally oriented intervention in crisis is indicated for many patients with acting-out tendencies whose illness began acutely, and whose illness was usually precipitated by a conflict situation formed by contradictory interpersonal relationships. The onset of the illness is generally acute, and most of the patients in this group suffer from schizo-affective or schizophreniform psychoses. Intervention in crisis is often sufficient to restore their equilibrium, though some patients may be in need of regular individual or family therapy after this stage.

The last group consists of the cases where the primary therapeutic concern comprises *extensive activities on both the patient and his closest interactional network and social environment, whose main purpose is to support the patient socially and to help him to cope better with his environment*. The different rehabilitative measures, including social clubs and other corresponding group activities – also needed by many other patients – are especially useful in this group. Most of the patients are relatively seriously ill, belonging to our diagnostic nuclear category, in addition to which they are characterized by poorer-than-average social starting-points and often a reluctant attitude towards treatment. Even so, the regular psychotherapeutic modes of treatment are not completely impossible even in this group of patients at a later stage. Psychopharmacologic treatment is more notable in this group than in the others, but it should be primarily aimed to support the patient's interpersonal relationships and rehabilitation and not be conceived of as treatment in itself.

The treatment of the patients of the schizophrenia group will always be carried out predominantly within the public psychiatric health care system for the very reason of the versatility of the functions associated with therapy and rehabilitation. At the end of our monograph, we present *some more general aspects of the prerequisites set by the development of need-specific therapy for the therapeutic system.*

The implementation of the psychotherapeutic functions requires that *both the management and the staff* are extensively *committed* and that both have internalized the therapeutic ideology accordant with the integrated model of illness and *created an atmosphere* where the work can be carried out cooperatively in a comprehensive way. Integrative case-meetings and consultations are important. This requires interest in and appreciation of the work of others. It should also be reflected in the possibility to participate in decision-making.

As far as we can see, quantitative resources are no hindrance for the development of a psychotherapeutic approach to the treatment of schizophrenic patients. A more crucial position is held by the *qualitative resources,* whose development naturally depends on extensive on-the-job training of the staff and associated development of a system of supervision and consultation. The future solution appears to be *multioccupational and versatile psychotherapeutic training of the psychiatric health care personnel*, with supervision for the need-specific therapeutic relationships the trainees are currently working on.

The development of *sectorized district psychiatry* has several advantages for the treatment of psychotic patients. The importance of out-patient care is emphasized, the continuity of the therapeutic relationships can be guaranteed better than at the present, and family-oriented work is facilitated as the services some closer to the population. The same is also true of the cooperation with the basic health care and the social welfare, which is important for the development of rehabilitation. From the viewpoint of the psychotherapeutic approach, however, it should be particularly underlined that it is exceedingly important to retain the qualitative level of the treatment even when the functions are decentralized. Knowhow must follow along: all of the smaller districts must have staff well capable of psychotherapeutic work, and all of the psychiatric teams must have an opportunity to receive psychotherapeutic supervision.

It would be necessary to integrate the *rehabilitative functions* with the psychotherapy of the schizophrenic patients earlier and more effectively than was done in our series, as they constitute one important part of global treatment.

An eight-year follow-up of our patient series is under way. We also continue to collect experiences of the need-specific treatment of schizophrenic patients within a state-wide project on the development of the investigation, treatment and rehabilitation of schizophrenic patients being carried out in Finland. The project on the development of the treatment of first-admission schizophrenics, which is part of the overall project, is being conducted in six different mental health districts in different parts of the country. The project also includes cooperation with Swedish, Norwegian and Danish investigators.

Appendix 1

The clinical and psychosocial variables defined in the basic examination

1. Diagnostic sub-category

1a) Typical schizophrenia	yes/no
1b) Schizophreniform psychosis	yes/no
1c) Schizo-affective psychosis	yes/no
1d) Borderline schizophrenia	yes/no

2. Ego-psychologic group

2a) Imminent ego disintegration	yes/no
2b) Acute ego disintegration	yes/no
2c) Regressive ego disintegration	yes/no
2d) Paranoid ego disintegration	yes/no

3. Presence of symptoms other than psychotic

3a) Neurotic symptoms	yes/no
3b) Depressive symptoms	yes/no
3c) Acting-out behaviour	yes/no
3d) Alcohol or other addiction problems	yes/no

4. Quality of the contact made by the patient

4a) Suspicious or reserved	yes/no
4b) Need for symbiotic reliance	yes/no

5. Presence of suicidal tendencies

   suicidal attempts or serious thoughts of self-destruction/no more than mild thoughts of self-destruction

6. Violence

   violent behaviour or serious threats of violence/no violent behaviour

7. Insight

   has some insight into one's own role in the development of one's problems or symptoms/no insight of this kind

8. Willingness to have therapy

   comes to have therapy of his own will/comes to therapy passively conforming or unwillingly

9. Judicial sanctions for admission

   admitted on the basis of judicial sanctions/admitted without sanctions

10. Refusal of therapy

    refuses some mode of therapy suggested/does not refuse

11. Previous therapies

    has been previously treated because of a psychic disorder (though not for psychosis in the public health care system)/no treatment of this kind

12. Time since the onset of psychotic symptoms

    under 1 mo./over 1 mo.

13. Manner of the onset of symptoms

    acute/slow

14. Age

    25 yr. or less/over 25 yr.

15. Sex

    female/male

16. Disorders of mother's personality

    psychotic or other severe ego disorder/no more than neurotic disorder

17. Disorders of father's personality

    psychotic or other severe ego disorder/no more than neurotic disorder

18. Social group of primary family

    I–II/III–IV

19. „Abnormality" of the social life course of the primary family:

    several changes of locality, inclusion of the family in a minority group, definite financial want, asocial or antisocial behaviours in family members, participation in the activities of labelled political or religious extremist movements/none of these factors

20. External family structure

    deviant external family structure in the patient's childhood/no such deviations

21. Patient's basic education

    junior secondary school or more/less than that

22. Patient's own social group

    I–II/III–IV

23. Psychologic separation from primary family

    at least ostensibly successful separation/strongly enmeshed or undergoing separation struggle

24. Marital status

unmarried/married, divorced or widowed

25. Social role

student, working, or working at home/unemployed

26. Occupational identity

at least ostensibly established occupational identity/occupational identity lacking or only taking shape

27. The patient has an empathic relative close to him

an empathic, understanding attitude in the spouse, mother or father/none of these are empathic

28. The patient has a non-understanding or hostile relative close to him

a non-understanding or hostile attitude in the spouse, mother or father/none of these are non-understanding or hostile

29. Psychosexual identity

the patient has an established heterosexual identity/psychosexual identity is delayed, chaotic, characterized by an identity crisis or homosexual

30. Way of dealing with aggressions

the patient avoids aggessive behaviour/impulsive or normal

31. Number of interpersonal relationships outside the primary family

the patient has no significant peer or friend relationships/the patient has at least one significant relationship

32. Quality of interpersonal relationships outside the primary family

the patient's interpersonal relationships are labile and short or characterized by recurrent conflicts/the patient also has fairly permanent interpersonal relationships

33. First therapeutic unit

33a) in-patient or day hospital ward of the Clinic of Psychiatry	yes/no
33b) Kupittaa Hospital	yes/no
33c) Out-patient unit	yes/no

Appendix 2

The psychological background variables

1. General assessment of ego-strength
2. Impulse-control
3. The style of primary-process thinking
4. The level of intellectual performance
5. Estimation of intellectual capacities
6. Intellectual deteriation
7. Stability of cognitive functioning
8. Coping with decompensation
9. Ego-boundary disturbance: self-object differentation
10. Tolerance for depression and related feelings
11. Psychological-mindedness
12. Emotional distancing in object-relations
13. Symbiotic relatedness in object-representations
14. Tendency to paranoiac/omnipotent control in object-representations
15. Chaotic or isolated object-images
16. Developmental level of object-representations
17. Withdrawal into autism or omnipotent fantacies
18. Quality of self-object relations
19. Quality of human dependency
20. The variety and flexibility of object-representations

Appendix 3

Treatment variables defined in the 5-year follow-up examination

1. Included in the group of psychotherapy cases yes/no
2. Has been given intensive individual therapy yes/no
3. Has been given intensive or less intensive family therapy yes/no
4. Has been given intensive therapy or intervention in crisis in a psychotherapeutic community yes/no
5. Neuroleptic medication during the follow-up period higher-than-average dose/ lower-than-average dose

The variable for medication was constructed by calculating the annual mean dose of neuroleptics on the basis of the analyses made in the follow-up examinations. The variable thus obtained was divided into two by cutting the scale half-way through.
For definition of the modes of psychotherapy, see pp. 93–94 and for the group of psychotherapy cases, see p. 109.

Appendix 4

Variables used in assessing the prognosis:

I Disappearance of the psychotic symptoms at the time of the 5-year follow-up

yes/no

II Decrease of the nuclear symptoms of schizophrenia during the 5-year follow-up period

fewer symptoms/equal number or more symptoms

The nuclear symptoms were defined thus:

- autism
- schizophrenic thought disorder
- hebephrenic affective disorder
- schizophrenic auditory hallucinosis
- somatic delusions of being influenced
- psychic delusions of being influenced
- catatonic symptoms (stupor and/or excitement)
- sensations of depersonalization and derealization

The numer of nuclear symptoms was classified with a three-step scale (4 or more nuclear symptoms, 2–3 nuclear symptoms, no more than 1 nuclear symptom) in both the basic examination and the follow-up examination. A shift of one step down on the scale was regarded as a decrease of nuclear symptoms.

III Maintenance of the working ability at the time of the 5-year follow-up

normal working capacity/working capacity reduced or lost

IV Avoidance of the disability pension at the time of the 5-year follow-up

not on pension/on pension

V Favourable development of the occupational identity during the 5-year follow-up time

favourable development/no favourable development

As favourable development was regarded a step upward a three-step scale:

- stable occupational identity
- developing occupational identity
- no occupational identity

VI Maintenance of the grip on life at the time of the 5-year follow-up

grip maintained/grip lost

VII Progressive development of the level of psychosexual development

progressive development/no progressive development

As progressive development was regarded a step upward a two-step scale:

- established heterosexual identity
- level of psychosexual development
  chaotic, delayed or characterized by identity crisis

VIII Progression of the patient's psychologic separation from the primary family during the 5-year follow-up period

progressive development/no progressive development

As progressive development was regarded a step upward a three-step scale:

- at least ostensibly successful separation
- separation struggle continued
- strongly enmeshed in the primary family

IX Favourable development of the quantity of the patient's interpersonal relationships outside the primary family during the 5-year follow-up period

favourable development/no favourable development

As favourable development was regarded a step upward a three-step scale:

- several significant relationships
- one significant relationship
- no significant relationships

X Favourable development of the quality of the patient's interpersonal relationships outside the primary family during the 5-year follow-up period

favourable development/no favourable development

As favourable development was regarded a step upward a three-step scale:

- stable and long-lived relationships
- relationships labile and short-lived or coloured by repeated conflicts

XI Increase of insight into one's problems during the 5-year follow-up time

increased/not increased

As indication of increased insight was regarded a step upward a three-step scale:

- sees one's problems and symptoms as part of oneself and makes efforts to solve the situation
- has some insight into one's own role in the development of the problems and/or symptoms
- lacks any insight into the connection between one's illness and the problems of one's life

XII The number of in-patient days during the 5-year follow-up period

less than 200 days/200 days or more

XIII Avoidance of in-patient treatment during the two last follow-up years

not in hospital/was in hospital

XIV The total outcome score according to the four-dimensional Strauss-Carpenter (1972) criteria at the end of the 5-year follow-up

12 or more/less than 12

Appendix 5

The statistical significances of the connections between the background variables and the treatment variables. The whole series.

Treatment variables	1 Psycho-therapy case	2 Intensive individual therapy	3 Family therapy	4 Psycho-thera-peutic community	5 Higher-than-average medication
1a	n.s.	n.s.	< .10	< .10	< .001
1b	< .05(−)	< .05(−)	n.s.	n.s.	n.s.
1c	n.s.	n.s.	n.s.	n.s.	n.s.
1d	n.s.	n.s.	n.s.	< .05(−)	< .05(−)
2a	n.s.	n.s.	n.s.	< .01(−)	< .01(−)
2b	n.s.	n.s.	< .05(−)	n.s.	< .05(−)
2c	< .05	n.s.	<0.5	< .001	< .001
2d	< .05(−)	n.s.	n.s.	= .10(−)	n.s.
3a	n.s.	< .05	< .10(−)	n.s.	n.s.
3b	< .10	n.s.	< .10	n.s.	n.s.
3c	n.s.	< .01(−)	n.s.	n.s.	n.s.
3d	n.s.	n.s.	n.s.	< .05(−)	n.s.
4a	< .05(−)	< .05(−)	n.s.	n.s.	.05
4b	< .05	< .05	n.s.	< .10	n.s.
5	n.s.	n.s.	n.s.	n.s.	n.s.
6	n.s.	n.s.	n.s.	n.s.	n.s.
7	< .10	= .001	n.s.	n.s.	n.s.
8	n.s.	= .01	n.s.	n.s.	< .01(−)
9	n.s.	n.s.	n.s.	n.s.	n.s.
10	n.s.	n.s.	< .05(−)	< .05(−)	n.s.
11	n.s.	n.s.	< .10	n.s.	< .10
12	n.s.	n.s.	n.s.	< .05(−)	< .10(−)
13	.10	< .05	n.s.	n.s.	n.s.
14	n.s.	n.s.	n.s.	n.s.	n.s.
15	< .05	n.s.	n.s.	< .01	< .05(−)
16	< .10(−)	n.s.	n.s.	n.s.	= .10
17	n.s.	n.s.	n.s.	n.s.	n.s.
18	n.s.	n.s.	n.s.	n.s.	n.s.
19	n.s.	n.s.	n.s.	n.s.	n.s.
20	n.s.	n.s.	n.s.	n.s.	n.s.
21	< .10	n.s.	n.s.	n.s.	n.s.
22	n.s.	n.s.	n.s.	n.s.	n.s.
23	n.s.	n.s.	n.s.	n.s.	n.s.
24	n.s.	< .05	n.s.	n.s.	n.s.
25	< .01	< .05	n.s.	n.s.	= .01(−)

Treatment variables					
	1 Psycho-therapy case	2 Intensive individual therapy	3 Family therapy	4 Psycho-thera-peutic community	5 Higher-than-average medication
26	n.s.	n.s.	n.s.	< .01	n.s.
27	n.s.	n.s.	n.s.	n.s.	< .10$^{(-)}$
28	n.s.	n.s.	n.s.	< .10$^{(-)}$	< .05
29	n.s.	n.s.	< .10	n.s.	n.s.
30	n.s.	=.10	n.s.	n.s.	n.s.
31	n.s.	n.s.	n.s.	n.s.	n.s.
32	n.s.	n.s.	n.s.	n.s.	n.s.
33a	< .05	n.s.	n.s.	< .05	< .01$^{(-)}$
33b	< .001$^{(-)}$	n.s.	n.s.	< .10$^{(-)}$	< .01
33c	n.s.	n.s.	n.s.	n.s.	n.s.

The numbers in the table refer to p-values. Those with a $^{(-)}$ sign indicate a negative connection. The background variables are numbered as in Appendix 1, the treatment variables as in Appendix 3.

Appendix 6

The statistical significances of the connections between the background variables and the treatment variables. Typical schizophrenics.

Treatment variables					
	1 Psycho- therapy case	2 Intensive individual therapy	3 Family therapy	4 Psycho- thera- peutic community	5 Higher- than- average medication
1a					
1b					
1c			The connections not calculable		
1d					
2a					
2b	n.s.	n.s.	n.s.	$<.10^{(-)}$	n.s.
2c	$<.05$	n.s.	n.s.	$<.01$	$<.05$
2d	$<.10^{(-)}$	n.s.	n.s.	$<.05^{(-)}$	n.s.
3a	n.s.	$<.10$	n.s.	n.s.	n.s.
3b	$<.05$	n.s.	$<.01$	$<.10$	n.s.
3c	n.s.	$<.05^{(-)}$	n.s.	n.s.	n.s.
3d	n.s.	n.s.	n.s.	n.s.	$<.05$
4a	$<.05^{(-)}$	$<.10^{(-)}$	n.s.	n.s.	n.s.
4b	$<.05$	$<.10$	n.s.	n.s.	n.s.
5	n.s.	n.s.	n.s.	n.s.	n.s.
6	n.s.	n.s.	n.s.	n.s.	n.s.
7	$<.05$	$<.05$	n.s.	n.s.	n.s.
8	n.s.	n.s.	$<.10$	n.s.	$<.10^{(-)}$
9	n.s.	n.s.	n.s.	n.s.	n.s.
10	$<.05^{(-)}$	n.s.	$<.10^{(-)}$	$<.05^{(-)}$	n.s.
11	n.s.	$<.10^{(-)}$	$<.05$	n.s.	n.s.
12	$<.10$	$<.05$	n.s.	n.s.	n.s.
13	$<.05$	$<.01$	n.s.	n.s.	n.s.
14	n.s.	n.s.	n.s.	n.s.	n.s.
15	n.s.	n.s.	n.s.	n.s.	$<.05^{(-)}$
16	$<.05^{(-)}$	$<.10^{(-)}$	n.s.	n.s.	n.s.
17	n.s.	n.s.	n.s.	n.s.	n.s.
18	n.s.	n.s.	n.s.	n.s.	n.s.
19	n.s.	n.s.	n.s.	n.s.	n.s.
20	n.s.	n.s.	n.s.	n.s.	n.s.
21	n.s.	$<.10$	n.s.	n.s.	n.s.
22	n.s.	n.s.	n.s.	n.s.	n.s.
23	n.s.	n.s.	n.s.	n.s.	n.s.
24	n.s.	n.s.	n.s.	n.s.	n.s.

Treatment variables					
	1 Psycho-therapy case	2 Intensive individual therapy	3 Family therapy	4 Psycho-thera-peutic community	5 Higher-than-average medication
25	n.s.	=.10	n.s.	n.s.	<.05$^{(-)}$
26	n.s.	n.s.	n.s.	n.s.	n.s.
27	n.s.	n.s.	n.s.	n.s.	n.s.
28	n.s.	n.s.	n.s.	n.s.	<.01
29	n.s.	n.s.	<.05	n.s.	n.s.
30	n.s.	n.s.	n.s.	n.s.	n.s.
32	n.s.	n.s.	n.s.	<.10	n.s.
33a	n.s.	n.s.	n.s.	<.10	<.10$^{(-)}$
33b	<.01$^{(-)}$	n.s.	n.s.	<.01$^{(-)}$	<.01
33c	n.s.	n.s.	n.s.	n.s.	n.s.

The numbers in the table refer to p-values. Those with a (–)-sign indicate a negative connection. The background variables are numbered as in Appendix 1, the treatment variables as in Appendix 3.

Appendix 7

The statistical significances of the connections between the background variables and major prognostic variables. The whole series.

Prognostic variables

Back-ground-variable	I	II	III	IV	VI	XI	XII	XIII	XIV
1a	.000$^{(-)}$	<.01$^{(-)}$	<.0.5$^{(-)}$	<.0.1$^{(-)}$	<.001$^{(-)}$	n.s.	<.001$^{(-)}$	.000$^{(-)}$	<.01$^{(-)}$
1b	<.05	<.10	<.05	n.s.	<.05	n.s.	<.10	n.s.	n.s.
1c	<.05	n.s.	n.s.	n.s.	<.10	<.10	n.s.	<.10	n.s.
1d	<.05	n.s.	n.s.	<.10	n.s.	n.s.	<.05	<.01	n.s.
2a	<.05	n.s.	n.s.	<.05	<.10	n.s.	<.05	<.01	<.01
2b	<.05	<.05	n.s.	<.10	<.05	n.s.	<.05	<.01	<.05
2c	<.05$^{(-)}$	<.10$^{(-)}$	<.05$^{(-)}$	<.01$^{(-)}$	<.05$^{(-)}$	n.s.	.000$^{(-)}$	.000$^{(-)}$	<.01$^{(-)}$
2d	<.01$^{(-)}$	n.s.	n.s.	n.s.	n.s.	n.s.	n.s.	n.s.	n.s.
3a	<.01	<.10	n.s.	n.s.	n.s.	n.s.	n.s.	n.s.	n.s.
3b	n.s.	n.s.	n.s.	n.s.	n.s.	n.s.	n.s.	n.s.	n.s.
3c	n.s.	n.s.	n.s.	n.s.	n.s.	n.s.	<.10$^{(-)}$	n.s.	n.s.
3d	n.s.	n.s.	<.05$^{(-)}$	<.10$^{(-)}$	n.s.	<.01$^{(-)}$	n.s.	n.s.	n.s.
4a	n.s.	n.s.	n.s.	n.s.	n.s.	n.s.	n.s.	<.05$^{(-)}$	n.s.
4b	n.s.	n.s.	n.s.	n.s.	n.s.	n.s.	n.s.	n.s.	n.s.
5	n.s.	n.s.	n.s.	n.s.	n.s.	n.s.	n.s.	n.s.	n.s.
6	n.s.	n.s.	n.s.	n.s.	n.s.	n.s.	n.s.	n.s.	n.s.
7	n.s.	n.s.	n.s.	n.s.	n.s.	<.10$^{(-)}$	n.s.	n.s.	n.s.
8	n.s.	n.s.	n.s.	n.s.	n.s.	n.s.	n.s.	n.s.	n.s.
9	n.s.	n.s.	n.s.	n.s.	n.s.	n.s.	n.s.	n.s.	n.s.
10	n.s.	n.s.	n.s.	n.s.	n.s.	n.s.	n.s.	n.s.	<.10$^{(-)}$
11	n.s.	<.10$^{(-)}$	n.s.	n.s.	<.10$^{(-)}$	n.s.	n.s.	n.s.	<.05$^{(-)}$
12	n.s.	n.s.	<.10	n.s.	n.s.	n.s.	n.s.	<.10	n.s.
13	<.01	<.05	<.10	n.s.	<.01	n.s.	n.s.	n.s.	<.05
14	n.s.	n.s.	n.s.	n.s.	n.s.	n.s.	n.s.	n.s.	n.s.
15	n.s.	n.s.	<.05	<.05	n.s.	n.s.	=.10	<.01	<.01
16	n.s.	<.05$^{(-)}$	<.05$^{(-)}$	<.05$^{(-)}$	n.s.	n.s.	n.s.	n.s.	<.01$^{(-)}$
17	n.s.	n.s.	n.s.	n.s.	n.s.	n.s.	n.s.	n.s.	n.s.
18	n.s.	n.s.	n.s.	n.s.	n.s.	n.s.	n.s.	n.s.	n.s.
19	n.s.	n.s.	n.s.	n.s.	n.s.	<.10	n.s.	n.s.	n.s.
20	n.s.	n.s.	n.s.	n.s.	n.s.	<.10$^{(-)}$	n.s.	n.s.	n.s.
21	n.s.	n.s.	<.10	n.s.	n.s.	n.s.	n.s.	n.s.	n.s.
22	n.s.	n.s.	n.s.	n.s.	n.s.	n.s.	n.s.	n.s.	n.s.
23	n.s.	<.01	n.s.	<.05	<.05	n.s.	<.05	n.s.	<.10
24	n.s.	<.10$^{(-)}$	n.s.	n.s.	<.10$^{(-)}$	n.s.	<.10$^{(-)}$	n.s.	n.s.
25	<.05	n.s.	<.001	<.001	.000	<.05	<.10	n.s.	<.001
26	n.s.	n.s.	<.05	<.05	<.05	n.s.	<.01	n.s.	<.10

Prognostic variables									
Back-ground-variable	I	II	III	IV	VI	XI	XII	XIII	XIV
27	n.s.	n.s.	< .05	< .01	< .01	n.s.	n.s.	n.s.	< .001
28	n.s.	n.s.	< .01$^{(-)}$	=.001$^{(-)}$	< .01$^{(-)}$	< .10$^{(-)}$	n.s.	=.10$^{(-)}$	< .10$^{(-)}$
29	n.s.	n.s.	n.s.	n.s.	n.s.	n.s.	< .10	n.s.	n.s.
30	n.s.	n.s.	n.s.	n.s.	n.s.	n.s.	n.s.	n.s.	n.s.
31	n.s.	n.s.	n.s.	n.s.	n.s.	< .10$^{(-)}$	n.s.	n.s.	n.s.
32	n.s.	n.s.	n.s.	n.s.	n.s.	< .05$^{(-)}$	n.s.	n.s.	n.s.
33a	n.s.	n.s.	n.s.	n.s.	n.s.	< .05	n.s.	< .01	n.s.
33b	n.s.	n.s.	< .10$^{(-)}$	< .01$^{(-)}$	< .05$^{(-)}$	< .10$^{(-)}$	n.s.	< .05$^{(-)}$	n.s.
33c	n.s.	n.s.	n.s.	< .05	n.s.	n.s.	n.s.	n.s.	n.s.

The numbers in the table refer to p-values. Those with a $^{(-)}$ sign indicate a negative connection. The background variables are numbered as in Appendix 1.

The prognostic variables are:

I	Disappearance of psychotic symptoms
II	Decrease of the nuclear symptoms
III	Maintenance of the working capacity
IV	Avoidance of pension
VI	Maintenance of the grip on life
XI	Increase of the insight ability
XII	In-patient days during the follow-up period
XIII	Avoidance of hospital treatment during the two last follow-up years
XIV	The total outcome score according to the Strauss – Carpenter criteria

Appendix 8

The statistical significances of the connections between the background variables and major prognostic variables. Typical schizophrenics.

Prognostic variables									
Back-ground-variable	I	II	III	IV	VI	XI	XII	XIII	XIV
1a									
1b									
1c	The connections not calculable								
1d									
2a									
2b	n.s.	n.s.	n.s.	n.s.	n.s.	n.s.	n.s.	$<.10$	$<.10$
2c	n.s.	n.s.	n.s.	n.s.	n.s.	n.s.	$<.05^{(-)}$	$<.05^{(-)}$	n.s.
2d	n.s.	n.s.	n.s.	n.s.	n.s.	n.s.	n.s.	n.s.	n.s.
3a	n.s.	n.s.	$<.10$	n.s.	n.s.	n.s.	n.s.	n.s.	n.s.
3b	n.s.	n.s.	n.s.	n.s.	n.s.	n.s.	n.s.	n.s.	n.s.
3c	$<.05^{(-)}$	n.s.	n.s.	$<.10^{(-)}$	n.s.	n.s.	$<.05$	n.s.	$<.05^{(-)}$
3d	n.s.	n.s.	$<.01^{(-)}$	$<.01^{(-)}$	$<.01^{(-)}$	$<.05^{(-)}$	n.s.	n.s.	$<.05^{(-)}$
4a	n.s.	n.s.	n.s.	n.s.	n.s.	n.s.	n.s.	n.s.	n.s.
4b	n.s.	n.s.	n.s.	n.s.	n.s.	n.s.	n.s.	n.s.	n.s.
5	n.s.	n.s.	n.s.	n.s.	n.s.	n.s.	n.s.	n.s.	n.s.
6	n.s.	n.s.	n.s.	n.s.	n.s.	n.s.	n.s.	n.s.	n.s.
7	n.s.	n.s.	n.s.	n.s.	n.s.	n.s.	n.s.	n.s.	n.s.
8	n.s.	n.s.	n.s.	n.s.	n.s.	n.s.	n.s.	n.s.	n.s.
9	n.s.	n.s.	n.s.	n.s.	n.s.	n.s.	n.s.	n.s.	n.s.
10	n.s.	n.s.	n.s.	n.s.	n.s.	n.s.	n.s.	n.s.	n.s.
11	n.s.	$<.10^{(-)}$	n.s.	n.s.	n.s.	n.s.	n.s.	n.s.	n.s.
12	n.s.	n.s.	n.s.	n.s.	n.s.	n.s.	n.s.	$<.10$	n.s.
13	$=.01$	$<.10$	$<.10$	n.s.	$<.10$	n.s.	n.s.	$<.10$	$<.05$
14	n.s.	n.s.	n.s.	n.s.	n.s.	$<.05$	n.s.	n.s.	n.s.
15	$<.10$	n.s.	$<.001$	$<.01$	$<.05$	n.s.	$<.05$	$<.01$	$<.01$
16	n.s.	$<.10^{(-)}$	$<.05^{(-)}$	$<.05^{(-)}$	n.s.	n.s.	n.s.	n.s.	$<.05^{(-)}$
17	n.s.	n.s.	$<.10^{(-)}$	$<.05^{(-)}$	n.s.	n.s.	n.s.	n.s.	n.s.
18	n.s.	n.s.	n.s.	$<.10$	n.s.	n.s.	n.s.	n.s.	n.s.
19	n.s.	n.s.	n.s.	n.s.	n.s.	n.s.	n.s.	n.s.	n.s.
20	n.s.	n.s.	$<.10^{(-)}$	$<.10^{(-)}$	n.s.	$<.10^{(-)}$	n.s.	n.s.	n.s.
21	n.s.	n.s.	$<.10$	n.s.	n.s.	n.s.	n.s.	n.s.	n.s.
22	n.s.	n.s.	n.s.	n.s.	n.s.	n.s.	n.s.	n.s.	n.s.
23	n.s.	$<.05$	n.s.	n.s.	n.s.	n.s.	$<.10$	n.s.	n.s.
24	n.s.	$<.10^{(-)}$	n.s.	n.s.	n.s.	n.s.	$<.10^{(-)}$	n.s.	n.s.
25	$<.05$	n.s.	$<.01$	$<.001$	$<.001$	n.s.	$<.05$	$<.05$	$<.001$
26	n.s.	n.s.	n.s.	n.s.	n.s.	n.s.	n.s.	n.s.	n.s.

Prognostic variables									
Background-variable	I	II	III	IV	VI	XI	XII	XIII	XIV
27	n.s.	n.s.	$<.10$	$<.05$	$<.01$	n.s.	n.s.	n.s.	$<.01$
28	n.s.	n.s.	$<.01^{(-)}$	$<.001^{(-)}$	$<.01^{(-)}$	n.s.	n.s.	$<.05^{(-)}$	$<.05^{(-)}$
29	$<.10$	n.s.	n.s.	n.s.	n.s.	$<.10^{(-)}$	n.s.	n.s.	n.s.
30	n.s.	n.s.	n.s.	n.s.	n.s.	n.s.	n.s.	n.s.	n.s.
31	n.s.	n.s.	n.s.	$<.10$	n.s.	$<.10^{(-)}$	n.s.	n.s.	n.s.
32	n.s.	$<.10^{(-)}$	n.s.	n.s.	n.s.	$<.05^{(-)}$	n.s.	n.s.	n.s.
33a	n.s.	n.s.	$<.10$	$=.10$	n.s.	n.s.	n.s.	$<.01$	$<.10$
33b	n.s.	n.s.	$<.10^{(-)}$	$<.001^{(-)}$	$<.05^{(-)}$	n.s.	n.s.	$<.05^{(-)}$	$<.10^{(-)}$
33c	n.s.	n.s.	n.s.	$<.10$	n.s.	n.s.	n.s.	n.s.	n.s.

The numbers in the table refer to p-values. Those with a $^{(-)}$ sign indicate a negative connection. The background and the prognostic variables are numbered as in Appendix 6.

Appendix 9

The statistical significances of the connections between the treatment variables and major prognostic variables. The whole series.

Prognostic variables									
Treat-ment variable	I	II	III	IV	VI	XI	XII	XIII	XIV
1	n.s.	< .10	< .05	n.s.	n.s.	< .01	n.s.	n.s.	n.s.
2	< .05	< .05	n.s.	n.s.	n.s.	< .05	n.s.	n.s.	n.s.
3	n.s.	n.s.	n.s.	n.s.	n.s.	n.s.	< .10$^{(-)}$	n.s.	< .10$^{(-)}$
4	n.s.	n.s.	n.s.	n.s.	n.s.	< .01	< .05$^{(-)}$	n.s.	n.s.
5	< .000$^{(-)}$	< .10$^{(-)}$	< .000$^{(-)}$	< .000$^{(-)}$	< .000$^{(-)}$	n.s.	< .000$^{(-)}$	< .000$^{(-)}$	< .000$^{(-)}$

The same statistical significances. Typical schizophrenics.

	I	II	III	IV	VI	XI	XII	XIII	XIV
1	< .05	< .05	< .01	n.s.	n.s.	< .001	n.s.	< .10	< .10
2	< .05	< .05	.05	n.s.	n.s.	< .001	n.s.	n.s.	< .01
3	n.s.	n.s.	n.s.	n.s.	n.s.	n.s.	n.s.	n.s.	n.s.
4	n.s.	< .10	< .05	= .10	< .01	< .01	n.s.	n.s.	n.s.
5	< .01$^{(-)}$	n.s.	< .001$^{(-)}$	< .000$^{(-)}$	< .001$^{(-)}$	< .05$^{(-)}$	< .001$^{(-)}$	< .000$^{(-)}$	< .01$^{(-)}$

The numbers in the table refer to p-values. Those with a $^{(-)}$ sign indicate a negative connection. The treatment variables are numbered as in Appendix 3, the prognostic variables as in Appendices 6 and 7.

Appendix 10

The statistical significances of the positive connections between the clinical, psychological and psychodynamic prognostic variables.

	I	II	III	IV	V	VI	VII	VIII	IX	X	XI
I	–	.000	.000	< .001	< .05	.000	< .01	< .05	< .10	n.s.	< .01
II	< .001	–	< .001	< .10	< .05	< .001	< .01	n.s.	n.s.	n.s.	< .05
III	< .001	< .01	–	.000	< .05	.000	< .001	< .05	< .01	< .01	< .01
IV	n.s.	n.s.	.000	–	n.s.	.000	< .01	< .05	< .01	< .05	< .05
V	< .01	< .01	< .001	< .01	–	n.s.	< .10	< .05	n.s.	n.s.	< .001
VI	< .01	< .05	.000	.000	< .01	–	< .05	n.s.	< .01	< .05	< .05
VII	< .001	< .01	< .001	< .05	< .05	< .10	–	< .01	< .05	< .05	< .05
VIII	< .05	n.s.	< .01	< .05	< .01	< .10	< .05	–	n.s.	n.s.	< .01
IX	< .1	n.s.	< .05	< .05	< .05	< .01	< .05	n.s.	–	< .001	< .05
X	n.s.	n.s.	< .01	< .01	< .10	< .05	n.s.	< .10	< .001	–	n.s.
XI	< .01	< .01	< .01	< .01	< .001	< .05	< .05	< .05	n.s.	n.s.	–

The numbers in the table refer to p-values. Those presented on the upper and right hand side of the table refer to the whole series, those presented on the lower and left hand side to the typical schizophrenic patients.

The prognostic variables included:

I	Disappearance of psychotic symptoms
II	Decrease of nuclear symptoms
III	Maintenance of working capacity
IV	Avoidance of pension
V	Favourable development of occupational identity
VI	Maintenance of the grip on life
VII	Farourable development of psychosexual identity
VIII	Progress of separation from the primary family
IX	Favourable development of the quantity of interpersonal relationships
X	Favourable development of the quality of interpersonal relationships
XI	Increase of insight ability

References

Aaku T, Rasimus R & Alanen Y O (1980): Nursing staff as individual therapists in psychotherapeutic community. Psychiatria Fennica 1980:9–31.

Aaltonen J (1982): Perhekeskeisen hoitoprosessin lähtökohdat psykiatrisessa avohoidossa. English summary: Basis for family-centered treatment process in psychiatric outpatient care. Ann Univ Turkuensis, Ser C, Vol 35.

Aaltonen J, Alanen Y O, Lehtinen K & Räkköläinen V (1984): Report of a family therapeutic part project connected with the Finnish programme to develop investigation, treatment and rehabilitation of schizophrenic patients. In Finnish.

Abasiekong E M (1981): Familism and hospital admission in rural Nigeria – A case study. Soc Sci & Med 15 B:45–50.

Achté K (1961) Der Verlauf der Schizophrenien und schizophreniformen Psychosen. Acta Psychiat Scand Suppl 155.

Achté K (1967): On prognosis and rehabilitation in schizophrenic and paranoid psychosis. Acta Psychiat Scand Suppl 196.

Achté K, Lönnqvist J, Piirtola O & Niskanen P (1980): Verlauf und Prognose schizophrener Psychosen in Helsinki. In Psychiatrische Verlaufsforschung. Methoden und Ergebnisse. Edited by G W Schimmelpenning. Huber, Bern.

Alanen Y O (1958): The mothers of schizophrenic patients. Acta Psychiat Neur Scand Suppl 124.

Alanen Y O (1973): Om familjeterapi av unga schizofrenipatienter. Nord Psykiat Tidskr 27:242–256.

Alanen Y O (1975). The psychotherapeutic care of schizophrenic patients in a community psychiatric setting. In: M.H.Lader (ed.), Studies of schizophrenia. Brit J Psychiat Spec Publ No 10.

Alanen Y O (1976): On background factors and goals in the family therapy of young schizophrenic patients and their parents. In: J Jorstad and E Ugelstad (eds.), Schizophrenia 1975. Oslo, Universitetsforlaget.

Alanen Y O (1978): Schizophrenia and the family. Psychiatria Fennica 1978:15–28.

Alanen Y O (1980): In search of the interactional origin of schizophrenia. In: The Family: Evaluation and treatment, edited by C K Hofling & J M Lewis. Brunner/Mazel, New York.

Alanen Y O, Kinnunen P (1975): Marriage and the development of schizophrenia. Psychiatry 38:346–355.

Alanen Y O, Laine A (1973): Development of a hospital centered community psychotherapy service for schizophrenic patients'. Evaluation of the first phase. In: J K Wing and H Häfner (eds). Roots of evaluation: An epidemiologic basis for lanning psychiatric services. London. Oxford University Press.

Alanen Y O, Montell R (1984): A national development and research programme for the investigation, care and rehabilitation of schizophrenics (Swedish, with English summary). Nord Psykiat Tidskr 38:401–407.

Alanen Y O, Rekola J, Stewen A, Takala K, Tuovinen M (1966): The family in the pathogenesis of schizophrenic and neurotic disorders. Acta Psychiat Scand Vol 42, Suppl 189.

Alanen Y O, Räkköläinen V, Laakso J, Rasimus R, Sourander C & Hyry A (1978 a): Psykoterapeuttisesti orientoituneen skitsofrenian avohoidon kehittäminen yhteisöpsykiatrian puitteissa. Teoksessa Psykiatrinen preventio ja kriisipsykiatria, ed. Y Alanen, R Järvi & V Lehtinen. (In Finnish). Ann Univ Turkuensis, Ser C:24.

Alanen Y O, Räkköläinen V, Rasimus R, Laakso J (1978 b): Psykoosipotilaiden sairaalahoito ja yhteisöpsykiatria. Suom Lääk l 33:1137–1142 ja 1215–1220. (In Finnish).
Alanen Y O, Räkköläinen V, Rasimus R, Laakso J (1979): Indications of different forms of psychotherapy with new schizophrenic patients in community psychiatry. In: Psychotherapy of schizophrenia, ed C Müller. Excerpta Medica, Amsterdam.
Alanen Y O, Räkköläinen V, Laakso J, Rasimus R (1980): Problems inherent in the study of psychotherapy of psychoses: conclusions from a community psychiatric action research study. In: Psychotherapy of schizophrenia, ed. J S Strauss et al. Plenum Press, New York.
Alanen Y O, Räkköläinen V, Laakso J (1982 a): Krankheitsmodelle bei der Schizophrenie und die Bedürfnisangemessenheit der Behandlung. Nervenarzt 53:150–153.
Alanen Y O, Räkköläinen V, Rasimus R, Laakso J, Järvi R (1982b). Developing the treatment of schizophrenia in a community psychiatric setting. Psychotherapeutic and family-centered approach. Psychiatria Fennica 1982:101–120.
Alanen Y O, Räkköläinen V, Rasimus R, Laakso J, Järvi R (1983): Psychotherapy of schizophrenia in community psychiatry. In: Psychosocial intervention in schizophrenia. Ed. by Stierlin et al. Springer-Verlag, Berlin.
Alanen Y O, Räkköläinen V, Rasimus R, Laakso J Kaljonen A (1985a): Psychotherapeutically oriented treatment of schizophrenia: Results of 5-year follow-up. Acta psychiat Scand 71, Suppl 319:31–49.
Alanen Y O, Räkköläinen V, Rasimus R, Laakso J & Kaljonen A (1985b): Psychotherapeutically oriented treatment of schizophrenia: Results of 5-year follow-up. Yale J Biol Med 58:383–402.
Alstrom C H (1942): Mortality in mental hospitals with special regard to tuberculosis. Acta Psychiatr Neurol Scand Suppl 24.
American Psychiatric Association (1980): Diagnostic and statistical, manual III. Washington, D.C.
Anderson C, Hogarty G, Reiss D (1980): Family treatment of adult schizophrenic patients: A psycho-educational approach. Schizophr Bull 6(3):490–505.
Anttinen EE (1983): Can the vicious circle of chronicity and institutionalization be broken? Psychiatria Fennica 1983:21–31.
Anttinen EE (1985): Chronicity and hospitalization: can the vicious circles be broken? In The long-term treatment of functional psychoses. Ed by T. Helgason. EMCR, Cambridge Univ Press, Cambridge, Great Britain.
Anttinen EE, Eloranta K & Stenij P (1971): Kotisairaanhoidon mahdollisuudet skitsofreniaa sairastavien jälkihoidossa ja kuntoutuksessa. English summary: The care and rehabilitation of schizophrenic out-patients with home-care. Kansaneläkelaitoksen julkaisuja. Sarja A:8. Helsinki.
Anttinen EE & Stenij P (1974): The care and rehabilitation of schizophrenic out-patients with home care. Psychiatria Fennica 1974:145–154.
Appelbaum SA (1977): The anatomy of change. Plenum Press. New York.
Astrachan B M, Beaver L, Harrow N & Schwarz C (1974): Symptomatic outcome in schizophrenia. Arc Gen Psychiat 31:155–160.
Astrup C, Fossum A, and Holmboe R (1962): Prognosis in functional psychoses. Springfield, III. Charles C Thomas.
Astrup C, Noreik K (1966): Functional psychoses, diagnostic and prognostic models. Springfield, III.: Charles C Thomas.
Beard J H, Malamud T J, Rossman E (1978): Psychiatric rehabilitation and long-term rehospitalization rates: the findings of two research studies. Schizophrenia Bull 4:622–635.
Beck J C, Golden S, Arnold F (1981): An empirical investigation of psychotherapy with schizophrenic patients. Schizophrenia Bulletin 7 (No 2):241–247.
Becker J (1963): "Good premorbid" schizophrenic wives and their husbands. Fam Process 2:34.
Bednar RL, Lawlis GF (1971): Empirical research in group psychotherapy In Handbook of psychotherapy and behaviour change: An empirical analysis. Edited by Bergin A, Garfield S. New York, John Wiley & Sons.

Bellak L, Hurvich M & Gedimann H K (1973): Ego functions in schizophrenia, neurotics and normals. Wiley, New York.
Benedetti G (1955): Psychotherapie der Psychosen in H Hoff: Lehrbuch der Psychiatrie, Benno Schwabe, Stuttgart.
Benedetti G (1975): Ausgewahlte Aufsätze zur Schizophrenielehre. Vandenhoeck & Ruprect, Göttingen.
Benedetti G (1983): Todeslandschaften der Seele. Vandenhoeck & Ruprecht, Göttingen.
Bernheim K F (1982): Supportive family counseling. Schizophr Bull 8:634–640.
Bishop Y M M Frenberg FE & Hollan PW (1975): Discrete multivariate analysis: Theory and practice. Cambridge, Mass., MIT Press.
Bland R C, Parker J & Orn H (1976): Prongosis in Schizophrenia. Arch Gen Psychiatry 33:949–954.
Bland R C, Parker J H (1978): Prognosis in schizophrenia. Prognostic predictors and outcome. Arc Gen Psychiatry 35:72–77.
Bland R C, Orn H (1980): Prediction of long-term outcome from presenting symptoms in schizophrenia. J Clin Psychiatry 41:85–88.
Blatt S & Ritzler R (1975): Disturbances in object representation in schizophrenia. Psycho-Anal Contemp Sci 4:235–288.
Bleuler E (1911): Dementia Praecox oder die Gruppe der Schizophrenien. Deuticke, Leipzig.
Bleuler M (1941): Krankheitsverlauf, Persönlichkeit und Verwandtschaft Schizophrener und ihre gegenseitigen Beziehungen. Georg Thieme, Leipzig.
Bleuler M (1972): Die schizophrenen Geistesstörungen. Georg Thieme, Stuttgart.
Bowen M R H, Dysinger W M, Brodey & Basamania B W (1961): The family as the unit of study and treatment. Amer J Orthopsychiat. 31: 40–86.
Bowers M B jr (1980): Biochemical processes in schizophrenia: an update. Schizophr Bull 6:393–403.
Breslow N E & Day N E (1980): Statistical methods in cancer research. Volume 1: The analysis of case-control studies. IARC, Lyon.
British Medical Journal (1980): 2 Feb: Schizophrenia in different cultures (editorial).
Brown G W, Bone M, Dalison B & Wing J K (1966): Schizophrenia and social care. Institute of Psychiatry, The Maudsley Hospital, London.
Brown G W & Wing J K (1972): Influence of family life on the course of schizophrenic disorders: a replication. British Journal of Psychiatry 121:241–58.
Buddeberg C & Kesselring V (1978): Ehen Schizophrener – Struktur und Dynamik. Psychiat Prax 5:118–126.
Burnham D L, Gladstone A I, Gibson R W (1969): Schizophrenia and need-fear dilemma. New York.
Carlsson A (1978): Antipsychotic drugs, neurotransmitters, and schizophrenia. Amer J Psychiat 135:164–173.
Carlsson A & Lindqvist M (1963): Effect of chlorpromazine and haloperidol on the formation of 3-methoxythyramine and normetanephrine in mouse brain. Acta pharmac 20:140.
Carpenter WT, McGlashan T H & Strauss J S (1977): The treatment of acute schizophrenia without drugs: an investigation of some current assumptions. Amer J Psychiat 134:14–21.
Carpenter WT, Bartko J J, Strauss J S, Hawk A B (1978): Signs and symptoms as predictors of outcome: a report from the international pilot study of schizophrenia. Am J Psychiatry 135:940–944.
Carpenter WT, Heinrichs D W, Hanlon T E (1981): Methodologic standards for treatment outcome research in schizophrenia. Am J Psychiatry 138:4:465–471.
Caton C (1982): Effect of length of inpatient treatment for chronic schizophrenia. Am J Psychiatry 139:856–891.
Ciompi L (1980): The natural history of schizophrenia in the long term. Brit J Psychiat 136:413–420.
Ciompi L & Müller C (1976): Lebensweg und Alter der Schizophrenen. Eine katamnestische Langzeitstudie bis ins Senium. Springer, Berlin.

Claghorn J L, Johnstone E E, Cook T H, et al. (1974): Group therapy and maintenance treatment of schizophrenics. Arch Gen Psychiatry 31:361–365.
Cohen J (1968): Weighted kappa: Nominal scale agreement with provision for scaled disagreement of partial credit. Psychological Bulletin 70:213–220.
Cole J O, Davis J M (1969): Antipsychotic drugs. In: The schizophrenic syndrome, edited by L Bellak and L Loeb. New York: Grune & Stratton.
Corder B F, Corder R F, Hendricks A (1971): An experimental study of the effect of paired-patient meetings on the group therapy process. Int J Group Psychiat 21:310–318.
Davis AE, Dinit S & Pasamanick B (1972): The prevention of hospitalization in schizophrenia: five years after an experimental program. Amer J Orthopsychiat 42:1375–1388.
Davis J M et al. (1980): Important issues in the drug treatment of schizophrenia. Schizophr Bull 6:70–87.
Davis J M, Janicak P, Chang S & Klerman K (1982): Recent advances in the pharmacologic treatment of the schizophrenic disorders. In Psychiatry 1982, Annual Review. The American Psychiatric Association, Washington.
Dupont R L, Ryder R G & Grunebaum H U (1971): An unexpected result of psychosis in marriage. Amer J Psychiat 128:735–739.
Early D C (1960): The industrial therapy organisation (Bristol). Lancet 2:754–757.
Engelke W, Haselbeck H (1980): Bilanz einer therapeutischen Wohngemeinschaft. Selbsthilfe und Versorgung. Psychiat Prax 7:72–80.
Esterson A, Cooper D, Laing R (1962): Results of family oriented therapy with hospitalized schizophrenics. Br Med J 2:1462–1465.
Falloon I R H, Boyd J L, Mc Gill C W, Razani J, Moss H B, Gilderman A M (1982): Family management in the prevention of exacerbations of schizophrenia. New England J Med 306:1437–1440.
Federn P (1943): Psychoanalysis of psychoses. Psychiat Quart 17:3–19, 246–257, 470–487.
Fenichel O (1945): The psychoanalytic theory of neurosis. Norton, New York
Fenton W S, Mosher L R & Matthews S M (1981): Diagnosis of schizophrenia: A critical review of current diagnostic systems. Schizophr Bull 7:452–475.
Fink P (1981): The relatives group: Treatment for parents of adult schizophrenics. Int J Group Psychoter 31:453–468.
Fleck S (1976): A general systems approach to severe family pathology. Am J Psychiatry 133:669–673.
Forssen A (1979): Roots of traditional personality development among the Zaramo in Coastal Tanzania. Central Union for Child Welfare in Finland. Publ. 54. Helsinki.
Fowler R C & Tsuang M T (1975): Spouses of schizophrenics. A blind comparative study. Comprehensive Psychiat 16:339–342.
Freud S (1915): Das Unbewußte. In Gesammelte Werke, Band X. Imago, London 1946.
Fromm-Reichmann F (1950): Principles of intensive psychotherapy. Univ Chicago Press, Chicago.
Fromm-Reichmann F (1959): Psychoanalysis and psychotherapy. Selected papers (ed by D. Bullard). Univ of Chicago Press, Chicago.
Furlan P (1984): Paper read at the VIII International symposium on psychotherapy of schizophrenia. New Haven, Conn. USA.
Gam J (1980): A 5-year retrospective investigation of all first admitted schizophrenics to Danish psychiatric institutions in the fiscal year from April ist, 1970, to April 1st, 1971. In Stringsen E, Dupont A, Nielsen J A: Epidemiological research as basis for the organization of extramural psychiatry. Acta Psychiat Scand Suppl 285, Vol 62 1980.
Garmezy N & Rodnick E H (1959): Premorbid adjustment and performance in schizophrenia: implications for interpreting heterogeneity in schizophrenia. J nerv ment Dis 129:450–466.
Gerlach H (1977): Tardive dyskinesier. Nord Psykiat Tidskr 31:394–399.
Giovacchini P (1979): Treatment of primitive mental states. Aronson, New York.
Glick, I D, Hargreaves W A Drues J, Showstack J A (1976): Short versus long hospitalization. A controlled prospective study. Amer J Psychiat 133:509–517.

Glick I D & Hargreaves W A (1979): Psychiatric hospital treatment for the 1980's. Lexington Books. Lexington, Mass. Toronto.
Goldberg S C, Schooler N, Hogarty G, Roper M (1977): Prediction and relapse in schizophrenic out-patients treated by drug and sociotherapy. Arch Gen Psychiat 34:171–184.
Goldstein M J, Rodnick E H, Evans J R, May P R A & Steinberg M R (1978): Drug and family therapy in the aftercare of acute schizophrenics. Arch Gen Psychiat 35: 1169–1177.
Gomez E A (1981): Small supportive treatment units and the problem of recidivism in indigent chronic schizophrenic patients. Psychiatr Quart 53:178–183.
Gralnick A (1963): Conjoint family therapy: its role in rehabilitation of the inpatient and family. J Nerv Ment Dis 136:500–506.
Grinspoon L, Ewalt J, Shader R (1972): Schizophrenia: pharmacotherapy and psychotherapy. Williams & Wilkins, Baltimore.
Gunderson J G & Carroll A (1983): Clinical considerations from empirical research in Psychosocial intervention in schizophrenia. Eds H. Stierlin, L.C. Wynne, M Wirsching. Springer, Berlin.
Gunderson J G, Frank A F, Katz H M, Vannicelli M L, Frosch J P & Knapp P H (1984): Effects of psychotherapy in schizophrenia: Comparative outcome of two forms of treatment. Sch Bull 10:564–598.
Gunderson J & Gomes-Schwartz B (1980): The quality of outcome from psychotherapy of schizophrenia. In: Psychotherapy of schizophrena, ed. by J. S. Strauss & al. Plenum Press, New York.
Gunderson J & Kolb J E (1978): Discriminating features of borderline patients. Am J Psychiat 135:792–796.
Hakkarainen A & Salokangas RKR (1985): Comparative data of the incidence and chronification of schizophrenic patients in different parts of Finland. In: National Board of Health in Finland (1985). In Finnish.
Harris A, Linker I & Norris V (1956): Schizophrenia: A social and prognostic study. Brit J Prev Soc Med 10:107–114.
Harrow M, Grinker R R, Silverstein M L, Holzman P (1978): Is modern-day schizophrenic outcome still negative? Am J Psychiat 135:1156–1162.
Hawk A B, Carpenter W T, Strauss J S (1975): Diagnostic criteria and five year outcome in schizophrenia. A report from the International Pilot Study of Schizophrenia. Arch Gen Psychiatry 32:343–347.
Hermansen L (1968): Suicider blandt skizofrene. Nordisk Psykiatrisk Tidskrift 4:324–337.
Hertz M I, Endicott J, And Spitzer RL (1977); Brief hospitalization. A two year follow-up. American Journal of Psychiatry 134:502–507.
Herz M I, Spitzer R L, Gibbon M et al. (1974): Individual versus group aftercare treatment. Am J Psychiatry 131:808–812.
Hogarty G E, Goldberg S C and the Collaborative Study Group (1973): Drugs and sociotherapy in the aftercare of schizophrenic patients. One year relapse rates. Archives of General Psychiat 28:54–64.
Hogarty G E, Goldberg SC, Schooler N R, Ulrich R F and the Collaborative Study Group (1974a): Drug and sociotherapy in the aftercare of schizophrenic patients: II. Two year relapse rates. Arch Gen Psychiat 31:603–608.
Hogarty G E, Goldberg S C, and Schooler N R (1974b): Drug and sociotherapy in the aftercare of schizophrenic patients III. Adjustment of nonrelapsed patients. Arch Gen Psychiat 31:609–618.
Hogarty G E, Schooler, N R, Ulrich R F, Mussare F, Ferro P, and Herron E (1979): Fluphenazine and social therapy in the aftercare of schizophrenic patients – relapse analyses of a two year controlled study of fluphenazine decanoate and fluphenazine hydrochloride. Arch Gen Psychiat 36:1238–1294.
Huber G, Gross G & Sheuttler R (1979): Schizophrenie. Eine verlaufs- und sozial-psychiatrische Langzeitstudie. Springer. Berlin.

Jackson D D & Weakland J H (1961): Conjoint family therapy: some considerations on theory, technique and results. Psychiatry 24. Suppl 2:30–45.

Jacobson O A (1967): A catamnestic investigation of schizophrenia with an observation period of 30 years. Acta psychiat Scand 217:44–45.

Jeste D V & Wyatt R J (1981): Changing epidemiology of tardive dyskinesia: An overview. Am J Psychiatry 138:297–309.

Johanson E (1958): A study of schizophrenia in the male. Acta psychiat neurol Scand Vol 33 Suppl 125.

Johansson A (1956): Psychotherapeutische Behandlung eines Falles von Schizophrenie. Psyche 10:568–587.

Johansson A (1985): Skitsofrenian analyyttisen psykoterapian ongelma. (The problem of analytic psychotherapy of schizophrenia) In Finnish with Swedish summary. Ann Univ Turkuensis, Ser C Vol 53.

Jones M (1953): The therapeutic community. Basic Books, New York.

Juel-Nielsen N (1985): Suicides and functional psychoses. In The long-term treatment of functional psychoses. Ed by T. Helgason. EMCR, Cambridge Univ Press, Cambridge, Great Britain.

Kaila K (1954): Presentation at the meeting of Finnish Psychiatric Association.

Kanter J, Lin A (1980): Facilitating a therapeutic milieu in the families of schizophrenics. Psychiatry 43:106–119.

Karon B P, VandenBos G R (1972): The consequences of psychotherapy for schizophrenic patients. Psychotherapy: Theory, Research and Practice 9:111–119.

Karon B P, VandenBos G R (1975): Issues in current research on psychotherapy vs. medication in treatment of schizophrenics. Psychotherapy: Theory, Research and Practice: 143–148.

Karon B P & VandenBos G R (1981): Psychotherapy of schizophrenia – Treatment of choice. Jason Aronson, New York.

Katschnig H & Konieczna T (1985): Social network and the long-term course of mental disorders – research needs. In the long-term treatment of functional psychoses. Ed by T Helgason. EMRC, Cambridge Univ Press, Cambridge, Great Britain.

Kaufmann L (1976): Long-term family therapy with schizophrenics. In Schizophrenia 75, ed. by J Jorstad & E Ugelstad. Universitetsforlaget, Oslo.

Kernberg, O (1967): Borderline personality organization. J Amer Psychoanal Ass 75:647–685.

Kernberg O (1975): Borderline conditions and pathological narcissism. Jason Aronson, New York.

Kernberg O (1976): Object relations theory and clinical psychoanalysis. Jason Aronson, New York

Kety S S, Rosenthal D, Wender P H and Schulsinger F (1971): Mental illness in the biological and adoptive families of adopted schizophrenics. Amer J Psychiat 128:82–86.

Klerman G L (1984): Idealogy and science in the individual psychotherapy of schizophrenia. Schizophr Bull 10:608–612.

Knight R P (1939): Psychotherapy in acute paranoid schizophrenia with successful outcome: A case report. Bull Menninger Clinic J: 97–705.

Langfeldt G (1937): The prognosis of schizophrenia and the factors influencing the course of the disease. Acta physiat neurol Scand Suppl 73.

Langfeldt G (1939): The schizophreniform states. Munksgaard, Kobenhavn.

Langfeldt G (1953): Some points regarding the symptomatology and diagnosis of schizophrenia. Acta psychiat Scand Suppl 80:7–26.

Langfeldt G (1956): The prognosis of schizophrenia. Acta psychiat neur Scand, Suppl 110.

Lansky MR, Bley C R, McVey G G & Brotman B (1978): Multiple family groups as aftercare. Internat J Group Psychother 29: 211–224.

Laquer H P et al (1964): Multiple family therapy: further developments. Internat J Soc Psych, Spedial Ed, Vol II.

Lassenius B, Ottosson J-O & Rapp W (1973): Prognosis in schizophrenia. Acta psychiat Scand 49:294–305.

Lazell EW (1921): The group treatment of dementia praecox. Psychoanal Rev 8:168–179.
Leff J, Kuipers L, Berkowitz R, Eberlein-Vries R & Sturgeon D (1982): A controlled trial of social intervention in the families of schizophrenic patients. Brit J Psychiat 141:121–134.
Lehtinen V, Salokangas RKR, Holm H & Laakso J (1980): Treatment prevalence in psychiatric out-patient care in Finland. Acta psychiat Scand 62:221–235.
Lehtinen V (1983): Regional variation of the incidence of mental disorders in Finland. Presented in Finnish in the symposium Research and Public Health, the Academy of Finland.
Levene H I, Patterson V, Murphy B G, Overbeck A L and Veach T L (1970): The aftercare of schizophrenics: An evaluation of group and individual approaches. Psychiat Quart 44:296–304.
Liberman R P, Wallace C J, Vaughn C E, Snyder K S & Rust C (1980): Social and family factors in the course of schizophrenia: Toward an interpersonal problem-solving therapy for schizophrenics and their families. In The psychotherapy of schizophrenia, ed by Strauss et al. Plenum, New York.
Liberman R P, Wallace C J, Falloon I R & Vaughn C E (1981): Interpersonal problem-solving therapy for schizophrenics and their families. Compr Psychiat 22:627–630.
Lichtenberg J D & Pao P N (1960): The prognostic and therapeutic significance of the husband-wife relationship for hospitalized schizophrenic women. Psychiatry 23:209–213.
Lidz T, Cornelison A R, Fleck S & Terry D (1957): The intrafamilial environment of schizophrenic patients. I. The father. Psychiatry 20:329–342.
Lidz T, Fleck S & Cornelison A R (1965): Schizophrenia and the family. Internat Univ Press, New York.
Lindberg D (1981): Management of schizophrenia. Psychiatrica Scand Suppl 289 63:100–112.
Lipton M A, DiMascio A & Killman K F (1978): Psychopharmacology. Raven Press, New York.
Luborsky L, Mintz J, Auerback A, Christoph P, Bachsach H, Todd T, Johnson M, Cohen M & O'Brien C P (1980): Predicting the outcome of psychotherapy. Arch Gen Psychiat 37:471–481.
Mahler M (1968): On human symbiosis and the vicissitudes of individuation. Int Univ Press, New York.
Marinow A (1972): Suicide among schizophrenics. Acta Psychiat Scand 8:1–16.
Markowe M, Steinert J, Heyworth-Davis F (1967): Insulin and chlorpromazine in schizophrenia: a ten-year comparative survey. Brit J Psychiat 113:1101–1106.
Marsh LC (1933): Experiments in group treatment of patients at Worcester State Hospital. Ment Hyg 17:396–416.
May P R A (1968): Treatment of schizophrenia. Science House, New York.
May P R A, Tuma A H, Yale C, Potepan P & Dixon W J (1976): Schizophrenia – follow-up study of results of treatment. Arch Gen Psychiat 33:474–486
May P R A, Tuma A H, Dixon W J (1981): Schizophrenia. A follow-up study of the results of five forms of treatment. Arch Gen Psychiat 38:776–784.
Mc Cormick D J and Broekema V J (1978): Size estimation, perceptual recognition, and cardiac rate response in acute paranoid and nonparanoid schizophrenics. J Psychol 87:385–398.
Mc Dougall J (1982): Alexithymia, psychosomatosis and psychosis. Int J Psychoanal Psychother 9:379–388.
Mc Glashan TH & Miller GH (1982): The goals of psychoanalysis and psychoanalytic psychotherapy. Arch Gen Psychiat 39:377–388.
Mc Glashan TH (1984): The Chestnut Lodge follow-up study. Arch Gen Psychiatry 41:573–601.
Mezquita J (1982): Half-way services in the rehabilitation of chronic mental patients. Acta psychiat Scand 65:245–252.
Miles C (1977): Conditions predisposing to suicide: A review. J Nerv Ment Dis 164:231–246.
Mosher L R, Keith S J (1979): Research on the psychosocial treatment of schizophrenia: A summary report. Am J Psychiatry 136:623–631.
Mosher L R & Keith S J (1980): Psychosocial treatment: Individual, group, family and community support approaches. Schizophr Bull 6:10–41.

Mosher L R, Menn A Z & Matthews S M (1975): Soteria: evaluation of a home based treatment of schizophrenia. Amer J Orthopsychiat 45:455–467.

Mosher L R, Menn A Z (1978): Community residential treatment for schizophrenia: two-year follow-up data. Hosp Commun Psychiatry 29:715–723.

Mosher L R, Menn A Z (1983): Scientific evidence and system change: The Soteria experience. In Psychosocial intervention in schizophrenia ed by Stierlin H et al. Springer. Berlin.

Müller C (1955): Über psychotherapie bei einen chronischen Schizophrenen. Psyche 9:350–369.

Müller C (1959): Das Senium Schizophrener. Karger, Basel.

Müller C (1961): Die Psychotherapie Schizophrener and der Zürcher Klinik. Versuch einer vorläufigen katamnestischen Übersicht. Nervenarzt 32:354–368.

National Board of Health in Finland (1985): National development and research programme for the care and rehabilitation of schizophrenia, a preliminary rapport (in Finnish). Lääkintöhallituksen julkaisuja No 69.

Niskanen P & Achté K A (1972): The course and prognosis of schizophrenic psychoses in Helsinki. A comparative study of first admissions in 1950, 1960 and 1965. Monogr Psychiat Clin Helsinki Univ Central Hosp No 4.

Niskanen P, Lönnqvist J & Achté K A (1973): Schizophrenic and paranoid psychotic patients first admitted in 1970, with a two-year follow-up. Psychiatria Fennica 1973:103–114.

Niskanen P & Pihkanen T A (1972): Attitudes of the relatives of schizophrenic patients. Acta psychiat Scand 48:174–185.

O'Brien C P, Hamm K B, Ray B A et al (1972): Group vs. individual psychotherapy with schizophrenics: a controlled outcome study. Arch Gen Psychiatry 27:474–478.

Olson R P, Greenberg D J (1972): Effects of contingency-contracting and decision-making groups with chronic mental patients. J Consult Clin Psychol 38:376–383.

Pao P N (1979): Schizophrenic disorders. Internat Univ Press, New York.

Parloff M B, Dies R R (1977): Group psychotherapy outcome research 1966–1975. Int J Group Psychother 27:281–319.

Paul G L. Lentz R J (1977): Psychosocial treatment of chronic mental patients: Milieu vs. social-learning programs. Cambridge. Mass, Harvard University Press.

Phillipson H (1955): The Object Relations Technique. Tavistock publ, London.

Pulkkinen E (1982): Paranoidisen ja ei-paranoidisen skitsofrenian kehittyminen ja kulku. English summary: Development and course of paranoid and nonparanoid schizophrenia. Academic dissertation, Helsinki.

Räkköläinen V (1976): Psychodynamic and interpersonal aspects of psychosis. In: Schizophrenia 75, ed. J Jorstad & E Ugelstad. Universitetspresset, Oslo.

Räkköläinen V (1977); Onset of psychosis. A clinical study of 68 cases. Ann Univ Turkuensis, Ser D:7.

Räkköläinen V & Alanen Y O (1982): On the transactionality of defensive processes. Int Rev Psycho-Anal 9:263–271.

Räkköläinen V, Salokangas R, & Lehtinen P (1979): Protective constructions in the course of psychosis, a follow-up study. In: Psychotherapy of schizophrenia, ed. C. Müller. Excerpta Medica, Amsterdam.

Raman A C, Murphy H B (1972): Failure of traditional prognostic indicators in Afro-Asian psychotics: Results of a long-term follow-up survey. J New Ment Dis 154:238–247.

Rapaport M, Hopkins H K, Hall K, Belleza T & Silverman J (1978): Are there schizophrenics for whom drugs may be unnecessary or contraindicated? Int Pharmacopsychiat 13:100–111.

Rennie T A C (1939): Follow-up study of five hundred patients with schizophrenia admitted to the hospital from 1913 to 1923. Archives of Neurology & Psychiatry 42:877–891.

Rieder R O, Mann L S, Weinberger D R, van Kammen D P & Post R M (1983): Computed tomographic scans in patients with schizophrenic, schizo-affective and bipolar affective disorder. Arch Gen psychiat 40:735–739.

Robins L N, Helzer J E, Weissman M M, Orvaschel H, Gruenberg E, Burke J D & Regier D A (1984): Lifetime prevalence of specific psychiatric disorders in three sites. Arch Gen Psychiatry 41:949–958.

Robinson M B (1970): A study of the effects of focused videotape feedback in group counseling. Comp Group studies 1:47–75.
Rockland L H & Pollin W (1965): Quantification of psychiatric mental status. Arc Gen Psychiat 4:23–28.
Rogers C R, Gendlin E G, Kiesler D J, et al. (1967): The therapeutic relationship and its impact. Madison, University of Wisconsin Press.
Rosenthal D, Wender P H, Kety S S, Welner & Schulsinger F (1971): The adopted-away offspring of schizophrenics. Amer J Psychiat 128:87–91.
Rosenthal D, Wender P H, Kety S S, Schulsinger F, Walner J & Rieder R O (1975): Parent-child relationship and psychopathological disorder in the child. Arch Gen Psychiat 32:466–476.

Salokangas R K R (1977): Skitsofreniaan sairastuneiden psykososiaalinen kehitys. Kansaneläkelaitoksen julkaisuja, Sarja AL:7. Turku. English summary: The psychosocial prognosis in schizophrenia.
Salokangas R K R (1978): Psychosocial prognosis in schizophrenia. Ann Univ Turkuensis, Ser D:9.
Salokangas R K R (1980): Hospital and outpatient care for psychotic patients during the last three decades. Acta Psychiat Scand 62:47–62.
Salokangas R K R (1983): Why psychotherapy works or does not work in the treatment of schizophrenic patients. Paper read in the XX Nordic Psychiatric Congress, Bergen.
Salokangas R K R (1985): Skitsofrenian hoito ja ennuste. Jälkitutkimus psykoterapeuttista yhteisöhoitoa saaneiden skitsofreniapotilaiden psykososiaalisesta enusteesta. Kansanterreystieteen julkaisuj M 89/85. English summary: Treatment and outcome in schizophrenia. A follow-up study of the psychosocial outcome in schizophrenic patients trented in a psychotherapeutic community.
Salokangas RKR & Räkköläinen V (1985): In National Board of Health (1985).
Salonen S (1975): The hospital ward from the standpoint of the patient's self-esteem. Psychiatria Fennica 1975:325–331.
Salonen S (1976): On the technique of psychotherapy of schizophrenia. In: Schizophrenia 75, ed. J Jorstad & E Ugelstad. Universitetsforlaget, Oslo.
Salonen S (1979): Psychotherapeutic studies in schizophrenia. Ann Univ Turkuensis, Ser D:12.
Sartorius N (1984): Personal communication
Sartorius N, Jablensky A & Shapiro R (1978): Cross-cultural differences in the short-term prognosis of schizophrenic psychoses. Schizophr Bull 4:102–113.
Schilder P (1936): The analysis of ideologies as a psychotherapeutic method, especially in group treatment. Am J Psychiatry 93:601–617.
Schindler R (1957): Zehn Jahre "bifokale" Gruppentherapie. Congress report of the II Internat Congress for Psychiatry, Vol III:379–386.
Schindler R (1959): Der soziodynamische Aspect in der "bifokalen Gruppentherapie". Acta psychother 7:207–220.
Schindler R (1980): Die Veränderung psychotischer Langzeitverläufe nach Psychotherapie. Psychiatria Clin 13 206 – 216 (1980).
Schneider K (1959): Clinical Psychopathology. Grune & Stratton, New York.
Schulz, C C (1963): A follow-up report on admissions to Chestnut Lodge: 1948–58. Psychiat Quart 37:220–233.
Schulz C G (1975): An individualized psychotherapeutic approach with the schizophrenic patient. Schizophr Bull, Iss 13:44–69.
Schulz C G (1976): Presentation of a clinical scale to assess self-object differentiation in psychotic patients. In Schizophrenia 75. Ed J Jorstad & E Ugelstad. Universitetsforlaget, Oslo.
Schwartz R, Biehl H, Krumm B & Schubart C (1980): Case-finding and characteristics of schizophrenic patients of recent onset in Mannheim. Acta Psychiat Scand Suppl 285, Vol 62, 1980.
Scott R D & Ashworth P L (1967): Closure at the first schizophrenic breakdown: a family study. Brit J Med Psychol 40:109–145.

Scott R D & Montanez A (1972): The nature of tenable and untenable patient-parent relationships and their connexion with hospital outcome. In: Psychotherapy of Schizophrenia, ed. by D Rubinstein & Y O Alanen. Excerpta Medica, Amsterdam.
Scott R D & Alwyn S (1978): Patient-parent relationships and the course and outcome of schizophrenia. Brit J Med Psychol 51:343–355.
Sechehaye M-A (1947): Die symbolische Wunscherfüllung. Huber, Bern 1955. (French orig 1947).
Selvini-Palazzoli M, Boscolo L, Cecchin G & Prata G (1977): Paradox und Gegenparadox. Klett & Cotta, Stuttgart.
Shellow R S, Brown B S & Osberg J W (1963): Family group treatment in retrospect: four years and sixty families. Family Process 2:53–67.
Sifneos P E (1972): Short-term psychotherapy and emotional crisis. Cambridge: Harvard Univ Press 1972
Silverman J (1967): Variations in cognitive control and psychophysiological defense in the schizophrenias. Psychosom Med 29:225–251.
Simon W & Wirt R D (1961): Prognostic factors in schizophrenia. Amer J Psychiat 117:887–890.
von Sivers E (1973): in Lindelius R and Kay D W: Some changes in the pattern of mortality in schizophrenia in Sweden. Acta Psychiat Scand 49:315–323.
von Sivers E (1983): En efterundersökning av 111 patienter vårdade för schizophreni första gången under åren 1961–65. Nord Psykiat Tidskr Vol 37 Suppl 7 (with English summary).
Sjöström R (1982): Psykoterapi vid schizofreni – en retrospektiv studie. Sv Läkartidningen 79:3183–3186.
Sluzki E (1981): Process of symptoms production and patterns of symptoms maintenance. J Marit Fam Ther 7:273–280.
Soskis D & Bowers M (1969) The schizophrenic experience. J. Nerv Ment Dis 149:443–449.
Speijer N (1961): The mentally handicapped in the sheltered workshops. Ministry of Social Affairs and Public Health, Hague.
Stanton A H, Gunderson J G, Knapp P H, Frank A F, Vannicelli M L, Schnitzer R & Rosenthal R (1984): Effects of psychotherapy in schizophrenia: 1. Design and implementation of a controlled study. Schizophr Bull 10:520–563.
Stephens J H (1970): Long-term course and prognosis in schizophrenia. Seminars in Psychiatry, 2:464–485.
Stephens J H (1978): Long-term prognosis and follow-up in schizophrenia. Schizophr Bull 4:25–37.
Stierlin H (1974): Separating parents and adolescents. Amsterdam. Quadrangle, New York.
Stierlin H (1976): The dynamics of owning and disowning. Fam Process 15:277–288.
Stierlin H (1983): Relations on the family therapy of schizopresent families. In Psychosocial intervention in schizophrenia, ed by H Stierlin, L C Wynne & M Wisrsching, Springer, Berlin.
Strauss J, Carpenter W (1972): The prediction of outcome in schizophrenia: I. Characteristics of outcome. Arch Gen Psychiatry 27:739–746.
Strauss J. Carpenter W (1974): The prediction of outcome in schizophrenia: II. Relationships between predictor and outcome variables. Arch Gen Psychiat 31:37–42.
Strauss J, Carpenter W (1977): Prediction of outcome in schizophrenia. Five-year outcome and its predictors. Arch Gen Psychiatry 34:159–163.
Strauss J & Frader M (1976): Justifying intensive psychotherapy for schizophrenia in a community psychiatric center. In Schizophrenia 75, ed by J Jorstad & E Ugelstad. Universitetsforlaget, Oslo.
Sullivan H S (1930): Socio-psychiatric research. Amer J Psychiat 87:977–991.
Sullivan H S (1931): The modified psychoanalytic treatment of schizophrenia. Amer J Psychiat 88:519–540.
Sullivan H S (1953): The interpersonal theory of psychiatry. Norton, New York.
Sullivan H S (1962): Schizophrenia as a human process. Norton, New York.
Suomen sairaalatalous (Finnish Hospital Economy) 1977.

Tanaka Y, Hazama H, Kawahara R & Kobaynski K (1981): Computerized tomography of the brain in schizophrenic patients: A controlled study. Acta Psychiat Scand 63:191–197.

Tepper S J & Haas J (1979): Prevalence of tardive dyskinesia. J Clin Psychiat 40:508–516.

Thornton J F, Plummer E, Seeman MV & Littmann S K (1981): Schizophrenia: a group support for relatives. Can J Psychiat 26:341–344.

Tienari P, Sorri A, Naarala M, Lahti I. Pohjola J, Boström C, Wahlberg K-E (1983): The Finnish adoptive family study: Adopted-away offspring of schizophrenic mothers. In Psychosocial intervention in schizophrenia, ed by H. Stierlin, L C Wynne & M Wirsching, Springer, Berlin.

Tienari P, Sorri A, Lahti I, Naarala M, Wahlberg K-E, Rönkkö T Pohjola J & Moring J (1985): The finnish adoptive family study of schizophrenics. Yale J Biol Med 58:227–237.

Towne R D, Sampson H & Messinger S L (1961): Schizophrenia and the marital family. J Ner Ment Dis 133:424.

Tsuang M T, Dempsey M, Woolson R F, Fleming J A (1979): Long-term outcome of major psychoses I and II: Arch Gen Psychiatry 36: 1295–1301, 1302–1304.

Ugelstad E (1978): Psykotiske langtidspasienter i psykiatriske sykehus – nye behandlingsforsok. Universitetsforlaget, Oslo.

Ugelstad E (1979): Possibilities of organizing psychotherapeutically oriented treatment programs for schizophrenia within sectorized psychiatric service. In Psychotherapy of schizophrenia, ed by C Müller, Excerpta Medica, Amsterdam.

Urist J (1980): Object relations. In Woody H (ed). Encyclopedia of clinical assessment. Jessey-Boss Publishers, San Francisco.

Vaillant G E (1964): Prospective prediction of schizophrenic remission. Arch Gen Psychiatry 11:509–518.

Vaughn C E & Leff J P (1976): The influence of family and social factors on the course of psychiatric illness. Brit J of Psychiatry 129:125–137.

Venables P H (1967): Partial failure of cortical-sub-cortical integration as a factor underlying schizophrenic behaviour. In The origins of schizophrenia, ed by J Romano. Excerpta Medica, Amsterdam.

Venables P H & Wing J K (1962): Level of arousal and the subclassification of schizophrenia. Arch Gen Psychiat 7:114–119.

Watt D C, Katz K & Shepherd M (1983): The natural history of schizophrenia: a 5-year prospective follow-up of a represential sample of schizophrenics by means of a standardized clinical and social assessment. Psychol Med 13:663–670.

Waxler N E (1979): Is outcome for schizophrenia better in non-industrial societies? J Nerv Ment Dis 167:144–192.

Wender P H, Rosenthal D, Kety S S, Schulsinger R & Welner J (1974): Cross-fostering: a research strategy for clarifying the role of genetic and experiential factors in the etiology of schizophrenia. Arch Gen Psychiat 30:121–128.

Whitehorn J C & Betz B J (1954): A study of psychotherapeutic relationships between physicians and schizophrenic patients. Amer J Psychiat 111:321–331.

Whitehorn J C & Betz B J (1960): Further studies of the doctor as a crucial variable in the outcome of treatment with schizophrenic patient. Amer J Psychiat 117:215–222.

World Health Organization (1973): The international pilot study of schizophrenia. WHO, Geneva.

World Health Organization (1979): Schizophrenia – An international follow-up study. John Wiley, Chichester.

Will O A jr (1961): Process, psychotherapy and schizophrenia. In Psychotherapy of the psychoses, ed by A Burton, Basic Books, New York.

Will O A jr (1967): Schizophrenia: the problem of origins. In: The origins of schizophrenia, ed. by J. Romano. Excerpta Medica, Amsterdam.

Wing J K (1960): A pilot experiment of long hospitalized male schizophrenic patients. Brit J Prev Soc Med 14:173–180.

Wing J K (1978): The social context of schizophrenia. Amer J Psychiat 135:1333–1339.
Wing J K, Bennett D H & Denham J (1963): The industrial rehabilitation of long-stay schizophrenic patients. Medical Research Council Mem No 42. HMSO London.
Winnicott D W (1960): The theory of the parent-infant relationship. Int J Psycho-Anal 41:585–595.
Wyatt R J, Cutler N R DeLisi L E, Jeste D Vet al (1982): Biochemical and morphological factors in the etiology of the schizophrenic disorders. In Psychiatry 1982, Annual Review. The American Psychiatric Association. Washington.
Wynne L C, Ryckoff I M, Day J & Hirsch S (1958): Pseudomutuality in the family relations of schizophrenics. Psychiatry 21:205–220.
Wynne L S, Singer M T & Toohey M L (1976): Communication of the adoptive parents of schizophrenics. In Schizophrenia 1975, ed by J Jorstad and E Ugelstad. Universitetsforlaget, Oslo.

Zigler E, Levine J & Zigler B (1977): Premorbid social competence and paranoid – nonparanoid status in female schizophrenic patients. J New Ment Dis 164: 333–339.

MIX
Papier aus verantwortungsvollen Quellen
Paper from responsible sources
FSC® C105338

If you have any concerns about our products,
you can contact us on
ProductSafety@springernature.com

In case Publisher is established outside the EU,
the EU authorized representative is:
Springer Nature Customer Service Center GmbH
Europaplatz 3, 69115 Heidelberg, Germany

Printed by Libri Plureos GmbH
in Hamburg, Germany